Making the Mexican Diabetic

D1478449

Making the Mexican Diabetic

Race, Science, and the Genetics of Inequality

Michael J. Montoya

UNIVERSITY OF CALIFORNIA PRESS
Berkeley · Los Angeles · London

University of California Press, one of the most
distinguished university presses in the United States,
enriches lives around the world by advancing scholarship
in the humanities, social sciences, and natural sciences. Its
activities are supported by the UC Press Foundation and
by philanthropic contributions from individuals and
institutions. For more information, visit www.ucpress.edu.

University of California Press
Berkeley and Los Angeles, California

University of California Press, Ltd.
London, England

Library of Congress Cataloging-in-Publication Data

Montoya, Michael J. 1965–
   Making the Mexican diabetic : race, science, and the
genetics of inequality / Michael Montoya.
      p.   cm.
   Includes bibliographical references and index.
   ISBN 978-0-520-26730-5 (hardcover : alk. paper)
   ISBN 978-0-520-26731-2 (pbk. : alk. paper)
   1. Non-insulin-dependent diabetes—Mexico—
Genetic aspects.   2. Mexican Americans—Health and
hygiene.   I. Title.
   [DNLM: 1. Diabetes Mellitus—ethnology—
Mexico.   2. Diabetes Mellitus—ethnology—United
States.   3. Genetic Research—Mexico.   4. Genetic
Research—United States.   5. Indians, North
American—ethnology—Mexico.   6. Indians, North
American—ethnology—United States.   7. Mexican
Americans—ethnology—Mexico.   8. Mexican
Americans—ethnology—United States.   9. Risk
Factors—Mexico.   10. Risk Factors—United States.
11. Socioeconomic Factors—Mexico.
12. Socioeconomic Factors—United States. WK 810]
   RA645.D5M66   2011
   362.196'46200896872073—dc22
                                        2010038017

Manufactured in the United States of America

19 18 17 16 15 14 13 12 11 10
10 9 8 7 6 5 4 3 2 1

This book is printed on Cascades Enviro 100, a
100% post consumer waste, recycled, de-inked fiber.
FSC recycled certified and processed chlorine free. It
is acid free, Ecologo certified, and manufactured by
BioGas energy.

For Johanna, Zoe, Eliah, and Sidra for accompanying me on this journey. I delight in the prospects of accompanying you on yours.

Contents

Acknowledgments

Research for this book would not have been possible without the financial support of the Ford Foundation, the Wenner-Gren Foundation, the National Science Foundation, and the Department of Anthropology at Stanford University. The School of Social Sciences and The Center for the Study of Latinos in a Global Society, both at the University of California—Irvine also supported this project financially. Additionally, there are a great many people who have assisted me with this project. I wish to thank the mutual support of colleagues at Stanford including Carole Blackburn, Rozita Dimova, Martha Gonzales-Cortes, Hideko Mitsui, Doug Smith and Miriam Ticktin for their feedback, encouragement, and solidarity through institutional and research challenges of one sort or another. To Nicolas De Genova, I am indebted to the unfettered use of his apartment on my frequent visits to Chicago, for challenging and provocative conversations during the data collection phase of this research, and for productive conversations during the revision phase of this book.

For their wisdom, solidarity and constructive feedback on many facets of this project, words of thanks are due to Deborah Heath, Linda Hogle, Chris Schofield, Joyce Kirk, Erin Koch, Barbara Ley, Paul Rabinow, Rayna Rapp, Alan Goodman, Karen-Sue Taussig, Jay Kaufman, Tom Lauderbach and to Vydunas and Jenny Morgan-Tumas. For reviews of all or portions of this manuscript, I am indebted to two anonymous reviewers, Stefan Helmreich and colleagues in the Departments of

Anthropology and Chicano/Latino Studies at UC-Irvine, especially Mei Zhan, Angela Garcia, Kris Peterson, Victoria Bernal, Susan Greenhalgh, Kaushik Sunder Rajan, Bill Maurer, and Leo Chavez. This project has also benefited from the conversations, formal and informal, with Sheena Nahm, Cristina Bejarano, Erin Kent, Connie McGuire and the students in Borders and Bodies and Proseminar courses in the department of anthropology as well as my medical students in the Program in Medical Education for the Latino Community (PRIME-LC) in the UCI School of Medicine. Jose Rea and Victor Becerra can never be repaid for their continued support and inspiration.

Portions of this book were presented at numerous venues and I am indebted to the questions and comments I received at each. Early drafts of chapter 4 were presented at the University of Minnesota Department of Anthropology and at the "Critical inquiries into race" panel of the American Sociological Association meetings. An early draft of chapter 3 was presented at "Nations, Bodies and Borders," a panel for the Canadian Association for Social and Cultural Anthropology. Portions of chapter 5 were presented at the American Anthropological Association, at the Stanford Center for Biomedical Ethics Works in Progress Series, and at the University of Wisconsin, Madison, Science and Technology Studies Program. Sections of this book were also presented at Portland State University School of Community Health (Portland, OR) the Five Colleges Faculty Seminar in Culture, Health and Science (Amherst, MA) the New England Regional Conference on Medical Anthropology (1995), and the "Culture, Medicine and Power" conference at the University of Minnesota. I have benefited also from the many thoughtful comments from colleagues at the University of Kentucky, University of Chicago, University of California–Los Angeles, University of California–Riverside, and University of California–Davis. I found the discussions held at the Genetics, Admixture and Identity workshop at the University College London organized by Sarha Gibbon, Monica Sans, and Carlos Ventura Santos especially useful in furthering my understanding of population genetics. I am also indebted to Yin Paradies and Malia Fullerton for their thoughtful criticisms and technical advice while I worked through sections of this manuscript.

Additionally, I thank Sylvia Yanagisako, Joan Fujimura, Nancy Chen, and Sarah Jain, for their insightful, challenging and always-helpful feedback and encouragement. I would also like to thank Renato Rosaldo, Jane Collier, Paulla Ebron, Akhil Gupta, Miyako Inoue, and Purnima Mankekar. Their influence is clearly evident throughout. Additionally, Troy Duster, Duana Fullwiley, Melbourne Tapper, Jonathan Kahn, the late Helen Montoya-Cox, Judy Treskow, Joyce F. Kirk, Carla Rodriguez Gonzalez, Cristina Bejarano, and Rachael Stryker have all influenced this project in ways great and small. I am also indebted to the careful guidance of Naomi Schneider, Kalicia Pivirotto, Kate Warne, and Mari Coates at University of California Press. The copy editor Norma McLemore and the production editor Christine Dahlin prevented a raft of grammatical and typographical embarrassments. I and my readers can thank J. Naomi Linzer, the indexer, for her skillful guide to key terms. All remaining errors and omissions, technical or conceptual, are mine alone.

Of course, this project would not have been possible without the countless scientists and research staff who agreed to be interviewed, observed and accompanied from Mexico, the United States, and the United Kingdom, but especially "Nora," "Gary," "Carl" and "Judi" (because of human subject requirements, pseudonyms have been used throughout this book). This book is surely better as a result of their insight. A special thanks go to Jim and Jean Morgan for their ever ready support and wise counsel. Finally, I want to thank Janet Walker and Ernest and Gayla Walker whose enduring support fueled more hours of work when sheer force of will did not.

Preface

My thinking for this project began with my encounter with the techno-sciences as a member of the research team for Mapping Genetic Knowl-edge, funded by the National Institutes of Health through its Ethical, Legal and Social Implications Research Program. Led by Deborah Heath, Rayna Rapp and Karen-Sue Taussig, the project was an anthropological venture into the basic scientific, clinical, and lay understandings of three heritable connective tissue disorders.[1] Along with two other research assistants, Barbara Ley and Erin Koch, I spent three years (full time dur-ing the summers) conducting ethnography in labs, online, and at confer-ences, learning from and with scientists, clinicians, and lay communities of affected persons. The world of science studies and of the anthropol-ogy of medicine had become flesh in my interviews, bench-side conver-sations and experiences, and interactions with three practicing an-thropologists. I learned the look and feel of scientific collaboration, interdisciplinarity, stratified knowledge products and networks, and arcane scientific debates of tremendous consequence. I explored the conundrum of multiple accountabilities in contexts in which the stakes for ethnographic knowledge were seemingly dwarfed in comparison to the discovery of the gene for a condition suffered by thousands, which was now rendered preventable. Additionally, I was humbled by the suf-fering, stamina, and vigor of those persons and families who dealt with the life-and-death uncertainties of these conditions. It is from here that I crafted my interests in the sciences of diabetes.

The scientific, social, and institutional contours of the diabetes research enterprise, with its fundamental reliance upon DNA labeled with race and ethnicity, proved exceptionally useful and in many ways an exemplary set of material and semiotic conditions for understanding race and ethnicity in the post-genomic era. Were the classifications similar, for example, when scientists and pharmaceutical marketing managers worked with and spoke of donors' bodies? Did the labels change as the DNA was refined for further experimentation and analysis or when researchers represented their results to audiences outside of the consortium? Following diabetes researchers would at least answer an anthropologically informed question: If race is a *social* category, how can it reasonably inform cutting-edge medical-genetics research on such complex diseases like asthma, heart disease, and diabetes?

After interviewing several researchers at the University of Texas in San Antonio, I flew to North Carolina, where I had arranged an interview with two researchers at Glaxo Wellcome, a molecular biologist and director of research and a key bioinformatician. The Texas and Glaxo researchers were members of the international consortium interested in the genetic analyses of type 2 diabetes. After these preliminary interviews, I was sure to ask permission to follow up and, if it felt right, to inquire as to the possibility of conducting long-term ethnographic research in their laboratories. During this preliminary fieldwork, everyone I interviewed in Mexico, Texas, and North Carolina verbally agreed to allow me to conduct sustained follow-up research should I desire to do so.

A year later, after another visit to Research Triangle Park in North Carolina, I was preparing the final approvals from Glaxo for my arrival and subsequent "deep hanging out," as Renato Rosaldo so aptly describes the ethnographic enterprise. Several carefully crafted e-mails were exchanged detailing my methods and the terms and conditions of my ethnographic presence. After much careful discussion about Institutional Review Boards and about the substance of interviews, participant observation, and laboratory life, I promised a low-impact ethnographic presence and agreed to sign a confidentiality statement. I was readying for fieldwork and getting nervous because I had not heard back from the director of research and the senior biostatistician, both of whom had agreed that Glaxo would welcome me for a year or so. I had carefully explained in writing—as agreed upon with the director of research—my methods (mostly participant observation and interviews) and my intellectual interests.

Through these e-mail and phone call volleys, I received permission, albeit lukewarm, to conduct ethnographic research in Glaxo's laboratories and was waiting for something in writing to "seal the deal." The seal would never be affixed. The director of research was promoted because a competitor company stole his boss, the biostatistician went on maternity leave, and the new director of research—formerly the head of the genetics lab—had not been informed of the negotiations between his colleagues and me. Two months prior to leaving for the field and after considerable effort at explaining anew my methods and motives, I was given a definitive "no" from Glaxo and began searching for a new field site.[2]

I didn't have to search long. I had originally found Glaxo through its membership in the consortium. Glaxo scientists were early participants in diabetes genetic research, and the collaborative ties between them and their academic colleagues predated the consortium. Glaxo's corporate research and development apparatus entailed a coordinated effort between their genetics laboratories (researchers who handle genetic material) and their quantitative analysis team (those who work exclusively with data sets). This "wet and dry" lab arrangement was unique at the time, and while I was disappointed that I would not be able to work in this environment, many labs in the academic sector were either formally or through collaborative networks institutionalizing similar coordinated wet and dry lab operations.

Fortunately, while waiting for permission to conduct field research with Glaxo, I had interviewed other scientists who were members of the consortium. I was particularly interested in the use of quantitative methods for genetic analyses of type 2 diabetes because I knew that the DNA came from diverse populations whose membership in ethnic groups was somehow arrived at quantitatively. I hypothesized that quantitative analyses would offer taxonomic systems for global populations that would range from the purely social, "Sun County Mexican Americans," to the hypercoded lexicography of single nucleotide polymorphic (SNP) clusters, for example, those sets of persons who share SNPs 26, 46, and 15 on chromosome 20. After a phone interview and a face-to-face interview at the American Diabetes Association Meetings in San Diego, "Nora," a quantitatively minded geneticist, generously agreed to host my deep hanging out.

When asked what I planned to do, what my project was, my reply was always the same. I was interested in learning about diabetes as a genetic disease, in the collaborative nature of the consortium science, and in the use of population DNA in diabetes research. In terms of genetics, I said I was interested in the changes—if any—brought about by the expansion of an endocrinological model of diabetes to one of genetics in this era of big genetic science. Included in this were my interests in the transition from standard incidence and prevalence patterns to genetic epidemiological analyses of type 2 diabetes. In terms of collaboration, I explained that I was interested in the mix of governmental, corporate, academic, and nongovernmental researchers representing a range of disciplines and national contexts all involved in the consortium. In terms of population-based data sets, I would say that I was interested in how and why social categories could inform biomedical research. As my relationships with my collaborator-informants developed, both the methods and premises of my research became clearer to both me and my interlocutors. The subjects/objects of my inquiry were in all honesty co-configured dialogically.[3] That is, my original intent and questions were educated attempts to enter the conversations about genes, illness, health, race, and technoscientific knowledge practices and claims making. As my engagement unfolded in situ, my questions, if not my intentions, were altered by what I was learning.

Committed to empirically sound ethnography, I kept open my own expectations and hypotheses. I wanted "the data" I collected to support whatever conclusions I might eventually make. One mark of anthropology is the provisionality of the initial hypotheses. I was prepared to accept that I was wrong about a lot of my initial hypotheses. In most respects, I was not wrong as much as I was underinformed. It is for this reason that I feel a word of acknowledgment must go to my collaborators in this project. What anthropologists previously called "informants," I prefer to call "collaborators." In Chicago, I was conducting participant-collaboration with Gary and Nora, but especially with Nora. This project is, in part, my version of their professional lives ethnographically documented and herein rendered. The terms of collaboration, within participant-collaboration, were still one sided, with me offering little up front save companionship, confessional space and time, and an occasional social analysis of some issue confronting the research. The social analyses were rarely accepted at face value because everyone thinks he or she is a social analyst, especially if the person is a highly educated and affluent biomedical researcher at the top of the field. What is more, the epistemological differences between anthropology and genetic epidemiology were insurmountable in the amount of undivided time I felt I could squeeze out of Nora, her lab, her immediate collaborators and the wide world of consortium members. Bridging this epistemological divide remains an unfinished project. To say the least, I am grateful for the hours of interviews, endless lurking, and innumerable questions about things big and small that were always answered and obliged by those whose world I had entered.

However, as collaborator, I am not positioning this project as aligned with the immediate goals and objectives of geneticists. Rather, I use the term "collaboration" to acknowledge that I, like my interlocutors, am interested in type 2 diabetes among Mexicano/a people. This project thus is part of the collective conversation about this disease, its epidemiological patterns, and the sociocultural implications of the search for its genetic foundation. Further, I consider the researchers and field workers with whom I worked as *my* collaborators because I am indebted to the gracious acceptance of the time and intrusion of my ethnographic practice that my collaborator/informants endured. Though I set forth an understanding of the disease different from their own, our projects are interconnected. To be sure, I have influenced, ever so modestly, the use of race in diabetes genetics just as I have been influenced by the lives of the genetic epidemiologists whose work I observed.

More than a collaborative orientation toward ethnographic practice contributes to the argumentation made available by this project, however. This book is a product of the a priori social and political commitments that I bring to my ethnographic practice. Thus, a scant intellectual-biographical disclosure is in order to further situate this book. I use "situate" to refer to the way I include myself within the frame of research itself, and the ways my presence in space and time are, as consciously as I can make it, part of the empirical record of this book. As Rabinow puts it, "to place oneself midst the relationships of the contending *logoi* (embedded as they are within problematizations, apparatuses, and assemblages) is to find oneself among anthropology's problems."[4] Of course such problems are always already part and parcel of the practices of knowledge production.[5]

My intellectual interests have always been in the in-between spaces. Neither geographic, social, nor conceptual boundaries ever seemed to satisfy my experience of the world. I was the first of my large, religious, multiethnic, working-class family to graduate from college. My experience of the powerful versus oppressed academic narratives of the 1970s and 1980s (e.g., gender, race, class, sexual orientation), while rich with experiential validation and political possibility, never accounted for the resilience and brilliance of the working people I knew and loved. Reading these academic texts was, for me, as if their—our—power was of no consequence. The era of resistance that closely followed these struggles also bore close grand narrative resemblance to the have–have not syndrome that came before. It was as if a liberal guilt motivated intellectual pursuit: a worthy one, but one in which I could not participate.

In spite of this, anthropology and science studies offered me a way to understand the in-between space, the place where meaning is produced by multiply positioned people. Race and disease was the ideal terrain for my kind of inquiry because I could ask questions that probed ontological certainties associated with social identity and with the unequal distresses of (post)industrial life. Since the reductive labeling of race, class, gender, and sexual orientation have never satisfied the social mobility and complex hybridities of my social position and affinities, the race debates in anthropology fit the bill. Especially since within those debates there existed frantic boundary banter that seemed altogether too simplistic.

What is more, I think there is work to be done to reconcile the ideological force of biology and race/ethnicity in terms that resonate outside of academe. For example, in 1997, the complications of type 2 diabetes took the life of my beloved tia Helen Montoya-Cox. This, in part, invited a full ethnographic investigation into the biology-identity-health equality complex, the subject of this book, which I find so vexingly interesting, inspiring, and irritating. Thus, in this project disease serves as the object of analysis that joins questions and positions of identity, family history, and biomedicine.

Given the personal affinities I bring to my topic, there are three ways I have worked to situate this project. By "situate," I mean, as Donna Haraway puts it, to create "partial, locatable accounts of the world that are both accurate and explicitly embedded within the contexts of its own production."[6] First, as I noted above, I situate the work of the scientists as my collaborators and strive to demonstrate the ways they themselves position their own work within fields of unequal power and institutional structures that are not always benign. Second, I explicitly interrogate the ways my discipline—anthropology—is implicated from within the moral economies of my project. This means that anthropology of race in its evolutionary and molecular iterations form part of the narrative of type 2 diabetes disease gene history. It also means that cultural anthropology and the race debates form part of the context of field-site construction. In this vein, I draw parallels between the biological prospecting of molecular science and the biographic prospecting of ethnographers. What are the differences between the taking of blood samples from Mexicanas along the border and ethnographically detailing the lives of biomedical researchers or of Mexicanas along the border? I submit that these are but different instances, situations if you will, of appropriation.

In addition, there are no innocent positions, and my account is no exception. I am empowered to conduct my ethnographic work by (dis) virtue of a field still rightly obsessed with race in its most pernicious iterations, and I have been funded by reviewers of my proposals who are worried about the direction of genetics and the use of racialized DNA therein. In this way I capitalize on the misfortunes of those who have directly suffered from racial supremacy in medicine (e.g., African Americans, Jews) and the scientific practices that it spawned.

Finally, I am "studying-up" in the sense first acknowledged by Nader.[7] Not only in the sense that I am mounting a repatriated anthropology studying powerful elites, but also in the sense that the estrangement and alienation that once served as the hallmark of ethnographic practice is re-created in my practice. In the inner-city neighborhood of my childhood, there were no professors, doctors, scientists, or professionals of any kind. We worked as pressmen, construction workers, brewery workers, postal employees, receptionists, hair stylists, and gas station attendants. That I now spend time learning about a privileged domain of knowledge production in order to engage in academic debates is, to put it bluntly, bizarre. It is so far removed from my own social location of origin that it is practically and literally impossible to justify my current occupation in a way that could satisfy the wildly ambivalent sentiments of my erstwhile kith and kin. My family of origin nods politely but never probes too deeply about what I do. For some, I have betrayed my ethnicity and class upbringing. Thus, this project deeply fits a pattern of social mobility and, oddly enough, of the classic anthropological practice of studying "the other." It is a pattern that includes both the conditions of the research endeavor but also the particular sensibility I bring to my work and my relationships with my ethnographic interlocutors.

To what ends such immodest intellectual and biographical contextualization cum reflection? This book was developed at a moment in which the problems of ethnographic interest must change the ethnographic practice if it is to be living, breathing, productive act, not a stale rehearsal of making an academic claim, ethnographically or otherwise. To avoid the telltale conundrum of an account that too neatly appeals to a superior view, a right way to think, requires an ethnographic practice that explodes the reductive tropes of a master narrative or, in this case, the bioreductionisms of race, genes, and disease. Faye Ginsburg expresses this sensibility as an extension of cultural critique wherein concerns about ethnographic writing shift to anthropological engagement with structural inequalities.[8] As she characterizes it, such ethnographically informed projects "call attention to the way people engage in self conscious mobilization of their own cultural practices to defend, extend, complicate, and sometimes transform both their immediate worlds and the larger sociopolitical structures that shape them."[9] I am also joining scholars such as Patricia Zavella who recognize the importance of social location as a means for readers to appreciate the diversity of approaches within Chicano/Latino studies, while at the same time affording a window into the presence of mind of the author.[10] It is the presence of mind that Kim Fortun reminds us is required of a cultural analysis relevant to the concerns that matter most.[11] Diabetes is one such concern.

CONTEXTS, COMMITMENTS, AND LOCATION WORK: IMMODEST INTENTIONS

Anthropology and the social and cultural studies of technosciences have concerned themselves with contemporary problems and situations within technoscientific milieus. This book is no exception. However, it is my hope that this project does more than create yet another account of a contemporary technoscientifically rich cultural formation. One aim of this project is that this ethnographic project might clarify, respectfully and modestly, some obscured sets of material and semiotic dynamics from which something else might emerge.[12] The immodest intent of this work is that what emerges might improve our understanding of the contemporary moment, but also point toward a more locatable, more situated account of diabetes and of diabetes genetic epidemiology. Further, I hope that such account might enable improved access to health care for research participants, an improved scientific accounting of social conditions within genomics research, an improved understanding of causes of chronic disease, and a definitive strike against the grooves of racialization that accompany so much population-based health research in the genomic era. After all, these are the stated aims of most if not all who shared their lives with me to make this project possible.

Location, beyond the spatial metaphor, describes something political. "Here and there" are sites constructed in fields of unequal power relations. Acknowledging their indebtedness to feminist scholarship, Gupta and Ferguson define "location work" as the ways in which as anthropologists we practice a "mode of study that cares about, and pays attention to the interlocking of multiple social-political sites and locations."[13] The topics we study are political, whether we like it or not. We should, therefore, offer a situated intervention based upon out attempts to achieve Haraway's "situated knowledge."[14] Our location as anthropologists must be called into question not only to perform a better description or explanation. Rather, it is my intent to convey to the reader the intellectual commitments to which I attempt to be held accountable.

My commitments as an interlocutor and author will be evident throughout this book and will be signified in places that attempt to disclaim this book as occupying privileged, more ethical and epistemologically objective positions. I will not rehearse the post-reflexive theories of contemporary anthropology except to acknowledge that an account can never adequately convey the substance of the matters at hand, no matter how gifted the presentation.[15] Rather, I seek to find the pressure points for movement[16] that, when pressed, will obligate new cultural formations. I take seriously Robyn Wiegman's cautions against presumptive emplotment of futures we can never predict.[17] Thus, my commitment to intervene requires creating the conditions for productive conflict.[18] That is, I hope to stimulate discomfort in the way diabetes is currently conceived such that the ensuing conflict over what might be done about it will produce a better collective and individual response to this public health and anthropological problem.

These commitments will be woven into the chapters and accompany the descriptions of my research methodologies (e.g., surveying an exhibit hall, traveling in a van across the border with genetic field workers, attending meetings, interviewing key informants, watching computational analyses). For it is in these relational interactions that I most attempt to do justice to learning the lives of my interlocutors. Additionally, the descriptions of the collaboration between ethnographer and interlocutor will appear as the need arises to accurately portray the events, behaviors, or knowledge products under study.

Situating Problems of Knowledge

The decades-long effort to sequence the human genome changed the way many people talk about human biology, disease, and difference. Genes were hailed as the ultimate medical solution to every kind of disease and unwanted behavioral condition. Popular media stories of criminals released from death row, genetic tests to find one's "true" ancestors, and science fiction movies all heralded a new genomic age.[1] It was the promise of the genomic revolution that led to the creation of the Human Genome Project. Formally launched in 1990 with funding from the Department of Energy and the National Institutes of Health (NIH), the costs to sequentially detail the patterns of proteins that DNA on each chromosome is reported to be more than $3 billion in public investment and likely much more from the private sector. While the advances in genomic sciences changed the way we talk about human difference, biology, and disease, its effect on the way we actually think about and act upon human difference remains to be seen. The ramifications of the use of genetics to think, talk, and solve the problems of type 2 diabetes, and of ethnoracial[2] differences in health more generally, is the subject of this book.

In many respects this book anticipates the end of the genomic era at precisely the moment many researchers have convinced funders such as the NIH and countless investors that the future of biomedicine rests squarely in genomic sciences. At the turn of the last century, interdisciplinary teams in universities and corporations were repackaging themselves to accommodate the post-genomic speculative promises for the mass genetic data sets soon to be at their avail in huge depositories called biobanks. Mapping new chromosomal regions, characterizing new informative bits of proteins called markers, and populating DNA data banks were the necessary preconditions for finding the genetic contributions for such common diseases as diabetes, asthma, heart disease, addiction, and hypertension. Researchers worldwide busied themselves with these foundational practices while finding susceptibility genes filled the research and popular cultural imaginaries as the most important and imminently doable task at hand.

The end of the genomic era has not arrived, however. The former director of the Human Genome Project, Francis Collins, has been appointed by President Obama as director of the NIH, and researchers daily report findings of suspected genetic contributions to this or that embodied or behavioral phenomenon. Little debate accompanies such findings; interdisciplinarity ends where epistemological interventions might begin. The new foundational practices of tooling-up labs and research networks have moved up the physiologic food chain to now include traits such as skin color and brain size and behaviors such as delinquency, gang membership, weapon use, arson, even bad driving, as well as a host of predisease bioindicators—those physiological conditions that are clinically implicated in a range of health outcomes (e.g., preterm birth, cancer survival, asthma).[3] Finding markers and querying the biobank infrastructures are now pointedly pressed into service in the enduring push to keep genomics at the cutting edge of biomedical research. These practices, while knowledge based, are not based on knowledge per se. They constitute what Greenhalgh describes as the problematization, assemblage, and micropolitics of science making through which we can trace "the political careers of scientific 'truths' and discover how science has gained its incredible power in the political and social realms."[4] This book examines the politics of knowledge claims about diabetes.

As it pertains to the human genome, politics and economics have modulated the genomic amplitude, tempered the optimism of most, and tested the patience of many. Anticipating the completion of the human genome, the NIH published its Roadmap in 2002, which charts the vision of the future of genomic sciences. This future, argue its authors, requires approaches that span the many divisions of the NIH and seeks public buy-in and thus acceptance from the lay (nonscientific) community. In this way, the Roadmap argues, we will be able to take full advantage of the genomic revolution, transform research practices, and accelerate clinical application. A year after the Roadmap was published, Francis Collins, then director of the National Human Genome Research Institute, published a vision of the role of genome research that shifted the focus to improving human health while also acknowledging the social and ethical frontiers the genomic era creates.[5] Expanding, as these official positions did, from the aims of finding the structure and function of the human genome to addressing cross-cutting interdisciplinary challenges with both clinical applications and social implications signaled that the human genome was not solely a basic scientific pursuit. It has application.

This bicameral basic and applied dimension is what gives "New Genetics" its cultural fraction.[6] New Genetics permeates our conceptions of life itself, of what it means to be a human, of who gets sick and why, and it is related to entire industrial and technoscientific apparatuses scarcely imaginable decades ago. As Palsson argues, we must "recognize the successes of the new genetics while exploring the implications of the gene centrism configured with and through them."[7] To this end, this book looks at the human genome as a cultural form of the most basic kind drawing upon—and in many ways constituting—new and old social and material orders. It is at this juncture, this confluence of basic, applied, computational, molecular, infrastructural, cultural, political, economic, and social assemblages, that I situate the story of diabetes genetic epidemiology.

DIABETES: A PUBLIC HEALTH PROBLEM

I began in 1998 to investigate the work of scientists searching for the genes that "cause" type 2 diabetes.[8] Diabetes is not one disease but many. More than 90 percent of all diabetics have type 2 diabetes, which is characterized by elevated blood glucose triggered by poor insulin production or insulin resistance in skeletal muscle and lipid tissue. Type 2 diabetes is also known as non-insulin-dependent diabetes because, unlike the rarer form of the disease, people with type 2 diabetes produce insulin and therefore seldom need therapeutic insulin at the initial onset of disease. Type 2 diabetes, hereafter referred to simply as diabetes, is, like heart disease, hypertension, and asthma, referred to as a complex disease because its putative risks lie in both environmental and biological domains. That is, diabetes is caused by an as yet unknown combination of factors that include lifestyle, diet, physical activity, and an array of physiological triggers, among which it is presumed that genetic susceptibility plays a part.

Diabetes is the seventh leading cause of death in the United States and is frequently referred to as a public health crisis in the government, academic, and popular press.[9] The World Health Organization has called diabetes an emerging epidemic with more than 16 million people affected in the United States and hundreds of millions more in the rapidly urbanizing Southern Hemisphere and China. According to the Centers for Disease Control (CDC), by 2025, 270 million people worldwide will have diabetes. If the current trend continues, over the next 50 years, one out of three Americans will develop diabetes in their lifetime. For the general population, one in three represents a 165 percent increase by the year 2050. Since 1987, the death rate ascribable to diabetes has increased by 45 percent, whereas the death rates due to heart disease, stroke, and cancer have declined.

Diabetes is a peculiar disease. Its symptoms have been likened to quantitative variation of normal physiology. Its causes have been attributed to genes (read errors), environment (read behaviors), and gene-environment interactions (read lifestyle, nutrition, physical activity levels, marriage practices, and ancestry). During the course of my research, not once did the living conditions for Mexicanas/os along the U.S.-Mexico border figure into a conversation about causality. Drug companies narrate diabetes as a biochemical error, and genetic epidemiologists frame the disease as a population-based syndrome. Because diabetes in indigenous populations has been criticized as a response to the onslaught of unhealthy Anglo values and lifestyles, social scientists have framed it as a disease of civilization or a disease of capitalism.[10]

The hallmark of the condition of diabetes is hyperglycemia, or high blood sugar, caused by the poor utilization of insulin. Insulin is a hormone released by beta cells in the islets of Langerhans of the pancreas. The hormones function to control blood sugar levels. Insulin regulates glucose transport into cells so they can produce energy or store glucose for later use. As food gets digested and transformed into simple sugars, the pancreas is stimulated to release insulin to be used by the muscles as energy, thus preventing hyperglycemia. Most people with diabetes suffer from elevated blood glucose because the insulin their pancreas produces is underutilized by their fat and muscle tissues. Diminished insulin uptake results in hyperglycemia, elevated blood glucose levels.

The pervasiveness of the rhetoric of diabetes as a public health threat is evidenced in the September 2000 issue of *Newsweek* magazine. The cover story, titled "An American Epidemic: Diabetes," tells of the rise of diabetes among Americans. It featured (in the online version) a photograph of Yolanda Benitez, a middle-aged woman with diabetes. The photo shows Benitez heating a tortilla on a cast iron *comal* (skillet). The front-page text reads, "Something terrible was happening to Yolanda Benitez's eyes. They were being poisoned; the fragile capillaries of the retina attacked from within and were leaking blood." The main health concerns for people with diabetes, as the story of Benitez illustrates, are the complications. According to the CDC, diabetes is the leading cause of blindness among people between the ages of 20 and 74. In fact the CDC estimates that when the costs of diabetes complications—eye disease ($470 million), kidney failure ($842 million), and lower extremity amputations ($860 million)—are added to the costs of controlling glucose ($100 million), the expenditure for type 2 diabetes exceeds $2.7 billion annually.[11]

Geneticists, epidemiologists, government analysts, and journalists frame diabetes as an ethnoracial disease. In fact, it is hard to find a discussion, popular or scientific, about diabetes without a discussion of its differential impact on people of color. A publication from the U.S. Center for Disease Control and Prevention reads:

> The burden of disease is heavier among elderly Americans—more than 18 percent of adults over age 65 have diabetes—and certain racial and ethnic populations, including African Americans, Hispanics/Latinos, and American Indians and Alaska Natives. For example, American Indians and Alaska Natives are 2.8 times more likely to have diagnosed diabetes than non-Hispanic whites of similar age.[12]

Similarly, a grant application submitted to the U.S. Public Health Service by one scientist I worked with begins its "Background and Significance" section with the differential prevalence patterns of diabetes in populations defined with ethnoracial labels. It reads, "Type 2 diabetes has an estimated prevalence of 6–8 percent in white populations, 10–12 percent in African Americans, and 15–20 percent in Mexican Americans." The proposal cites an array of scientific references for each population. Additionally, the *Newsweek* story describes Benitez as a "representative victim" of diabetes, citing the usual ethnoracial statistics, a claim that we will return to in chapter 5.

Schooled in the critique of genetic determinism, I was concerned with this scientific practice that, from the outside looking in, appeared to actively transform DNA labeled with historically specific folk taxonomies (Mexican American, Asian, European) into substances with biological significance. Through participant-observation and text-based analyses, I tracked the use of race/ethnicity within an international consortium of scientists who had formed a transdisciplinary and transnational academic-, corporate-, and state-funded alliance. Some of the 33 institutional members include the University of Chicago, the University of Texas, the NIH (including Francis Collins, the director of the Human Genome Project), the American Diabetes Association [ADA], Harvard University, and GlaxoSmithKline.[13]

In the early stages of project development, I traveled to Mexico, Texas, and North Carolina to interview researchers who were in one way or another interested in an aspect of diabetes. In Mexico, I spoke with a population geneticist at the Instituto Nacional de Nutrición, Salvador Zubiran; a geneticist at the Universidad Nacional Autonomia de México; and a clinical researcher at a children's hospital in Mexico City. The population geneticist had biologically characterized some samples used by the clinical researcher who was a coauthor with a University of Texas epidemiologist involved in a San Antonio–based family study. The transnational and cross-disciplinary collaboration of my ethnographic interlocutors figured prominently in the development of the methodological and theoretical foundations of my research. In addition to my interest in race and ethnicity, I was interested in the nature of this scientific collaboration. To understand it would require attending to the transient investigators, data sets, DNA samples, and institutional arrangements that assembled the diabetes enterprise and the locally derived social relations that brought forth the cultural form at each collaborative node. Additionally, I set about to characterize the breadth and depth of scientific cooperation and how such communal research practices could thrive amid the hype about intellectual property.

DIABETES: AN ANTHROPOLOGICAL PROBLEM

Analytically, the type 2 diabetes enterprise is productively understood as an anthropological problem of the first order. In saying this, I am influenced by Ong and Collier's definition of anthropological problems as those involving a confluence of "forms and values that bear directly upon individual and collective existence through which technological, political, ethical reflection and intervention occur."[14] This is Anthropological with a capital A, that which Rabinow calls appropriately, *an-*

thropos.[15] Diabetes is not merely to be understood as an object of human sciences through which we come to locate an instance of population governance.[16] Rather it is also a cultural form that requires attention to humans as both biological and social beings. By confluence, I think not of a noun, a mixture, but a verb, a process of merging together old and new ways of conceiving illness, disease, human variation, biology, society, knowledge, and so on.

Take, for example, diabetes scientists' use of human DNA. Intervening into the value-laden and context-bound configurations of human bodies, the type 2 diabetes enterprise enlists research subjects by virtue of their perceived membership in ethnic groups. Mexicano/as, blacks, Asians, and a host of other groups were enrolled as if these groups made sense sui generis. I was curious as to why the race or ethnicity of a population was important for research into disease given the conviction within anthropology that race is a social construct.

I demonstrate in the pages that follow that my interests in the diabetes enterprise at times sharpened and at others blurred as the "conversation" I was having required me to reflect anew upon my understandings. For example, I began by wondering how race could be biologically meaningful if it is a social construct. I ended, through a series of dialogical conversations,[17] with a clearer explanation of the meanings of "race" and of "social" and of "constructions" that emerge within this technoscientific cultural form. In this way, this project befits Annelise Riles's conceptualization of fieldwork as "an act of circling back, of engaging intellectual and ethical origins from the point of view of problems that now begin elsewhere.[18] That is, the dialogics of my ethnographic practice required me to return to what I had thought I understood. More important, however, as my understanding changed and I came to understand the logics of pragmatism, of antipolitics, of value generation, of service to humanity, the problems of race and diabetes and genetics came to be imaginable as mere markers of larger cultural assemblages with histories and trajectories well beyond my field site and interlocutors.

The problems of diabetes science certainly do not originate in the social worlds of diabetes genetic epidemiology. The disease, and its attendant medical-scientific enterprise are co-configured by the context of their production.[19] The idiom of co-configuration parallels Jasanoff's idiom of coproduction in several important ways. First, diabetes as a material and semiotic assemblage is conceptualized as irreducible to either the material or the semiotic. As Jasanoff remarks, "The co-productionist idiom stresses the constant interplay of the cognitive, the material, the social and the normative."[20] Second, the diabetes genetic enterprise as a technoscientific formation is unpacked as a means through which researchers order knowledge about a chronic epidemiological problem, while at the same time ordering Anglo-Mexicano relations. Jasanoff keenly observes of the interplay of society and science, "Science and technology operate, in short, as political agents."[21] In the coproductionist vein, then, this book demonstrates the means through which a technoscientific project co-configures disease, populations of affected groups, and social orders more broadly. However, I do not adopt Jasanoff's idiom of coproduction wholesale.

This book demonstrates that something unique occurs when we examine the embodied inflections of a natural or cultural assemblage such as "the Mexican diabetic," in which the materiality and meanings of the ethnic body and diabetes are freighted with structural violence and inequality. While I share Jasanoff's resistance to a reductionist social science that finds reproductive social forces in every (scientific) claim or artifact, the case of the "Mexican diabetic" in this postgenomic moment articulates squarely with the racially structured social formations that co-configure well-worn relations of domination and subordination.[22] Far from a coproductionist account of a technoscientific ordering that rejects "a priori demarcations,"[23] the diabetes enterprise, it will be shown, asserts its recombinatory force in the midst of incredible social inequalities. Thus the diabetes enterprise must be unpacked for its ideological work, which at times reinforces and at others resists the reproductive articulations of racial domination. In other words, the diabetes enterprise does reproduce social forces but not unidirectionally or in isolation of the context of its production. The practices that co-configure Mexicanos as diabetic, type 2 diabetes as an inherited condition, and diabetes science as delinked from the sociohistorical orderings of the U.S.-Mexico border are the site of the articulation between racially structured social formations and science and technology. The challenge before me is to account for pronounced structural inequalities within the co-configurations without sullying our understanding of the operations of nature and culture within these same co-configurations. Such is my hope for this book.

In many ways, the diabetes research enterprise is a product of the promises and perils associated with the height of the human genome project, the speculative futures of biotech and other markets, the historic demographic and geopolitical shifts in the United States and

Europe that enabled and required frequent contact—and often conflict—between ethnically diverse peoples. The question becomes, What role does the diabetes genetic enterprise play in this constitutive process today and can we learn anything new about the problems of race in science and the broader sociocultural forces through an ethnographic engagement with this scientific enterprise? At an even finer resolution, what happens to the semiotic status of the materials (genes, blood samples, DNA donors) when they become the building blocks of a technoscientific enterprise? And, further, in what ways do these artifacts themselves inflect the social worlds out of which they were fashioned?

This book presents a more comprehensive and complex presentation of my questions and conclusions than I have heretofore been able to discuss with those with whom I studied. In that, it is still conventionally one sided and unavoidably at times presentist if not disciplinist in it representative prejudices.[24] That is, it is my account of events and their meanings. Still, it is my hope that this book illustrates the important sociocultural work that diabetes scientists carry out in the name of finding the genetic bases of disease. I hope also that it reconfigures anthropological problems as neither utilitarian puzzles that our analyses can piece together nor as enactment of the revelatory moment of discursive emergence—modes of analysis that have been attributed to Dewey and Foucault, respectively.[25] And both the puzzle solved and the revelation fall short of capturing the entangled contingencies of anthropology's problems when we honestly acknowledge our historical and institutional emplacement within the contesting apparatuses of knowing and versions of making and understanding human beings and our world.[26] This ethnographic investigation of diabetes genetic epidemiology, which occurred in the twilight of the completion of the human genome, offers just such problems.

THE BIRTH OF THE DIABETES ENTERPRISE

In 1993, the American Diabetes Association (ADA) launched the GENNID study. The acronym GENNID stands for the Genetics of Non-Insulin Dependent Diabetes. The GENNID study aims to acquire, test, store, and analyze blood samples from "African American, Japanese American, Hispanic and non-Hispanic white" families. At the time, the

GENNID study was predominantly a DNA-collection project. Acquisition centers were set up in university hospitals throughout the United States and were organized by folk taxonomies of ethnicity and race. For example, white samples were gathered in Utah and St. Louis, African American samples in Arkansas and Chicago, Hispanic samples in Texas, and so on. By 1998, more than twelve hundred individuals from 220 families had contributed DNA to the study. The ADA's Web site directs interested researchers to an online catalogue of these samples.[27] Following the link takes one to the Coriel Cell Repository. Coriel started in 1953 as a public nonprofit clearinghouse and storage facility (biobank) for a variety of biological samples and cell cultures. DNA samples were added later. The catalogue includes a reference population and various human variation panels along with their respective price tags. The GENNID samples are not publicly available, however. To access these requires an NIH grant or an arrangement with the ADA.

A few years after the GENNID study began, a consortium of clinical epidemiologists, geneticists, statisticians, and molecular biologists working on the genetics of type 2 diabetes formed an informal alliance to analyze the growing body of DNA samples acquired from diabetic individuals and their families. It was the height of the Human Genome Project, and the organizers of the alliance anticipated the next stage in genetics-based research: making sense of the human genome for disease research. It was a forward-thinking approach. Finding the genetic contribution to chronic disease such as type 2 diabetes would be an intellectual and financial gold mine. The alliance, which soon became the International Diabetes Genetic Analyses Consortium, was formed because each researcher realized that his or her few samples could never reach the statistical significance required for genetic analyses of a complex condition like diabetes. Several consortium members remarked, "Everyone had to fail a few times before coming to see the importance of joining the consortium." Herein, I refer to the "diabetes consortium" as a constellation of people, technology, tools, and biological and chemical materials involved in the production, circulation, and consumption of diabetes knowledges. This constellation of human and nonhumans will hereafter be referred to as key actors, or actants, in the making of diabetes knowledges in this postgenomic era.[28] I refer to the "diabetes enterprise" as a broader and even more heterogeneous constellation of actants involved in diabetes research and product development. In short, the consortium involves knowledge while the enterprise involves products, potential or realized, that the knowledge has in some way enabled.

The research for this book is anchored within a subset cluster of the consortium consisting of scientists from the University of Chicago in collaboration with the University of Texas Health Sciences. The head of the analysis team and arguably the coordinator of the consortium is at Chicago and the director of the sampling operation for the principle data set is in Texas. I interviewed and observed these and other consortium scientists in their places of work, at scientific meetings, and during their collective conversations about the power of their data sets and experimental results. Inspired by actor network theory, I follow DNA samples analytically and physically as they are drawn from a donor's body and processed along the pathways of scientific research. The latter, the following of DNA samples and the sociocultural formations they enable, is the central organizing trope of this book.

I found the consortium by following the GENNID samples from the ADA to the pharmaceutical giant then called Glaxo Wellcome. The company's researchers partner with academic and clinical researchers because Glaxo does not have access to diabetic patients. To identify drug targets, Glaxo acquires samples and conducts genomic scans and linkage analyses to help its partners identify potential genetic causes for disease. In fact, the populations drive the partnerships. Glaxo, for example, was allowed to join the consortium because of its contract with the ADA to genotype and analyze the GENNID data. As the head of the Department of Human Genetics at Glaxo's U.S. headquarters told me, "You can't do genetics without family materials." The relationship between populations and partnerships will be explored in detail in chapter 4.

Over a period of 21 months of field research from 1998 to 2000, I conducted research at the University of Chicago School of Medicine, at scientific meetings and workshops, and at a genetic epidemiology field office on the U.S.-Mexico border. Following a collaborative pathway extending out of the Chicago laboratories, I also visited the labs and research field sites of collaborators in the United Kingdom. Blending empirical research methodology from anthropology and the social studies of science, I followed a cluster of researchers in their labs, field offices, conferences, and other venues of knowledge production. I physically followed DNA data sets through the pathways of research in Mexico,

Texas, and Chicago. As will be shown in the chapters that follow, my method of following blood samples required that I accompany research field workers on home visits, to places of work, and anywhere a sample donor was to be sampled. I followed donors as they worked their way through the field office research stations, then followed the vials of their blood to the field office laboratory. I then tracked the samples as they were shipped to collaborators and moved back and forth between the places that the sample had occupied, from Chicago to Texas and to the United Kingdom.

I observed more than 80 formal and informal meetings between collaborating investigators. I listened to conversations, both formal and casual, noted the population labels in use, and documented other discussions about population DNA, data sets, and collaboration. This included conversations in phone calls, impromptu meetings between colleagues, formal journal club and lecture presentations, lunch conversations, corridor talk, bench banter, one-on-one and small group meetings, consortium meetings, meetings with guest lecturers, and between research participants and research field workers. Additionally, I conducted more than 20 interviews with diabetes researchers from public, private, and corporate institutions[29] and attended five national scientific conferences.[30]

Further, I analyzed manuscripts, conference presentations, journal club reports, grant proposals, laboratory materials, newspaper articles, and drug company promotional materials to document the ways population labels are codified in writing for an array of audiences. Together, these methods help produce an understanding of how race and ethnicity, two social constructs with complicated scientific registers, are constituent elements in the configuration of biogenetic studies and explanations of a chronic disease like diabetes. In fact, in the conclusion of this book, I show that race and ethnicity in technoscientific use are reconfigured into "bioethnicity," which is a hybrid concept that attains meaning through the confluence of natures and cultures.[31] Further, this project elaborates the empirical claims that scientific practices shape and are shaped by the social context of their production and explains the role of genetic research in the persistent use of race to divide populations in society at large.

RACE, DISEASE, AND THE PRODUCTION
OF KNOWLEDGE: A LAYERED PROBLEM

Taking as its main problem the axiomatic (non)existence of distinct human racial groups and the heterogeneous meanings of race, this book explains how the social constructs of human variation (white, Mexican, African American, etc.) inform the work of scientists looking for genetic susceptibilities to type 2 diabetes. Diabetes affects ethnic groups disproportionately. For decades, biomedical researchers have collected demographic and genetic information taken from racialized populations. In this book, I focus on the use of information and material taken from Mexicans and Mexican Americans specifically. The use of DNA from other groups also informs the work of researchers, professionals, and others who are interested in postgenomic diabetes. However, the arguments put forth here centrally revolve around the principal data set taken from the U.S.-Mexico border.

Placing DNA acquisition within the sociohistorical context of the U.S.-Mexico border, the processes and products of genetic epidemiological research can be understood as founded upon long-standing racialized social and economic inequalities. Yet, this project does not advance new theories or instances of overtly racist science. On the contrary, the type 2 diabetes genetic epidemiological enterprise—hereafter simply the diabetes enterprise—illustrates how the science of diabetes and social inequality are co-configured in spite of the acts of socially responsible scientists. For this project, I foreground the connections between medical science, a highly codified and privileged social practice, and the larger social forces that link political economy with race and ethnicity and, to a degree, gender. Further, under the persistent history of violent conflict, exclusion, enmity, and threat, Mexicanos/as on the U.S.-Mexico border who participate in genetic research fulfill an embodied role as racialized objects of research in a manner wholly consistent with such histories.

Understood in this context, the case of the diabetes enterprise demonstrates that DNA donors serve as global human capital for genetics-based medical research. The state and academe are revealed as privileged domains of sociocultural production that promote the generation of value for some and not others. Yet I have worked to ground the contributions of state and academic institutions by presenting how the work that emanates from a university is inseparable from the lives of the actors who operate these institutions. Furthermore, as intended beneficiaries and necessary actors within the pathways of research, DNA donors become transformed into transnational protogenetic subjects of state-capital interpellation. Readers interested in the use of human subjects will learn that in this enterprise, donor populations and their DNA become silenced commodities through the quantitative SNP-based genetic research practices. Donors' samples are part of the larger reworking of "the biological" through regimes of exchange and ultimate profitability. Further, I came to appreciate that scientists do not unconsciously re-create racial typologies, but instead carefully press the social formations of ethnic identity into the service of the biogenetic research enterprise. As a consequence, diabetes research conflates the descriptions of affected populations with the attributes of those populations, thus pathologizing the ethnicity of DNA donors.

I begin with an outline of the problem of population labels. This is intended to introduce the reader to issues addressed in detail in the chapters that follow.

Race/No Race: Public Debates

At its most rudimentary, this project seeks to answer the following question: How do diabetes researchers resurrect empirically defunct biological separations between populations? Does the use of Mexicano/a DNA in biogenetic research convert ethnicity into biological race? The answer lies in the difference between ethnicity and race. If the labels do not reference race, a fictive biological construct, then they must refer to ethnicity. Ethnicity is not discernable at the level of the phenotype—visible empirical types, presumed to be an expression of underlying genetics. This is because ones' ethnicity is a complex of ascriptive and descriptive elements derived from geographic, political, historical, and socioeconomic factors. The differences between "white" and "Hispanic white" or "Latino" and "Mexican" are just two examples. The fundamentally social and historical nature of ethnicity is all the more apparent in labels like Islamic, Black Arab, American, non-Hispanic African American, and Japanese Brazilian, to name a few appearing in research abstracts. Clearly these are not biological nomenclatures in any simple sense. But the race-and-no-race debates deserve a closer examination, for they orient much of this book.

Race, some have argued, is an unstable category subject to contestation.[32] Race cannot be understood as a free-standing metalinguistic taxonomic system because it is always mediated through human actors that are caught up in discourses of social location, identity, class, nation, culture, science, sexuality, and nature-biology. Yet when the biology of human variation is at issue, the discussion often gets simplified as an either/or debate. On the one hand, there are those who argue that distinct biological racial groups do not exist at all.[33] Biological anthropologist Jon Marks writes:

> Biological variation exists within the human species, and some of it is structured geographically. But this component of our biological variation is (1) very small relative to the total and (2) not patterned in such a way as to permit the formalization of a reasonably small number of natural "races." To the extent that we popularly identify such clusters, they are the result of cultural impositions of meaningful distinctions on nature, a classically anthropological example of a "folk taxonomy."[34]

These researchers argue that there is no biological justification for racial groupings. They draw upon decades of research to note that most variation, approximately 95 percent, exists *within* so-called racial groups, that racial groups are not biological clusters, and that biological variation is a function of the evolutionary effects of geographic distance.

Though race has been a contested topic for decades, this most recent debate can be linked to the emergence of the Human Genome Project. In 1990 the United States Human Genome Project began the coordinated efforts to map and sequence the human genome. Among the assemblage of scholars involved in launching this effort was a working group charged with evaluating the ethical, legal, and social implications (ELSI) of the project. In 1996, seven years after the project began, this advisory group was the only group whose work to initiate the project was not complete.[35] Sociologist Troy Duster, then chair of the group and the leading critic of "race" in medicine, explained to a national blue ribbon panel that the group's charge was as pertinent as ever because "as genetic discoveries are made, they affect people of varying social positions, cultures, religions and genders differently."[36] The group would be needed in perpetuity, he explained, because it was the only entity able to evaluate the effect of genetic advances on groups rather than on individuals or individual bodies.

The distinction between the consequences for human groups rather than individuals is central to the cultural work of the diabetes enterprise and of this project. In this vein, the effect (good or bad) of genetic advances on an individual diabetic is a different set of issues from the ways categories of diabetic groups (e.g., Mexican diabetics) are effected.

It is understandable, then, that issues involving groups defined by such labels as "Black, Native American, Asian, Mexican" would be one of the most salient themes in determining the social, legal, and ethical implications of the Human Genome Project. The ELSI working group remains to this day, and a portion of the genome project's research budget is devoted to the group's original charge.

That charge addresses a long-standing debate in medicine, public health, epidemiology, and the social sciences that calls into question the dubious applicability of racial groupings in studies of health outcomes, interventions, and disease etiologies.[37] For example, Duster's work documented the ways that the genetics of sickle-cell anemia led to the pathologization of African Americans.[38] He illustrated how public health campaigns that encouraged African Americans to get screened for the disease in effect curbed African American birthrates.

Other studies critiqued the labels used in public health research, the discordance between biology and race, and unequal treatments based upon race and sex. For example, R. Hahn, Mulinare, and Teutsch examined infant mortality in the United States between 1983 and 1985 and found highly inconsistent coding of race and ethnicity of infants at birth and death.[39] Their research sheds doubt on all racial and ethnic labeling in medical research. A subsequent national study of funeral directors found similar taxonomic instabilities.[40] Related problems for forensic identification have been identified by Goodman.[41] A study by Schulman and colleagues demonstrated that the race and sex of a patient influenced the rates at which physicians referred individuals for cardiac catheterization.[42] This landmark study confirmed that race and sex operated independently of differences in the clinical presentation of the patients.[43] Similarly, a report issued in March 2002 by the National Academies of Science, Institute of Medicine, reviewed more than one hundred studies and reaffirmed these patterns in health care.[44] The report found that minorities, irrespective of access, education, and income, were discriminated against in health care.

Since 2000, there has been a steady stream of editorials and special commentaries reiterating that race is a social construct and not a biologically meaningful taxonomic system. In various ways and from an array of biomedical or other academic disciplines, authors warn against the improper use of race in research or clinical practice.[45] Parts of the debate have spilled onto the pages of the *New York Times*. Psychiatrist Sally Satel, for example, boldly proclaimed in the *Sunday Times Magazine*, "I Am a Racially Profiling Doctor" (May 5, 2002). At the end of the first paragraph she writes, "When it comes to practicing medicine, stereotyping often works." Satel is critical of the no-race position because in her practice and among her colleagues, race (defined as genetic differences based on ancestral geography), she says, should not be ignored. Citing diagnostic anecdotes and research into variable drug efficacies by race, Satel argues that attention to racial or ethnic differences can help patients. The *New York Times* science reporter Nicolas Wade came to similar conclusions in his reporting on a study that supports the continuation of racial or ethnic self-identity in biomedical and genetic research.[46] Citing a National Cancer Institute researcher who claims that critics are unqualified, Wade champions a study by Neil Risch and colleagues that argues that a race-neutral approach to human categorization in biomedical research is statistically less valid than racial self-identification. Wade presents the Risch study as if it were a definitive end to the no-race critique ("Race Is Seen as a Real Guide to Track Roots of Disease," July 30, 2002).[47]

Reardon's astute analysis of the Human Genome Diversity Project articulates the crux of this debate.[48] That project was an attempt to collect the genomes of isolated and often indigenous peoples in an effort to preserve a genetic record of human biodiversity and thus enable an understanding of human evolution. The project died almost as soon as it began and has morphed into numerous other biobanking projects.[49] In assessing the controversies that surrounded the Human Genome Diversity Project through much of the 1990s, Reardon observed that the scientific issues of human genetic differences were inextricably linked with social and ethical issues of North-South relations, colonialism, intellectual property rights, and human origin narratives of particular groups. The failure to implement the project was a result of epistemological differences between geneticists and their critics and a priori political encumbrances of human genetics research itself. Scientists argued over the appropriate and ethical units of analysis (populations, individuals, groups, bodies), while activists and community groups critiqued the assumptions that social and cultural groups could ethically or accurately map onto genetic groups in the first place.

Like the conundrum presented by the Human Genome Diversity Project, when we examine closely the development of genetic knowledge derived from epidemiological research into type 2 diabetes, the problematic ontological incongruities of race and genes come into view. That is, *races are not biological categories discernable through genetic frequencies.* Beyond the difficulties of navigating the socioethical alongside the scientific, as suggested by the coproduction framework,[50] the ways genetics is used to explain population differences for medical purposes are at odds over what constitutes a person. On the one hand, a race-neutral perspective sees no link between a blood sample and the person from whom DNA has been extracted. There is only DNA, bits of genes, not persons. On the other hand, critics of race see people whose bodies are interpellated by a dominant ideology of genetic reductionism and groups of people whose genetic information is the telegraphic proxy for their bodies and the personification of their group. Within the Human Genome Diversity Project, Reardon describes this conflict as an understanding that "imagines a 'population' corded off from modernity; what makes these 'populations' genetically interesting is precisely what defines them as not part of modern Western social orders."[51] Key to the project and the collection of genetic materials for disease research are the presumed concordance between genes and race and, even more important, between genes and disease.[52]

Some scholars remain deeply skeptical of any use of social taxonomies in the biosciences. They argue against any racial or ethnic classification based on evolutionary or biological phenomena between or within populations.[53] Molnar, for instance, writes in his textbook *Human Variation: Races, Types, and Ethnic Groups*, "I shall use, where necessary, the term *race* to mean a group or *complex* of breeding populations sharing a number of traits."[54] The no-race school of thought is also opposed to work that seeks to establish the concordance between genetic variation and racial groupings.[55] Some no-race theorists charge that the use of race or racial typologies as a means to define populations is, simply, racist.[56] Anthropologist Harrison defines racism as "the nexus of material relations within which social and discursive practices perpetuate oppressive power relations between populations presumed to be essentially different."[57] It is the "presumption of essential difference" and the consequences of those presumptions that are at the core of the race–no-race debate.

Populations in Research

Genetic data affirm that neither geographic circumscription nor distinct evolutionary lineages can support population or individual taxonomies as we currently construe them.[58] Further, more human variation can be found within than between geographically, linguistically, and culturally categorized groups.[59] Patterns of variation do correlate with geographic distributions, but these variations do not directly correspond to U.S. racial categories. Anticipating a steady stream of spurious claims about the existence of biological race, in 1998 the American Anthropological Association commissioned a statement on race authored principally by Audrey Smedley and carefully reviewed by a working group of distinguished anthropologists.[60] The American Anthropological Association Executive Board adopted the position that "most physical variation, about 94 percent, lies *within* so-called racial groups." In the AAA statement, the authors argue that biological indices cannot be used to differentiate human groups labeled with conventional taxonomies of race because race is fundamentally an ideology about human differences. The statement argues that medical research derived from such groups thus inaccurately portrays biological differences between peoples.

At first glance, diabetes researchers seem to be the perfect example of the inaccurate use of racial taxonomies in biomedical research. An example will illustrate. The premier venue for presenting research findings for diabetes is the American Diabetes Association Scientific Sessions. The 1998, 1999, and 2000 ADA's Scientific Sessions Abstract Books parsed research according to 23 distinct investigative areas. The areas garnering the most research attention at the meetings include, in order, metabolism, clinical diabetes, macrovascular complications, insulin action, immunology, islet biology, genetics, and epidemiology. On average, the meetings publish nineteen hundred abstracts each year with posters representing more than half of all reports. Oral presentations constitute 16 percent of abstracts, with reports of research published only for the abstracts books accounting for the remaining 31 percent.

An analysis of the abstracts indicates that the use of ethnoracially labeled groups in diabetes research is on the rise. Between 1998 and 2000, the different kinds of population labels used by researchers jumped 17 percent, from 153 to 179 distinct ethnoracial labels. During this same period, there was a 60 percent increase in the overall use of data with ethnoracial labels, from 191 uses to 305. The greatest increase in ethnoracially labeled populations occurred among geneticists whose use of such labels jumped 60 percent, followed by epidemiologists whose use jumped 30 percent over the three years surveyed. And even though type 2 diabetes researchers deploy ethnoracial labels approximately four times as often as those conducting research on type 1, ethnoracial labels frequently appear in complications research, which crosses both diabetes domains. The trend as indicated in research abstracts suggests that at the very moment "race" is pronounced scientifically dead, diabetes researchers increasingly use population-based specificity to advance their research agendas.

Admittedly, race and ethnicity present a conundrum for medical researchers. On the one hand, since conservatively 96–99 percent of human genetic material is common to all human beings, there is minimal biological basis for parsing populations by genetic differences. On the other hand, there are different frequencies in the distributions of genetic material that some researchers believe may prove important in finding genetic contributions to diabetes and other complex diseases, frequencies in which leading researchers claim ethnic membership plays an important role. The pertinent question is how can the two propositions be explained without resorting to academic one-upmanship, or by simply amplifying old arguments in increasingly dismissive or inflammatory language?

For this project, the question is not whether population-based data is informative, but rather, informative of what? For some kinds of research, population specificity is explained as a way to control for heterogeneous research variables. For genetics, for example, research protocols based on the fine-grained single nucleotide polymorphism (SNP; see the glossary) require population specificity to help reduce the "noise" in their data. In other words, the reduction in gene variants supposedly afforded by a carefully selected group of human subjects significantly shrinks the size of the haystack through which researchers must sift in looking for a needle.[61] Finding a genetic component to type 2 diabetes, for example, facilitates the more difficult task of identifying physiological triggers and pathways by localizing molecules of interest.

There are related advantages afforded by population-based research in epidemiology, investigations of patient or practitioner behavior, and analyses of health care delivery. For example, collecting ethnic-specific data can help document health disparities, practitioner biases, or unequal access to health care.[62] It is less clear, however, that the use of ethnoracial labels is helpful in clinical trials, treatment protocols, and non-epidemiological research into complications.

The labels used by diabetes researchers reveal the profoundly social nature of population identifiers. For example, in the more than 460 ADA research abstracts analyzed, there are seven labels for African Americans, including Afro-American, non-Hispanic black, black, and non-Hispanic African American. For Latinos there are eight labels, including Latin, Latino, Mexican American, and Mexican. However, most interesting anthropologically are the increases in the frequency and the population

Portuguese
Native Canadian

Tukano (Amazonian Jungle, Colombia)
Ingeneria, Urbanization, Lima (Peru)
American White
North European
Alaskan Native
Pirutapuyo (Amazonian Jungle, Colombia)
Indian Asian
Western European
First Nation

Islamic
Norwegian
North Dakotan
Hispanic American
Non-Hispanic Black
United States Black
Filipino
European
White European
Asian American
British Caucasian
Finnish
South Indian Inuit
Non-Hispanic
Italian
Afro-American
Caucasian (White)
Pakistani
"Other"

Vietnamese
Ghanian
Indian
British
Saudi Arabian
(French)
Western (French)
Mexican
Native Caribbean
Afro-Caribbean
Fijian
Sardinian
Maori
Huaras, Ancash (Peru)
"Race"
American
Nigerian
North Indian Asian
Lebanese
Scottish
Scandinavian
United States Caucasian
Non-Hispanic African-American (Virgin Islands)
Hispanic White
United States
Amish
Swiss
Chilean
Chinese
Swedish
American Indian
Israeli, Arab
Slavic
Asian Indian
Puerto Rican
Ontario, Canada
Non-Hispanic Black
South Indian Asian
Turkish
Mapuche
Ashkenazi Jewish
United Kingdom Caucasian
Black
Wayko, Lamas, San Martin (Peru)
Dominican
Mexican-American
Japanese
Canadian
San Antonio
French Caucasian
Japanese-American
United States White
Icelandic
Pacific Islander
United Kingdom Origin (In Australia)
Egyptian
Belgian
Native
Cherokee
Non-White
South Asian
Non-Caucasian
North American
Dutch
Muslim
Desano (Amazonian Jungle, Colombia)
Singaporean
Spanish (Mediterranean Caucasian)
Romanian
Asian
West African Ancestry
Yemenite Jew
West Indian Hispanic
Bedouin-Arab
West Indian
Brazilian
United Kingdom
Arab
North European Caucasian
White Caucasian
North African
Malay
Latin
"Ethnicity"
Saudi
Trinidad, West Indies
Ethiopian
Eastern European
Jewish
Hispanic Black
Native American
North Indian
German
Cunumbuque, Lamas, San Martin (Peru)
Tohono O'odham
Pima Aboriginal
Nauru
Mexican-Born
Castilla, Piura (Peru)
Tarapoto, San Martin (Peru)
East Canadian First Nation
Taiwanese
African
French
Mauritian
Korean
Anglo
New Zealander (European Descent)
Muslim/Bedouin
Polish
African American
Danish
White
Non-Hispanic White
French Canadian
Montana/Wyoming
Caribbean Latino
Danish Caucasian
United Arab Emirates
Japanese-Brazilian
Western
labels

FIGURE I. Complete list of population labels used in ADA abstracts, 1998–2000.

breadth of monikers used to describe so-called white people. In 1998 there were only two uses of the label "Caucasian (white)"; by 2000 there were 31. The current range of ethnic labels for people of northern European ancestry is quite diverse, including white, British Caucasian, Hispanic white, North American, Western, and a nonstatistical reference to a population labeled simply "United States." In all, there are at least 30 different population labels that could fit in the "white" category. Continents, nations, and religions are also represented including Jewish, Islamic, Muslim, African, Asian, Amish, French, German, Japanese, and Europid. Based upon the classificatory moving targets represented in diabetes research abstracts, it is clear that diabetes researchers' labels are fundamentally social constructs founded upon social history, geopolitical boundaries, or census categories.

Notably, the journal *Nature Genetics* banned the use of population labels on its pages unless the science requires it. In an editorial the journal notes, "Race might be a proxy for discriminatory experiences, diet or other environmental factors."[63] But to conduct research designed to exploit the purported genetic differences between populations identified with ethnoracial labels raises a host of ethical questions that go beyond questions of scientific accuracy.

RACE, SCIENCE, AND DISEASE

Because the production of knowledge is the object and subject of this book, it is also concerned with productively discomforting academic discourses and narratives. These include (1) theories of race, (2) theories of science and society, (3) political economy of the body and health, and (4) studies of the historical and contemporary lives of Latinos, predominantly Mexicano-identified peoples in the United States and elsewhere. It draws upon these discussions in an effort to initiate conversation between them and to thereby extend these theories in productive ways.

Critical theories of race figure heavily in the context of this project. Since Boas first problematized the relationship between one's phenotype and one's character by showing that the ethnological and sociological evidence did not support the prevailing assumptions of his day, social prejudices based upon biological race have been thoroughly rejected in anthropology as elsewhere.[64] Still, the arguments for and against biological differences between human groups remains contested terrain. The very existence of biological race has surfaced as a contested issue again and again.[65] In genetics, Lewontin, Rose, and Kamin are arguably the most emblematic of the critiques of biological race and of reducing everything to a biological problem.[66] Equally groundbreaking and productively discomfiting are philosophers of technosciences who skillfully sully the determinisms, biologisms, and geneticizations in gendered and racialized ideologies within scientific texts.[67]

Research that states that the characteristics of individual health are the consequence of biology are adroitly critiqued by Duster and Krieger, whose accounts, respectively, of passive eugenics and of the embodiment of inequality point to the power of the social analytic on matters of human biology and health.[68] Lewontin and colleagues trace the development of race from its original concept of a different "kind" to that of a species and subspecies to subgroups defined by blood and geography or by outward appearances. Current debates, which will be examined within the context of medical and genetics research in chapter 1, have centered on the differentiation made possible through analysis of shared genetic frequencies.[69] As the chapters that follow will show, the resurgence of the race debate in science and medicine are linked with the political changes of the past and present social relationships forged within, through, and among ethnic groups. What is important is not merely that race is an ever-changing political construct.[70] The present case particularly, though not exclusively, highlights racial relations between Anglos and Mexicanos on the U.S.-Mexico border and beyond. The racial category called "Mexicano" is understandable as a political construct and as a biological one intimately tied to the conditions of its production, in the laboratory, and in the lives of those whose DNA makes possible the diabetes scientific enterprise.

Hannah Arendt, for example, argued that Jews and modern anti-Semitism were part of the development of the modern nation-state. Aspects of Jewish history and the societal roles of Jews over the last few centuries were important influences on the configuration of Jewishness and prejudices toward them. She argues that Jews were not scapegoats or millennial victims; most, of course, were impoverished laborers rather than cosmopolitan merchants or financiers. Yet their occupation of an "ethnic" niche in such fields made Jews easy targets as imperialism weakened the need for their financial role in service to states whose social and economic policies had worked to create Jews as a special social class. Mexicanos also occupy an ethnic niche related to the labor that they provide. However, beyond the manual labor so commonly associated with Mexicanos, the donation of DNA affords a further articulation of the role for Mexicanos as an ethnic group. It is a role, I argue here, that articulates in embodied form specific social and economic policies toward Mexicanos since before the Treaty of Guadalupe Hidalgo in 1848.

Omi and Winant similarly argue that state apparatuses such as economic and social policies shape the racial order.[71] Examining the United States from the 1960s to the 1990s, they argue that race is an autonomous historically situated ideological field of social and political organization and as such must be understood as simultaneously experiential, embodied, and structural. Several other authors have examined the ways race as a biological notion has been transformed by social factors.[72] Building on these theorists, this book illustrates that the racialization of Mexicanas/os and other groups taken up in genetic epidemiological research is, indeed, part and parcel of specific historical, political, and social situations. Yet attention to the specificities of Mexicana/o DNA, DNA donation, participation in research, and rates of disease demonstrates the resilience of racialized inequality even within the social world of curing disease. Hence this case also accentuates the conundrum of technoscientific idealism when placed within a space of great conflict and oppression. To be sure, Mexicana/o racialization everywhere is intimately tied to the constructs of race, space, and legal strictures of U.S. nationalism and global capitalism.[73] As such, this ethnography of the diabetes genetic enterprise is notably inspired by the everyday hopeful act of DNA collection, processing, circulation, representation, and consumption.

This book also details the problem of race and of racialization of Mexicanas/os as intimately linked to the political economy of the U.S.-Mexico border. Such structural forces as agribusiness, immigration reform, war, dispossession, drug commerce, and trade agreements and disagreements all shed light on the peculiar stranglehold on the conditions of living for Mexicanas/os along the border. To understand those conditions, which are the same forces that enable DNA acquisition, it is important to anchor the transfer of biological samples within the very same sets of systemic racialized inequalities that characterize the U.S. treatment, governmental and lay alike, of the Mexicana/o residents along the border. Racialized inequalities that are inseparable from social orders of white supremacy have historically served U.S. global capital expansionism in the region.

Current questions of race, its existence or its utility, are thus not a scientific coincidence. The findings of the genetic epidemiologists studied are herein evaluated in terms of the actors and networks involved in their production. Following Callon and Latour, this book uses actor network theory to explore the role DNA samples themselves play in the claims making processes of diabetes knowledge production.[74] Callon and Latour's notion of actor network theory proposes that only by examining the ways persons and things work together can we understand how one scientific claim gains purchase over another. No fact stands alone, they infer, because nature and society lie behind facts after they are made, never behind facts in the making. The proof of a claim's success is its ability to enroll allies (persons and things) in its support. This is neither conspiratorial, competitive alliance making nor strategic maneuvering.[75] Rather, it is an analytical approach that enables, as it has herein, the inclusion of an accounting of the human and nonhuman actors, actants, involved in the scientific process.[76]

In this book, it is demonstrated that the rise of the genetic epidemiological approach to type 2 diabetes is embedded in a particular social and historical context that is understandable through an assessment of the key racialized actant, DNA. Arguing that diabetes is at once a biological and a political construct, this book expands actor network theory by grounding it explicitly into the nuanced positioned interests of Mexicanas/os and those who genetically study them. I argue that (complicating Callon and Latour) nature and society are indeed behind the facts in the making, for "nature" and "society" constitute the processes and products of scientific fact. My argument is akin to that of Latour and Fujimura, who argue that a scientific claim is coproduced with the problems that initiated its examination in the first place.[77] As Haraway argues of the ways race, class, sexuality, and gender are produced, "Both the facts and the witnesses are constituted in the encounters that are technoscientific practice. Both the subjects and objects of technoscience are forged and branded in the crucible of specific, located practices some of which are global in their location."[78] Hence the race debates in medicine and the ethnographic case study herein, are co-constituted with the particular technological developments of genomic science and of population genetics. In other words, this book and the range of topics it addresses must be conceptualized in tandem with the national social agendas to make the United States a color-blind society, a land of equal opportunity, and a place free of inequalities of health.[79] The research for this book occurred while the U.S. Supreme Court was deliberating on an affirmative action case involving the University of Michigan, during the referendum preparations of the California Racial Privacy Initiative, and under the publicity generated by the U.S. government's Healthy

People 2000 and 2010 initiative. The aims of the latter are to end the inequalities of health burdens patterned along racial and ethnic lines.

As it pertains to health, medicine, science, and diabetes, context matters in this book. First, within these chapters, health, disease, risk, and the embodiment of ethnicity are simultaneously theorized such that both the co-constituted cultural meanings and political economies of diabetes and the U.S.-Mexico border are revealed. Scheper-Hughes and Lock argue that we must carefully scrutinize the kinds of bodies evoked in specific contexts if we are to explain how certain bodies and the "cultural sources and meanings of health and illness" are produced.[80] The use by diabetes scientists of bodies identified with racialized labels thus affords an opportunity to examine the cultural work that occurs when people are treated as individuals, as diabetics, as research participants, as humans, and as Mexicanas. It also enables us to observe and assess the manner in which we are all increasingly conscripted into various pathological states.[81] In the chapters that follow, there appear many instances in which the social body and the individual body are reworked through the metaphors of Mexicana/o ethnicity. A more general application of this process is advanced in the concept of bioethnicity (see chapter 5), which is the resultant product of the ways ethnicity comes to be constructed as meaningful for scientific research.

This book also converses with social epidemiological analyses that examine disease and illness within their environmental, historical, and political contexts. Pertinent to this book are those authors who argue for the inclusion of social class as a predictor of health outcomes.[82] These analysts examine life expectancy as a conditional aspect of social inequality, presenting evidence that societies with the greatest income disparity also evince the greatest health disparities. Further, classic studies by epidemiologists Cooper and David and Krieger and Fee argue that cultural history, not genetic history, produces human disease.[83] Cooper and David assert that making a genetic claim for ethnic differences in disease "accepts as given precisely the thing to be explained,"[84] and Krieger and Fee argue that within-group comparisons would be a more informative means of examining the biological and social patterns of disease than are between-group comparisons.[85] Similarly, social epidemiological analyses have critiqued the use of race in the medical and epidemiological literatures, arguing that race is both an inaccurate and misleading research variable.[86] In particular, medical anthropologist Robert Hahn's seminal analysis of racial classifications between birth and death illustrate the fluidity of folk taxonomies used for vital statistics and by extension all epidemiological research.[87] Taking seriously these epidemio-logics, the case of diabetes within the Mexicana/o community exemplifies the embodiment of social inequality along the U.S.-Mexico border. The diabetes genetic enterprise thus affords a glimpse at how global technoscientific knowledge production plays out in local cultural contexts through the appropriation of embodied expressions of sociopolitical configurations.

This book is principally dedicated to an interrogation of the persistent enrollment of Mexicanas/os into genetics-based medical research practices. This project is not an ethnography about Mexicanos, however. The approach differs from the wealth of analyses of *maquiladoras*, of migration, Latino cultural citizenship, of *frontera* identity and *mestizaje*, of development and modernity, or of *indigenismo*.[88] Instead, I invert the ethnographic lens to examine the people who examine and produce (biologically and socially) those who make up the largest U.S. minority group, Latinas/os.[89]

However, the contingency of population taxonomies presented in the chapters that follow raises questions of central importance to understanding Anglo-Mexicano relations and Mexicano experiences. In what ways do changes in agricultural production along the U.S.-Mexico border determine the availability of a class of ready-made research subjects for Anglocentric scientific enterprises?[90] How can scholars account for the pernicious effects of the configurations of Mexicanas/os as an admixed biological race while preserving the cultural force of *indigenismo* and *mestizaje* inherent in critical counterdiscourses? How can the critique and understanding of capitalist hegemony be improved by an inclusion of Mexicana/o participation in capital-intensive research enterprises? And in what ways can a critique of the dominant rhetorics of Mexicano culture as fatalistic, unhealthy, superstitious, unserious (*relajo*) be fortified through an understanding of the embodiment of Mexicanos' susceptibilities to disease? These are all questions that are taken up to varying degrees, implied rather than directly addressed, and thus are not the central themes of this book.

The theoretical orientations and commitments outlined above are beginning points for understanding the analyses and arguments that follow. Shared by theories of race, social and cultural analyses of science, and social epidemiologists is the critical contextualization of the phenomena of race, disease, health, and Mexicano ethnicity. There exists a common thread in these constellation of terms that are mutually composed through biological research and sociocultural conditions. It is the aim of this book to extend these theoretical conversations by offering an empirical foothold for making critical contextual connections and thereby resist the reductionist limitations of viewing this constellation of phenomena in isolation of one another or as either predominantly sociological or predominantly biological.

BEYOND REDUCTIONISMS

One set of recurrent sociocultural processes that make the case of the type 2 diabetes genetic enterprise especially vexing is the reductive and deterministic discourse of biology and genetics in particular. Simply put, the epistemic authority[91] of genes and biology reconfigure all things racial, ethnic, and pathological as if they were at their most fundamental level biological or genetic phenomena. Hubbard, and Hubbard and Wald, have critiqued the field of genetics for its reductive and deterministic biases.[92] In genetics, genes get endowed with tremendous and entirely unfounded powers of causation. However, Hubbard and Wald remind us that genes do not make proteins. Genes are DNA segments that, in concert with a concatenation of other metabolic apparatuses within cell formation, work to synthesize a protein.[93] The consequences of reductive reasoning make highly individual (gene or organism or person) what is best understood as a dynamic interaction within a specific environment.

Hubbard and Wald demonstrate that the idea that genes cause disease not only creates a context in which solutions get constructed as technical problems rather than as social or environmental ones, but additionally places the person affected by a disease in a double bind of being both blamed for the behavior that caused the condition (e.g., sedentary lifestyle for diabetes) and deprived of agency.[94] So, for example, when field office worker Judi is asked why her community has such high rates of diabetes, she remarks, "It's in our blood." Judi's acceptance of a genetic (blood heredity) explanation of diabetes etiology illustrates the process of geneticization characterized by Lippman.[95] Geneticization occurs when social, behavioral, and physiological problems are defined as genetic and when solutions to those problems are presumed to rely upon genetic expertise.

To be sure, the mechanisms of determinism and reductionism at work in the diabetes enterprise are similar to those that deal in representations of sex and gender and of geneticization writ large. The racially deterministic impulse states that the characteristics of the individual are a consequence of their biology. Determinism fits the prevailing social order, Lewontin and colleagues assert, because its practitioners always try to change the population to fit the environment.[96] In the case of race, the differences between populations (skin color, language, or clusters of gene polymorphisms) have been used to explain criminality or intelligence without having to critically examine the organization of society itself. Like the earlier work of Boas, who tried to use the science of biological race to critique the "psychological origin or the implicit belief in the authority of tradition,"[97] Lewontin and colleagues use genetic determinism to critique capitalist society for the ways certain questions about human variation are never asked.

Deterministic and reductionistic science are not unique to disease science, nor are racializing discourses. Cartmill analyzed the use of racial categories in physical anthropology from 1965 to 1996.[98] He found that such racial categories as australoids and Negroid were used consistently about 40 percent of the time for the entire thirty-year period. This large minority shares with the rest of physical anthropology "the general conviction that human behavior is significantly channeled, constrained and determined by human biology."[99] We all have to eat and sleep, for example. However, Cartmill points out that there is a danger of using biology as justification for social order. Race, for example, is often conflated with blood heredity. This essentialist notion leads to arguments about the superiority or inferiority of one biologically delimited group or another. He argues that while Tay-Sachs disease for evolutionary and sociocultural reasons may be more common among Ashkenazim, this does not mean that Ashkenazim are inferior. Membership does not equal Tay-Sachs, and Tay-Sachs cannot be used as proxy for membership. Rather, certain combinations of genes in certain environments can lead to Tay-Sachs disease. Like other social constructs, Cartmill writes, races are real in their consequences.

More pernicious than the consequences of using biological concepts to explain social phenomenon are the ways reductionism, determinism, and geneticization configure the way knowledge is produced. For example, feminist scholars of science have shown the ways that primatology and embryology imagined women, from the outset, only vis-à-vis their biological differences from men.[100] Similar conceptual and institutional prefigurations reinforce dubious distinctions between humans from nonprimates, and cleave illness from disease.[101] In each case, it is shown how cultural logics shape the ways researchers observe and interpret data and diagnose, manage, or treat human suffering with a priori assumptions about the very phenomenon they seek to understand.

A recurrent theme within this book, therefore, is the ways the objects of interest resist ontological assimilation into the bifurcations of difference and the reductionism that occurs when difference itself is left unexamined. I thought this project was going to easily enable a taking of sides, epistemological at least, related to the matter of race, disease, and human variation. Instead, I found that the dualisms that shaped the conceptualization of the project did not fit. Race, as a kind of differentiation within the diabetes enterprise, was simultaneously many different things, practices, and processes with many different consequences. To be sure, as I will show throughout this book, race, Mexicano, ethnicity, genes, and diabetes can be mapped onto familiar patterns of social reproduction. They also map onto other questions, problems, and logics that are not easily traced in the dystopias of modernity, advanced capitalism, neoliberalism or their often violent histories.

Moving beyond the dualisms that are inherent in reductionistic thought, I argue that the contests between race as social or biological reinforce both sides of the argument while maintaining a hold on the modernist logics of divide and conquer. Thus the challenge I have set forth here is to think about race as an idea, as a thing, as a practice, as a system in a way that does not lead to the grooves of either-or thinking. Thus throughout this book, you will read instances of confluences between natures, cultures, and other binaries. What would race look like had Descartes not successfully mechanized the body, divorcing it from the soul? What would disease look like if health were not its opposite? What would a knowledge making, or an accounting of one epistemological approach to the body look like, feel like, and produce if I resist the temptation to racially place everything about the diabetes enterprise as either social or biological?

Surely this will leave some uncomfortable seeking to locate this work along a continuum of "race" and "no race." Yet I share with Gravlee the desire to push beyond discussions that reiterate that race is a social construct about which biology can tell us little.[102] While true, this insight closes rather than opens the conceptual terrain about race and how it relates to biology. Although I reproduce these debates here, I do so only to orient the reader to the epistemological field in which I situate this project. I find it more productive, more faithful to my field encounters, to resist the dualistic side-taking of biology versus society in examining the diabetes enterprise.

Eschewing reductionistic thinking leaves us with a far more interesting and productive set of approaches to disease, human variation, and race. I draw upon Margaret Lock's keen insights that "biological difference—sometimes obvious, at other times very subtle—molds and contains the subjective experience of individuals and the creation of cultural interpretations. A dialectic of this kind between culture and biology implies that we must contextualize interpretations about the body not only as products of local histories, knowledge, and politics but also as local biologies."[103] Local biology, like biocultural and ecosocial approaches to human health, requires the simultaneous acknowledgment that diet, physical activity, stress, labor relations, forced migrations, poverty, and a host of other sociohistorical factors shape and are shaped by experiences that can have biological outcomes.[104]

On the other hand, attempting to explain a particular configuration of biogenetic and medical knowledge requires an acknowledgment that science is a practice that is a product of the lived experience of people who are powerfully influenced by local contexts. Karen Sue Taussig's work on genomic knowledge and practice demonstrates the "multiple ways the local production of scientific and medical knowledge of genetics and its application in practice intertwine with history, religion, geography, and political economy."[105] Ethnographers of technoscientific sociocultural forms who ignore the context of knowledge production and, I would add, its consumption and reception do so at the risk of clinging to the fictions of a monolith of Western science. As Taussig argues, technoscience unfolds in ways deeply bound to geographic, temporal, local, and global concerns, very few of which travel as "universal scientific objects and events."[106] To assess the meanings and significance of emergent technoscientific claims, let alone to contribute to the understandings of the problems scientists seek to understand, requires that we move beyond old dichotomies and simplistic epistemological tournaments.

For the diabetes enterprise, this postreductionistic approach does not mean that racialization does not occur within my ethnographic encounters or that old, patterned conscriptions of social difference are not made to do biological work and that biological differences are not made to do sociocultural work. Indeed they do. Rather, what I have found confounds simple binaries. Annemarie Mol describes this as mutual inclusion.[107] Drawing upon Michel Serres, she notes the Aristotelian logic that proposes difference as mutual exclusion, A and not A, creates a dichotomy where it did not necessarily exist.[108] The arguments about race as biological versus race as a social construct operate in similar fashion. Building upon the logics of exclusion in the making of categorical difference, dare I say ontological difference, by thinking "race" is an either-or proposition, as a taxonomic system of mutual exclusions of membership and nonmembership, or as natural or as social, conceals more than it unmasks.[109] More than unmasking, however, this book explains how diabetes and social difference are both locked in epistemological approaches that incommensurably trap the social and the biological aspects of blood sugar regulation and population differences in a zero-sum reductionistic claim to the right way to think.

This problematic is beyond matters of representation in which faithfully accounting for the ethnographic materials takes precedence over authority, domination, mastery, or unitary points of view.[110] While important, thinking race ethnographically and anthropologically is akin to creating an integration of a disparate range of facts,[111] in which the cultural milieu is the epistemological field of contest over the ontological status of certain facts, such as What is diabetes? What are genes? What is the environment? What is race? Put another way, the diabetes enterprise is best examined, experienced, understood as totiontological. More than "a multiple" in Mol's formulation, totiontology is meant to describe the ways race and diabetes, just two of the subjects or objects of interest here, are not ontologically fixed.[112] They, like many "things," are and have always already been inorganic, material semiotic actors in a complexly integrated cosmology.[113]

Whereas Haraway's famous cyborg resists the logical bifurcations inherent in Western ontological premises by and through transgressions, the totiontological conceptualization I seek resists the bifurcations of nature/culture and biology/society by my act of integration, which is meant to imply a form of "doing justice" by making whole and partial all at once.[114] Imagining the subjects/objects of this book in the totiontological vein requires us to keep our conceptualizations open and fluid. Things like race, diabetes, genes, environments, just like bodies, people, groups, concepts, and so on, are always already not fixed in their potentials. Like the totipotency of stem cells, they and we have the near-infinite capacities of differentiating or joining materially or semiotically and thus for affecting life worlds, cell worlds, concept worlds, epistemes, and the complicated systems through which we or they all swim.[115] This appears transgressive only to the Cartesian in us all who seek the habitual comforts of stasis and certainty.

Insisting that diabetes is social and biological and political and historical and material and cultural and behavioral and the list should rightly go on and on, I attempt to situate the ethnographic materials and my account of them as they possibly are. Not as I want them to be, or as I need them to be, or as I necessarily encounter them to be. This requires that I acknowledge, as I have sought to do in this introduction, the "debates" and their limits but to do so in a way that might transform our understandings. This is not a claim to greater authentic perspective or truth. Rather, it is an attempt to bring our attention back to diabetes by loosening the hold on our imagination and not the epistemological traps that characterize our episteme.[116]

These political-theoretical orientations are important for understanding the problematics of race within the diabetes enterprise. Simply pointing out the ways disease is reduced to biology, the ways "Mexicanness" is presumed a biologically reliable category, the ways genes are fetishized as having superordinate agency albeit after an environmental trigger, merely restates the old arguments. What I am after here is a more situated account of the diabetes enterprise that explains why race is configured as it is while at the same time illustrating ways that race as a cultural form is not static or simplistically socially reproductive. "Race" generally and "Mexicanness" specifically, after all, are lively cultural forms[117] that are wholly dependent upon the assemblages that cohere within the diabetes enterprise.

In this, I am building upon and extending the works of critical analyses of technosciences that have shown how socially reproductive processes constitute the technosciences. However, I have tried to avoid language that portrays these processes as overdetermined, originating within technoscientists, or technoscentific practices and claims. Such overdetermination runs at odds with the work of Arendt, Omi and Winant, and the findings of this project, which demonstrate that race operates through political and historical forces that constituted the technoscientific claims from the outset.[118]

Further, while explicitly mentioned in the arguments of antireductionists, the causal links between genetic reductionist thought and the negative consequences of racial stratification are implied rather than demonstrated. For instance, similar to Duster's claims, Lewontin and colleagues and Hubbard caution that biological reductionism and determinism *necessarily* leads to negative consequences on certain populations.[119]

Like Cartmill (1998), this book counters this reproductive trope by analyzing the distinction between the representations *within* science and the social constructs that are operating in the larger social context.[120] Biology, in this light, is a social science whose constructs, theories, and categories can only be understood within the context of the production, representation, and consumption of its ideas.

Critics of race in science often gloss the heterogeneous approaches within the biological sciences. Many geneticists and biologists with whom I engaged, for example, are critical of the assumptions within their own fields and do not blindly reproduce social categories through their scientific practices. However, to test the assumptions about biological reductionism requires empirical evidence that both situates a set of concrete technoscientific practices within a social and historical context and also traces the scientific use of social categories through time and space.

In the chapters that follow, I have been empirically mindful of the distinction between race and ethnicity. As a result, we see that the labels in diabetes research reference social conditions that form ascriptive and descriptive group identifiers such as Latino, Mexicana/o, and African-American. Hence, the conclusions derived from data from populations so parsed must, in fact, implicate the social conditions from which the ethnic groups are derived rather than any etiological information directly pertinent to an individual's or group's biology. Furthermore, the uncareful use of ethnic labels distances diabetes researchers, clinicians, and others affected by this disease from the important work of finding the social determinants for the multiple diseases that fall under the diagnostic umbrella of diabetes.[121] Uncareful use of ethnicity and race in clinical conditions also has been shown to falsely associate ethnic groups with a particular form of the disease and to perpetuate racial stereotypes.[122]

The problematic assemblage of race, ethnicity, and diabetes science is quite similar to the seminal work of sociologist Troy Duster, who detailed the sociology of sickling blood cells, the anemia it sometimes causes, and the scientific and political pursuits for its prevention.[123] Duster demonstrates that even the presumption of the condition was used to discriminate against African Americans in the 1970s. Because the condition was wrongly attributed to African American bodies, such government agencies as the Air Force used it to deny African Americans pilot training. Sickled cells do not automatically lead to anemia. They are a result of genetic inheritance that confers resistance to malaria in some people whose ancestors came from mosquito-friendly environments (e.g., Africa, southern Europe, parts of Southeast Asia, China, and parts of the Americas). Most troubling, from Duster's account, were the efforts by well-meaning public health agents and community groups alike to conduct genetic testing on African Americans to prevent reproductive transmission of the disease. The costs versus benefits seemed clear to the Anglo professionals. However, the social consequences for the state-sponsored screening of African Americans recalled eugenics practices of the early 1900s. Whether diabetes for Mexicanas/os ultimately results in parallel consequences depends on a number of factors, some epistemological, others ontological, that are detailed in the chapters that follow.

Type 2 diabetes, though much more complex both genetically and environmentally than sickling, occurs in populations subjected to specific environmental, historical, social, and political pressures—pressures that shaped the formation of the ethnic group in the first place. I will argue in chapters 2 and 5 that ethnic population labels, if at all informative, reference the biological effects of a specific population's social history.[124] That ethnicity appears natural, and thus worthy of a label in medical research, is the degree to which the fallacy that humans can be biologically separated into racial groups is accepted. Researchers and clinicians compound this fallacy when they are unable to deeply question the assumptions about ethnic risk factors of disease and thus use data derived from ethnic groups as a freestanding independent variable. Hence, as it pertains to ethnic variations in disease, discussions of informed consent in genetic research, the medical mainstreaming of genetics, or even an explicit acknowledgment of the past relationship between human variation and political oppression, take for granted the appropriateness of the use of ethnoracial population DNA in the first place and imply that this time around, human variation research will be different. Further, the fields of epigenetics and developmental-systems biology complicate the search for susceptibility genes, candidate markers, or other molecular-based approaches to human health.[125]

Ethnically classifying research subjects is the result of a complex set of technoscientifically infused social relations, the explication of which is the subject of this book. More than implying that such taxonomies have some biological meaning in their own right, I argue that the use of populations for genetic studies of medical conditions is part of the fabric of race and racialized inequalities in the United States. The study of the diabetes knowledge production enterprise is an important means to assess the relationship between the material conditions that make knowledge about disease possible and the meaning systems created to explain those material conditions. Diabetes knowledge production enables a further elaboration of the workings of key metaphors of human difference as they are tied to the acquisitive thrust of the biogenomic capitalist moment. This project seeks, thus, to explain how we have come to think about race, capital, science, medicine, and disease in the particular way that we do and, in the process, to learn about the material and semiotic processes that make high blood sugar and the knowledges crafted to explain it, possible in the first place.

FOLLOWING DATA SETS: CHAPTER DESCRIPTIONS

The chapters that follow explore the use of populations and racial or ethnic labels in diabetes research to understand the relationship between genomic medicine and racial differentiation in U.S. society. Will genetic research into complex diseases like type 2 diabetes advance initiatives to end the common practice of dividing people by biological race? Or will they further reify categories of difference? We will analyze the cultural consequences of this research through a study of the use of populations in the diabetes research enterprise. The diabetes research enterprise is multifaceted and multisited and is carried out by a broad spectrum of people representing many academic disciplines. In this project, I have tried to account for as complete a list of human and nonhuman actors as possible while remaining focused upon the analytic category of human population research as crafted in diabetes science. This has required an ethnographic exploration of the different types and scales of activities that constitute the diabetes enterprise.

The chapters are organized around the processes of data set development. With the exception of chapter 1, which situates the diabetes research practices within the long-standing debates about the existence of race as a set of biological categories, the chapters follow a processual schemata. I ethnographically characterize the diabetes enterprise by following the use of Mexicana/o DNA at various stages of its acquisition, conversion to genotypic data sets, and through instances of its representations along its circulatory and consumptive pathways. Chapters 2 and 3 explore and contextualize the acquisition of DNA samples from the U.S.-Mexico border. Chapter 4 examines the movement and use of those samples to distant collaborators. Chapter 5 examines further the consequences of the circulation of samples throughout the enterprise. And chapter 6 draws together all the insights and analytical strategies of earlier chapters to offer a more nuanced explanation of the use of what is called "race" in medical research.

Chapter 1, "Biological or Social," problematizes the de facto split between race as a concept founded upon biological evidence and ethnicity as a concept constructed of social identities and political forces. I argue that neither race nor ethnicity account for the ethnoracial classificatory iterations found in genetic epidemiological research. Carefully examining the ways scientists actually use and produce ethnoracial taxonomic schemata in single nucleotide polymorphic research, I problematize the simplistic race/no-race binary and highlight the political and social consequences of the summary dismissal of population based medical genetics research.

In chapter 2, "Genes and Disease on the U.S.-Mexico Border," I detail the array of actors involved in acquiring DNA samples, present the sampling practices required to collect DNA, and analyze the context of DNA sampling along the border. By examining the political economy of the border and the competing explanations of the causes of diabetes, I critique the epistemological foundations of the geneticization of the disease. I argue that research protocols genetically diagnose Mexicana/o bodies and thus discursively construct Mexican American bodies as biologically predisposed to diabetes. I also argue that the social relations of DNA sampling along the border align the scientific enterprise with the state enterprise of continued capital accommodation and expansion in the region.

In chapter 3, "Purity and Danger," I juxtapose the representations of diabetes as a racialized disease with the ideologies of research participation and humanitarian service found within the sampling apparatuses along the border. This discursive juxtapositioning reveals that a transnational protogenetic subject is crafted through the biological embodiment of Mexicana/o ethnicity as an admixed biological group. Such embodiment is social, biological, and political, and it configures Mexicana/o and Mexicanness in a manner that is consistent with the recurrent Latino threat narrative.[126]

This ethnography of diabetes research also required an exploration of the work of an array of people in numerous places and the ways they articulate their multiple theories, methods, and collaborative practices one with another to make their science work. Thus, in chapter 4, "Collaboration and Power," I explore the networked practices of scientists with special attention to collaborations across computational platforms, conference tables, and nation-states. Charting the complex topography of collaboration provides a diverse collection of scientific narratives about diabetes and diabetes research. These narratives are at once predictably discipline specific but also reveal reconceptualizations of bodies, borders, and technosciences crafted through translations across social and disciplinary boundaries.

Inspired by feminist scholarship of technoscience, the material I present in this chapter reveals the interface of human and machine embodied in the computational practices that bring the diabetes enterprise to the fore. I present an ethnographically detailed account of the metaphors and narratives of quantitative diabetes science. It is a complicated account in which we are encouraged to think of ourselves as cyborgs—simultaneously organic and synthetic.[127] Quantitative analysts in the diabetes enterprise continuously deploy technology to translate the DNA data set from the material (sampling practices on the border, blood samples, and genotyped DNA) into symbolic code.

Exploring the relationship between collaboration and power, I argue that the search for a statistically powerful signal erases the social conditions of DNA donors' lives. In the present case, pure and powerful data sets are narrated in terms of standardized packages of variables that are "quiet," docile, and numerous.[128] I argue that when situated within the broader context of the disease and the social relationships necessary for DNA acquisition, the characteristics of a good data set serve as proxy for the characteristics of a good donor population. Yet, just as Haraway calls for increased attention to—if not embrace of—the liberatory possibilities of cybernetic sociality as a counterbalance to its undeniably oppressive consequences, I argue that the internal debates by those who use or make racial and ethnic variables in quantitative analysis show the self-corrective possibilities of diabetes analytical science.[129]

Chapter 5, "Recruiting Race," details the ways in which racialized DNA samples operate as value-generating cultural artifacts. I argue that samples are the currency in the marketplace for fundable projects, the keys to collaborative opportunities, and the objects through which the symbolic, material, and cultural contests for value surface. I examine the life history of a sample as a way to bring to the fore the tripartite nature of the diabetes enterprise and thus the analytical orientation of this project. That is, I explore the diabetes enterprise through three phases: (1) production (2) circulation, and (3) consumption of knowledge generally and race and ethnicity in particular.

Following Appadurai and Kopytoff, I argue that it is the exchangeability of samples that creates its value, not some quality inherent to the

DNA.[130] I also argue that at each phase of research, the sample acquires added value for those involved in its exchange. Commodification occurs out of the confluence of many processes: the career needs of researchers, the codification of the structures of possessive individualism within the practices of making and representing the processes and products of scientific knowledge, and the structure of competitive funding that virtually requires patent protection.

In chapter 6, "Bioethnic Conscription," I examine all three of these phases in the diabetes enterprise to illustrate how genetic epidemiologists, because they collaborate across disciplinary and national boundaries, are required to overtly position their knowledge within the sociohistorical context of its production. I focus on the representation of diabetes knowledge and present data that illustrate the principle of situated knowledge in "mainstream" scientific practice.[131] I argue that scientists who use ethnoracial taxonomic systems are far from simple-minded thinkers on matters of race and the potential social consequences of their claims. Their work evinces a critically nuanced reiteration of biological human variation that blends past and present arrangements of social inequality into future-oriented scientific knowledge.

Further, I argue that the representations of race and ethnicity in academic publications, government reports, and pharmaceutical marketing materials conscript the sociohistorical conditions that make ethnicity into the biological narratives of disease etiology. Pressing ethnic identities into the service of the biological in this way simultaneously constructs and exploits racialized social inequalities.

The practical applications for the present project, though not explicitly pursued here, are to aid in answering the following questions: What do the lives of those used in research tell us about the social conditions that underlie variation in disease? What conclusions about human biology and medicine are configured through the ways population variation is currently deployed? Does the use of ethnoracially parsed populations, or an obligatory assignation of labels after the fact, hinder the purported rationale for the research, to wit, discovering the causes of disease? Are the social etiology of diabetes and its complications misrecognized by using ethnoracially labeled populations? It is to these questions we now turn.

CHAPTER 1

Biological or Social

Allelic Variation and the Making of Race in Single Nucleotide Polymorphism–Based Research

On a hot Chicago day, I work with Pedro, a graduate student from Texas, as he retrieves samples from the 12-by-12-foot walk-in cooler. It is a welcome retreat from the Midwest heat. Pedro's lab space is across the hall from the cooler. After shuttling a few times with Pedro as he replaces his samples and places the Styrofoam boxes onto the shelves, I notice that the shelves are loaded with such containers. Upon closer examination, I noted the inscriptions on the boxes presumably corresponding to their respective contents: "Jap 2/78," "MexAm," "Black," "Utah," "Af-Am." Many of the boxes are more than ten years old. The array of nomenclature used to describe the populations mirrors the elasticity of ethnic identity in the United States over time and the general ambiguities of ethnic labeling. For example, labels for people of African ancestry change from "Black" to "African American" while other samples are labeled "MexAm," "Hispanic," or "Texas."

The lab, I soon discover, is teeming with what I will call "racial discourse." Racial discourse includes, among other things, labels on containers, abbreviations on reports, utterances from researchers, detailed and shorthand descriptions of human groups, and metalinguistic discussions about the origins of DNA samples. Racial discourse is productive and creative in Foucault's sense. That is, it is not simply "groups of signs (signifying elements referring to contents or representations)," discourse consists of "practices that systematically form the objects of which they speak."[1] This book is a record of the processes of racial discursive formation that are produced, circulated, or consumed by the complex concatenation of people, places, and things that make up the diabetes enterprise.

On my first day at the lab, I phone Nora from the security desk, and she comes down to meet me. We wend our way through the maze of corridors and elevators to the endowed endocrinology research wing. Set off by richly grained wooden railings and distinctive wall and flooring color schemes, the wing houses the laboratories of Gary and three other scientists. Nora is a white woman in her mid-forties who started in Gary's lab as a postdoc after receiving her Ph.D. in human genetics from Yale. She was Gary's first postdoc. That was in 1982. She is now an associate professor in the departments of human genetics and medicine. Gary is a white middle-aged man who was trained in biochemistry at the University of California—San Francisco during the 1970s. He is now a professor in the departments of biochemistry and molecular biology, human genetics, and medicine.

The capital improvements of the wing are announced by gold-lettered signage that pays homage to the donor. I arrive at 11 A.M., and thirty minutes later Nora is in her first meeting of the day. A colleague from the genetics department arrived to discuss a project using "a big Mormon family"[2] and a Hutterite[3] data set. The scientist came to Nora to discuss typing methods, genetic markers to be used, and genotype and phenotype issues related to heritability of genes hypothesized to cause polycystic ovarian syndrome (PCOS, which is sometimes associated with diabetes) in these groups.

At 12:10 P.M., two other colleagues arrive to talk with Nora. One is an endocrinologist whose office is down the hall, a few doors away from the endowed wing, and the other is a postdoc from Nora's dry lab. Carrying over her earlier conversation, Nora asks the endocrinologist if he would genotype a PCOS polymorphism in his samples. The researcher says it will take about a week, and talk moves to another project. Nora's postdoc had been running statistical tests for the endocrinologist, who remarks that the findings suggest a racial admixture, which, as will be revealed, is a common theme among diabetes researchers. In this encounter, no specific ethnic label is used, and the talk quickly turns to results from another study.

Twenty minutes later Nora and I are dashing through the hospital for her next meeting. A senior colleague, a pediatric endocrinologist, sought Nora's advice on his research. This colleague is new to research in general and newer still to genetics and statistics. He, too, is searching for PCOS genes, but the genotyping results of his ten subjects contained multiple errors. Of these ten, there are "five black samples" (which were referred to also as "African American"); the rest are "Caucasians." After explaining the errors[4] and encouraging the colleague to go back and have his genotyping redone, Nora concludes the meeting. On the walk back to the lab, Nora explains that while the pediatric endocrinologist, whom I would not see or hear about again, is likely an outstanding diagnostician and thus able to make phenotypic connections that most could not, he is not familiar with the basics of research design. He had, for example, found in his workup high levels of testosterone in his female subjects and thus spent some time trying to convince Nora (unsuccessfully) that the resultant increased musculature would confer evolutionary advantage that could be an important factor in the heritability of PCOS.

Back at her office I ask about PCOS, about the Hardy-Wienberg test, about the pediatric endocrinologist and his evolutionary theories, and about admixture. On the latter point, Nora offered the following explanation:

> If we were to do a collaboration with Penn [University of Pennsylvania] using Philadelphia's Italians and Chicago's eastern Europeans and Poles, they could have differences based upon geographic clines [in the United States] east to west and north to south. Maybe it would be due to migration out of Africa or selective advantages. It doesn't matter why they differ, but if you don't control for population genetics you will miss it if one heterozygote is preferentially passed on. . . . Africans and African Americans or black samples from Europe are most likely north-to-south clinal variations. The increased similarity in allele frequency decreases the chances of clinal differences.[5]

Later in the day Nora has other meetings including her usual back-and-forth with Gary and responses to my queries. Most of Nora's days consist of scheduled and impromptu meetings and phone calls, e-mails, and mail from across the corridor, the campus, the country, and continents. The volume of interactions between Nora and her collaborators make the pace of life in the lab, and thus following her physically and intellectually, very challenging. I was, at first, reluctant to intrude. Yet within days the novelty of my presence wore off, and Nora no longer introduced me as the anthropologist—à la J. K. Rowling "wearing a cloak of invisibility"—whom they should all ignore.

From this first day, the complexity of racial discourse in the diabetes enterprise was evident. The admixture narrative above reveals that the racial discourse of the lab draws upon population genetics, biological anthropology, evolution, statistics, human genetics, and physiology. Yet Nora's use of Euro-American ethnic groups and three diverse groups with African ancestry suggests that additional knowledges inform the racial discourse of the diabetes enterprise as well. While Nora's explanation of admixture that first day was simplistic and general—most likely for the benefit of her audience (me)—I would soon observe the complex scientific narratives about Africans, African Americans, European blacks, and a host of other groups. In fact, as I discuss in the sections and chapters that follow, Nora and her international colleagues in the diabetes enterprise routinely practice a racial discourse that troubles any notion that scientists are isolated from the social, cultural, and historical particularities of humans in the present moment. That is, racial discourse is shot through with contemporary social and historical realities.

By examining the racial discourse in the Chicago lab, my aim is to critically evaluate the race–no-race debates by elaborating the specific ways social constructions of race and ethnicity permeate the use of populations in the diabetes enterprise. This chapter sets the stage for those that follow by arguing that (1) race is not simplistically rebiologized; (2) words that describe groups are inherited from outside the labs; and (3) the rhetoric of danger that circulates in the ethical discussions about race in science and medicine is a discursive battlefield in which contested futures of racial stratification compete with one another using as evidence narratives of past abuses of medico-scientific power. To begin this discussion, I will attend to the ways scientists use and rationalize their use of ethnically labeled groups for diabetes genetics research. The racial discourse they use will be assessed for its reiteration of biological notions of racial difference in comparison with that of forensic sciences. Then I will return to the race–no-race debates to examine the ways the debates themselves stumble upon the presumption that science and society are somehow separate.

DIABETES GENETIC EPIDEMIOLOGY:
UNIQUE AND THRIFTY GENES

The racial discourse of the diabetes enterprise must be understood as a series of interlocking processes that involve production, circulation, and consumption of knowledges of and about disease, human biology, and ethnicity or race. Following scientists and blood samples through these discursive phases—the methodological and analytical strategy used for this research—is necessary to witness how racial discourse in the diabetes enterprise is constituted by social and material formations that are neither exclusively social nor bioscientific. By disaggregating these discursive phases we are able to see that the separation implied in the social/biological opposition is itself an artifice of a particular time and place, the explication of which is the aim of this book. We begin with the production of racial discourse as discerned in the Chicago laboratories of Gary and Nora.

In 2000, after several years of work, the main cluster of collaborator-informants with whom I work announced in the journal *Nature Genetics* the discovery of a polygene that confers susceptibility to type 2 diabetes. A polygene is an inherited set of genetic material from multiple chromosomes that together influence a phenotype. The report is significant for several reasons. First, it is the culmination of years of collaborative work across national, institutional, and disciplinary boundaries. Researchers from an array of disciplines and from state, corporate, and academic settings on three continents contributed to its production. Equally important is that the researchers reported having found a combination of genetic material that confers susceptibility to type 2 diabetes. As such, it was the first published report of a genetic association with disease susceptibility for a multigene disease with a rich environmental etiology. The report was so significant that it was accompanied by two commentaries, one on the methodological complexity of the report and the other a critique of the general merit of looking for genetic causes for diseases such as type 2 diabetes, which is well known to have environmental causes. The latter editorial reflects an open debate within diabetes sciences about the cost-benefit ratio of researching the genetics of complex diseases in light of the methodological complexity and immense uncertainty that the findings will result in any beneficial outcomes. The polygene finding is anthropologically interesting because the different bits of genetic material are thought to be variably found in different ethnoracial groups, which forms an important basis for the ways racial and ethnic admixture figures in diabetes science. Some diabetes scientists debate the appropriateness of using race and ethnicity at all by arguing that doing so detracts from closer scrutiny of gene locus-phenotype-trait interactions as opposed to noninteractive models. The stakes of these debates will become clearer as we examine the complex methodological approach used by researchers within the diabetes enterprise.

Genetic analysis is generally considered to be the process of drawing inferences from genetic data.[6] The genetic analysis used by diabetes genetic epidemiology researchers is a statistical, computer-assisted, highly codified, and abstracted practice whereby the quantitative distribution of genetic variation is used to infer ways that known genetic material affects a phenotype.[7] It is also used to hunt for genes or genetic material that affect a phenotypic group, such as diabetics, or for diabetes-specific genetic material in particular ethnic or racial populations.[8] The selection of particular populations for genetic analysis is the subject of this discussion.

The process of diabetes genetic analysis, which I will unpack below, involves increasingly finer grained localization of genetic material. Imagine the levels of analysis as follows: humanity, subpopulation, diabetic versus nondiabetic, genetic material, specific bits of genetic material, combinations of specific bits of genetic material. It is complicated because researchers are looking for code within code. Whereas some diseases are caused by single genes that are always present in affected persons—that is, they follow standard Mendelian inheritance patterns—most common diseases do not follow this standard. The genetic contributions to common diseases remains elusive because they are thought to involve multiple genes or multiple variants of genes that, compared with those found in the general population, are believed to put an individual at increased risk. Complicating things further are the heterogeneous factors external to the physical body that significantly affect who gets sick and who does not. This makes complex disease gene research exponentially more complicated than research into monogenetic conditions. Because genetic analysis is principally concerned with interpreting genetic information, the practice of analysis occurs after samples have been collected and the genetic information has been extracted.

While the process is not entirely linear, it is useful to distinguish between sampling, genotyping, analysis, physiological research, drug target studies, and translational studies. Table 1 outlines the process in linear form from sampling to developing therapies. For each research practice, there are numerous steps, methods, techniques, histories, and controversies. Because diabetes genetic epidemiology is a collaborative venture requiring the participation of scientists involved in any number of areas of research, the controversies are largely glossed over until a problem arises.

The acquisition and use of population DNA is the first requirement for this kind of science. It is the raw material from which the genetic data are derived. When queried, scientists say that the rationale for the use of ethnically and racially classified populations in diabetes research has little to do with the population per se. When asked why the South Texas Mexicana/o group was used, for example, one scientist remarked,

TABLE I DEVELOPMENTAL MODEL OF MEDICAL GENETIC RESEARCH: SAMPLING
TO THERAPY

Sampling	Populations are identified, and DNA samples are secured.
Genotyping and mapping	DNA samples are scored according to the pattern of genetic markers that appear in their DNA. An array of DNA segments with known locations, genetic markers, are used to locate and identify segments of DNA of interest.
Analysis (Association)	Multiple gene segments in multiple individuals and groups are statistically analyzed to make inferences about the association of the gene or gene segment with disease susceptibility.
Physiological research	Once gene segments are identified, their function is determined in an effort to understand their role in disease pathology.
Drug target studies	Once researchers suspect a physiological function for the gene segments, research can focus on biochemically altering that function.
Translational studies	Once researchers target a physiological mechanism responsible for disease, research can focus on the efficacy of therapies that specifically address that physiological function, e.g., drugs, diet, exercise, exposure avoidance.

"We're not going to learn everything we need to know about the genetics of type 2 diabetes from our studies of Mexican Americans, but it's a useful population in which to work." Other scientists report the reasons are public health concerns. When asked why low-income Mexican Americans were sampled in a randomized way, another scientist explained, "That's where the highest rates of diabetes are . . . and lower-income Mexican Americans have a higher rate than the suburbanites. It's a huge public health problem." Other reasons for the use of Mexican Americans are more pragmatically oriented to collecting samples. One geneticist remarked, "We were looking for a county in which the population was small enough that we could legitimately go in and characterize the whole county."

When asked what the specific advantages are to sampling Mexican Americans or other groups, researchers gave more technical replies. Describing the ways scientists compare differences in the frequencies of versions of genes called "alleles," one geneticist described it as follows:

The reason it [race/ethnicity] matters for genetic studies, why we have to really do the classification, is the following: The DNA markers that we use for these linkage studies can have markedly *different allele frequency distributions in different racial and ethnic groups.* If we had perfect data, where every member of the family was genotyped for our markers, it wouldn't matter what the precise allele frequencies were because everybody would be tied [related], but for a late-onset disease like type 2 diabetes, when we collect data on a family we don't usually have the parents, so *we have to make assumptions about what the allele frequencies are in order to do our analyses.* And the results of the analyses will depend on what we assume for those allele frequencies. And they can markedly affect the results, so if we think an allele is rare because, say, in the Caucasian population where we have a big survey of the allele frequency it is rare, and we say it's rare, and we analyze data in an African American population and it's common in that population, it may look like we have evidence for linkage there, because lots of the affected will have that allele, but it's not shared identically by descent. *It's just because that's a common allele in that population, and we didn't know it was common because we used the wrong allele frequency estimated from a different racial or ethnic group* [italics mine].

In other words, the use of racial or ethnic populations is explained as a means to control for the vast genetic variation that exists between and within human populations. Using populations, and, still better, members of the same families within these populations, reduces the number of variations that geneticists must contend with. Fewer allelic variations among the samples means that there is less genetic information to sift through. Further, the genetic markers used to highlight the genetics of those sampled have been developed with samples from specific populations. In short, researchers believe that racial- and ethnic-specific genetic information may ensure that important variations are not missed or, a related matter, that some populations are especially informative for some diseases.[9]

While the number of disease-related conditions for which the biomedical literature reports positive indications of genetic contributions increases weekly, diabetes has enjoyed a relatively long history of geneticized explanations. Neel's thrifty genotype hypothesis, for example, postulated that such populations as North American Indians, Australian Aborigines, and Micronesian Nauru are at increased risk of diabetes because they carry genes that conferred selective advantage in times of famine.[10] Now, according to the hypothesis, these peoples who have recently undergone a shift from hunter-gatherer mode of life to a modern sedentary lifestyle with concomitant energy dense food intake do not need the "thrifty genes" to rapidly convert sugars to fat. Thus, the "Coca colonization" hypothesis, as it is sometimes called, posits that recently "primitive" groups have undergone a "domestication of lifestyle" as they have moved to urban areas or lost their old way of life or both.[11] According to this hypothesis, these populations have, over time, evolved genetic traits that could metabolically compensate for periods of food scarcity. Because such scarcity is no longer the norm, the theory contends, the phenotypic consequence of thrifty genes in combination with the abundance of food and sedentary lifestyle typical of contemporary urban living make for impaired metabolic regulation of glucose. In other words, diabetes, like sickle-cell anemia, is thought to result from a genetic anachronism.[12]

Neel's hypothesis is predominantly environmental, that is, that the differential environments of certain groups confer significant risks. His published statements evince an uncanny reflexive modesty. For example, in revisiting his hypothesis 20 years later, Neel concludes that, "although incorrect in (physiological) detail, it may have been correct in (evolutionary) principle."[13] Neel concludes his revision with the following cautionary invitation: "All these speculations may be utterly demolished the moment the precise etiologies of NIDDM [non-insulin-dependent diabetes mellitus] become known. Until that time, however, devising fanciful hypotheses based on evolutionary principles offers an intellectual sweepstakes in which I invite you all to join."[14] The thrifty genotype hypothesis has captured the scientific imagination and underlying assumptions for why ethnically and racially identified populations have increased rates of diabetes.

The evidence for Neel's hypothesis remains elusive, however, and likely does not exist. Among the reasons for the paltry evidence for the thrifty genotype hypothesis are false assumptions pertaining to cycles of famine and to population structures of racially labeled groups. Famine cycles did not just occur among ancestral populations of contemporary minorities: they occurred among many groups the world over. Further, the peoples referred to as indigenous hunter-gatherers (e.g., Amerindian, Nauhuatl, Aztec, Zapotec, Aborigine, etc.), are not biological but social groups. The term "Mexican" is all the more complicated to apply the thrifty genotype hypothesis to because it refers to a national group that is the result of a rich combination of many peoples. Most pertinent, the failure of genetic scientists to control for environmental factors when those factors provide stronger explanatory evidence for global prevalence patterns among ethnoracial peoples has greatly frustrated the search for genetic reasons that some believe explain higher rates of diabetes among minorities than nonminorities.[15]

Social epidemiological evidence points to radical lifestyle disruptions, dispossession, poverty, and other hardships particular to minority groups as strongly linked to their diabetes.[16] Neel anticipated as much. In perhaps his last written statement on the thrifty genotype hypothesis, Neel writes that there is "no support to the notion that high frequency of Non Insulin Dependent Diabetes Mellitus (NIDDM) in reservation Amerindians might be due simply to an ethnic predisposition—rather, it must predominantly reflect lifestyle changes."[17] In spite of this, genetic *epidemiologists* argue that genetic differences, not lifestyle, explain rates of diabetes among different global populations. Drawing on research with Mexicanos/as, one diabetes consortium member writes, "There is strong evidence that Mexican Americans living in the barrio have considerably more Native Amerindian genetic admixture and as a result may have higher genetic susceptibility to diabetes."[18] And as Gary said of the protein implicated in the polygene discovery, "It smells and tastes like a thrifty gene in terms of its metabolic function."

It would be easy to dismiss these scientists as simply behind the curve, ill informed, or somehow compromised. However, the belief that diabetes within minorities is a genetic condition and that a thrifty genotype is responsible is the dominant view among scientists and clinicians alike. This book is an attempt to explain the reasons scientists continue to pursue genetic explanations in spite of the obvious limitations of the model.

FROM MEXICANA/O POPULATIONS TO MEXICANA/O SINGLE NUCLEOTIDES

The process used to find the diabetes polygene began with the traditional epidemiological profile of diabetes. Standard clinical epidemiology was used to identify the Mexicana/o population for study. In the late 1970s, an evolutionary biologist who had been doing work in South America moved his research to Texas. He "was looking for a more local population and a disease," recalled one geneticist. Death certificates from all 254 counties in Texas had been assessed. From this research and reports from physicians that "eighty percent of [their] patients were diabetic," the epidemiological hot spots appeared to be clustered all along the Rio Grande. "The mortality [for this area] was about three times higher than the general population of Texas," explained Carl, a middle-aged white human geneticist from the University

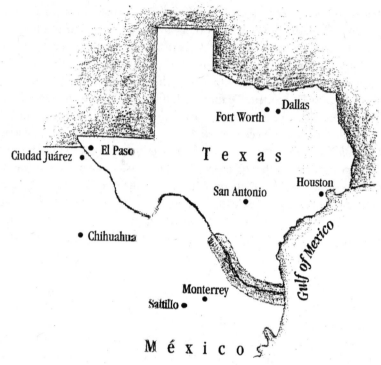

MAP 1. Image from El Camino Chamber of Commerce (2001).

of Texas and the director of the DNA collection field office along the border.

Over the ensuing five years, population surveys and blood samples were taken from as many family members as possible. The samples were then, as now, genotyped— that is, scored according to the pattern of genetic markers that appear in their DNA. An array of DNA segments with known locations ("genetic markers") were used to determine what genetic material the person with diabetes shares with his or her parents and siblings. This sharing pattern is then compared with known quantified patterns of inheritance to estimate which bits of genetic material are inherited together and thus are physically next to each other. This is an analytical method known as "linkage analysis."

Linkage analysis determines this physical proximity by tracing the genetic material's movement across generations. Linkage is important because the goal of genetic analysis is to find the position, identity, and, eventually, the function of the genetic material responsible for a particular disease.[19] The discovery of the diabetes susceptibility polygene reported in the journal *Nature Genetics* was derived by a combination of positional cloning and statistical simulation.[20] By tracking the inheritance patterns of known markers with those whose location is unknown, researchers could localize regions that may affect diabetes. Statistical tests determine whether two markers are likely to lie near each other on a chromosome and are therefore likely to be inherited together.

"Linkage disequilibrium" refers to patterns of inheritance of genetic material that do not occur randomly, as expected. Each person's haplotype (shared pattern of genetic material expressed in single nucleotide polymorphisms [SNPs]) is ascertained through linkage analyses. A SNP (pronounced "snip") is a place along a chromosome where there is allelic variation of just one nucleotide.[21] Central to this concept is that there are several versions of the "same gene" that could have been inherited from a person's parents. SNP analysis determines which version a person inherited and thus offers more specific genetic information about each individual. So, for example, a person could inherit one of two different versions of the same gene or the same version of the gene from each parent. Yet the objective of genetic analysis is to identity the precise bits of genetic material that confer susceptibility to disease. Therefore, the specific version of each gene of interest is important, since one or a combination of versions may be the culprit.

For researchers looking for clues to complex diseases, SNPs are a refinement of the gene concept. The statistical testing of inheritance patterns of SNPs between diabetics and nondiabetics, between diabetics and their affected and unaffected siblings, and between diabetics and their parents enables researchers to find the specific allelic variation that confers susceptibility to diabetes. Alleles are bits of genetic material with known effects upon a person's body. So, for example, a gene for the color of hair is determined by the alleles one inherits from one's parents. Diabetes genetic analysis attempts to identify the allele for diabetes by characterizing the single nucleotide variations that exist between diabetic and nondiabetic populations. For the case of type 2 diabetes polygenes, researchers first found the region(s) with the most linkage disequilibrium (nonrandom inheritance), then set about sifting through those region(s) to find the SNPs that were most closely associated with diabetes.[22]

At this point in the research process, the data set has been transformed from blood samples taken from individuals into graphic depictions of genetic sequences generated by computers attached to sequencing machines. Once the samples arrive at the lab, the DNA has to be purified and carefully placed in arrays of tiny wells on a plastic tray designed for use with the sequencing machine. The output from the sequencers is then entered into one of several statistical software programs created to localize genes and estimate inheritance patterns. Analysts continually tack back and forth between data sets or between multiple "runs" on the same data set to test the linkage between nucleotide markers. The analysts often run multiple data sets through multiple programs. Results come in the form of a ratio that expresses the likelihood that two markers are linked divided by the likelihood that they are not. These ratios rank the probability that nucleotides are inherited together. Anything higher than 1,000 to 1 is considered a positive indication of linkage. Those SNPs that are likely to be inherited with markers common to diabetics constitute the polygenes.

The SNPs implicated in the diabetes polygenes are from an intronic region (an allegedly noncoding region) of a gene that acts in combination with SNPs on other chromosomes. The inheritance of two different versions of the same gene is called "heterozygosity." However, to complicate things further, what the diabetes researchers found was a model of susceptibility that consists of heterozygosity for two different patterns of genetic code. The heterozygous pattern is a result of different versions of the same allele being inherited from each parent. For the susceptibility hypotheses to hold true, each haplotype must contain the same single nucleotide polymorphism (SNP).

There is a twist to all the doubles, couples, two genes, and two versions of the same haplotype model promulgated by this admittedly complicated example. Two genes, one the heterozygous haplotype and the other located on another chromosome altogether, interact. The heterozygosity is important, say the scientists, because this model of inheritance is presumed to be the result of ethnic admixture—one part from the Mexican American's Asian Native ancestry and the other from the Spanish Caucasian ancestry.[23] The susceptibility is common in Mexican Americans, hypothesize researchers, and uncommon in Finns and Germans because the allelic frequencies of the "Caucasians" reflect homozygosity more often than the heterozygosity required for the diabetogenic affect. While the precise identities and functions of the polygenes are still unknown, the location now enables further experiments to specify their molecular and biochemical characteristics and function, which is necessary before effective new drugs can be developed to treat diabetes.

THE REEMERGENCE OF RACE À LA SNPS?

The positional cloning technique described above, in which ever finer and finer regions on chromosomes are sifted, deploys SNPs as candidate genetic material for disease susceptibility. That the groups who have donated their DNA have been classified with racial and ethnic taxa prior to their selection and sampling and thus prior to the use of SNPs makes possible what sociologist Duster has argued is "the re-emergence of race in molecular biological clothing."[24] Duster is a vocal critic of scientific practices that parse populations. He argues that the wedding of SNPs with rapid genotyping technology makes racial profiling once again imaginable, scientifically and popularly. Scientifically, the technology that enables SNPs as the units of measurement affirm another case of what Fujimura terms a "theory methods package."[25] For diabetes research, this means that theories about genetic susceptibility are made, remade, and tested through SNP technology.

What matters for the present analysis are the processes whereby racial phenotypes are presumed as real evidence for biological differences between the ethnic groups they putatively represent. The presumption of biological difference now fortified with SNP-based research will, in Duster's view, have "real biological and social consequences."[26] Duster's trenchant vigilance against the making and remaking of biological race and its social consequence is now, as before, right on the mark.[27] Before we get too carried away with the latest tools for the genetic revolution, he cautions, the tools must be understood. Duster exposes the tautological basis of population differentiation based upon SNP analyses. "When researchers claim to be able to assign people to groups based on allele frequency at a certain number of loci, they have chosen loci that show differences between the groups they are trying to distinguish."[28] Yet, are these differences biological reiterations of racial groups?

The concern that allele frequency estimates reiterate racial typologies rests on the premise that when scientists find different frequencies in human groups that those groups come to be defined by those allele frequencies. In its raw form, the belief that humans can be grouped through meaningful biological traits requires adherence to an evolutionary theory that posits that different populations evolved in isolation of one another and hence are in fact related but different subspecies. The position that races are human subspecies maintains that humans started with common *erectus* ancestors, migrated out of Africa as *erectus* and evolved into *sapiens* independently of one another. Evolutionary biologist and

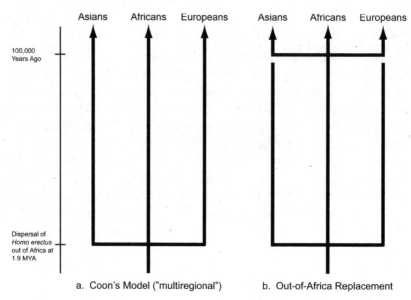

FIGURE 2. Candelabra model of evolution. Courtesy of Alan Templeton, *Evolution,* July 2007, 1507–1519.

zoologist Alan Templeton refers to this as the distinct evolutionary lineages definition of "race."[29] He argues that race as a subspecies of *Homo sapiens* is not supported by the evidence.[30]

Instead, Templeton offers a trellis model of continual cross-breeding between populations before, during, and after the outward migration from Africa. His critique of the out-of-Africa replacement hypothesis[31] includes statistical analyses of allelic variation,[32] genetic distance analyses, and various population and haplotype trees. For each kind of analysis, Templeton builds his case by weakening the data used for the candelabra evolutionary models. The candelabras are the three-pronged phylogenic model representing the three "races"—Asians, Africans, Europeans—whose origins are joined at the base by a crossbar on a single stand, the *Homo erectus* of Africa (fig. 2). The latest and most widely accepted version of the candelabra depicts a *Homo sapiens* takeover of the *Homo erectus* with the temporal crossbar repeated some hundred thousand years ago. But the three-pronged evolutionary pathways remain intact.

The differentiation depicted in the candelabra models are de facto biological races, argues Templeton. His trellis model (fig. 3) and the nested clade analysis (a statistical analysis of the variations on specific

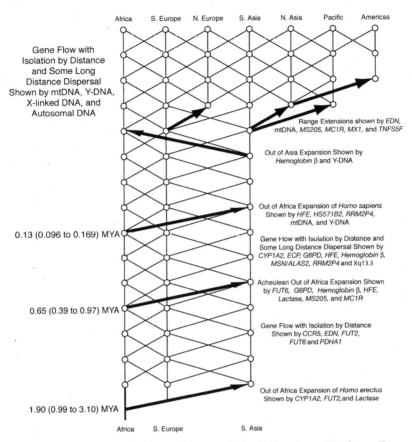

FIGURE 3. Trellis model of evolution. Courtesy of Alan R. Templeton, "Haplotype Trees and Modern Human Origins," *Yearbook of Physical Anthropology* 48 (2005): 33–59.

branches of a treelike diagram of genetic differences) of human genetic variation from which it is derived do not support the subspecies conclusion. Templeton's trellis model shows the multiple prongs joined by continual crossbars connecting the vertical prongs. Hence, the trellis hypothesis does not support a race-as-a-subspecies proposition since through drift and flow[33] we evolved together at about the same time.

However, just because genetic scientists draw upon ethnoracial groups does not mean that they adhere to a subspecies theory. In fact, to argue that scientists are simplistically re-creating "race as subspecies" is unsupported by those studies, including the present one, where direct observation of scientific use of DNA acquired from racial and ethnic groups occurs.[34] For example, anthropologist Duana Fullwiley found that there is a slippage between scientists' understanding of evolutionary human difference resulting from migration, geographic isolation, food, disease, toxins, diseases, and social histories and those population monikers set forth by the U.S. Census, lay taxonomies, or self-identifiers.[35] When queried directly, Fullwiley finds that scientists' use of race is either a source of confusion or a reiteration of "five human types"[36] corresponding to fractional percentages of genetic similarity. However, the closer one examines these genetic similarities, the more troubled with taxonomic uncertainty they become. Racial taxa become molecularized when intergroup genetic variation comes to stand in for intergroup difference along categorical lines set forth by U.S. government policies.[37]

OLD AND NEW: WORLDS AND POPULATIONS

Fullwiley (2008) details the way genetic scientists seeking to care for the health needs of their own ethnically defined communities craft biologistical constructions of race by selectively packaging DNA markers to craft composite populations.[38] The populations scientists compose, Fullwiley writes, are comprised of Old World races and assembled to fit New World populations that map specifically onto U.S. categories of human difference (e.g., black, Puerto Rican, Hispanic, Native American, and so on). The theory method package is called ancestry informative markers (AIMs), and it is used in the emergent industry of recreational genomics and the older industry of forensic genomics.[39] Fullwiley demonstrates how in the face of molecular-based evidence to the contrary, scientists' commitments to the idea that there are three or five races of humans remain through a process of reframing—that is, by making the data fit a priori commitments. The conceptual distinction between human types and human subspecies is best understood as a linguistic sleight of hand wherein Fullwiley's clearest interlocutor references typological difference, suggesting a mere linguistic convenience, when his definition of those typologies rest upon biologic human variation. Hence, while the overt reference to subspecies is avoided, the de facto definition of human types indeed reiterates these premises of difference.

Drawing upon Templeton and Fullwiley, the remainder of this chapter will refer to race as the representation of humans as if genetically distinct groups, subspecies, or types when such representation occurs (a) without reference to a definition of race or ethnicity, (b) without a qualification that such differences are estimates only, and (c) without the qualification that the genetic distinctions that can be estimated must be understood as variation along a continuous gradual geographically patterned clinal distribution of genetic variation.[40] In other words, not merely subspecies counts as "race." Rather, it is the unqualified use of biogenetic variation as if the populations represented anything more than the group from whom the DNA was taken. This will be the operational definition of race that will be used to tease out the dynamic meaning(s) of such words as "Mexican," "black," "Caucasian," "Polish," "Italian," "Amish," or "Hutterite" within the racial discourse of the diabetes enterprise.

The analyses of American Diabetes Association abstracts presented in the introduction demonstrates the profoundly social basis for the definition of the populations even before their DNA is used for the hunt for "meaningful" loci. However, what still requires an explanation is if a single nucleotide variant comes to be coded for "race" in the first place. Nor is it clear that biological race is what is meant when SNPs are used to identify populations. Careful scrutiny of the use of SNPs derived from racially and ethnically classified populations reveals a more complicated use of race.

At issue is whether the very use of race and ethnicity in medical science reiterates biological differences among *Homo sapiens*. Over the 20-month period I studied genetic epidemiologists at their benches, in their computer labs, at their DNA acquisition centers in Texas, and at numerous formal and informal meetings, I heard no one claim that his or her use of Mexicanas/os or African Americans or whites constituted evidence of differences between populations. However, the definition of race was never made explicit, and the clinal distributions of nucleotide variants were rarely noted. A notable exception was when Nora used clines in her description of why population admixture is important. Most of the time, however, qualifications of estimates and clines were absent, and definitions of "race or ethnicity" never occurred. Researchers were, after all, convinced of the relative homogeneity of Sun County Mexicanos through the admixture estimates reported in the literature. That these admixture profiles were estimates was the only consistent qualifier within the discussions of genetic variation. This occurred almost exclusively in the quantitative analyses and rarely if ever by Carl, his workers for the Sun County field office, or clinicians familiar with the diabetes enterprise. Similarly, the molecular biologists and clinical researchers spoke of population and group genetic differences without qualifiers of "estimates," geographic clinal distributions, or definitions of race or ethnicity. For all but the most careful researchers, diabetes is spoken about as a genetic condition, and specific SNPs as proxies for evidence of differences between populations labeled with ethnoracial taxa. Much of this racialization can be explained through the Janus-faced definition of Genetic Epidemiology, the field to which Nora and colleagues belong.

> *Genetic* Epidemiology: The use of populations to understand the genetics of disease.
> Genetic *Epidemiology*: The use of genetics to understand disease in populations.

The difference between these two formulations, albeit simplified, is best understood by reexamining the reasons that researchers give for the use of population DNA. Duster argues that SNPs have their racializing potential because race is a biological classification that persists, in Marks' words, as a "way of thinking."[41] Duster cites several examples of the socially objectionable ways this "way of thinking" could be bolstered by SNP-based research. His examples include forensic identification, blood quantum indices, and the making "of *arbitrary* [emphasis mine] groupings of populations (geographic, linguistic, self-identified by faith, identified by other by physiognomy, etc.)" with statistically significant allelic variations.[42]

On this last point I build upon Duster's conclusions by pointing to the fact that population groupings are far from arbitrary. It is the conditions rendering these social groupings possible that make the biogenetic reiteration of race imaginable in the first place. That is, it is precisely because the populations used in diabetes research have an a priori ethnic identity that SNPs can be imbued with their racializing potential. Had the DNA used for diabetes research not been labeled with the population taxa, the SNPs would have no upstream ethnic or racial group to be attached to, nor would it matter for the "discovery" of the diabetes polygenes. Duster reveals that the use of SNPs for group identification is founded upon allelic variations already selected to show group identification—a logical tautology. SNPs A, B, and C are (found in) X group. SNPs A, B and C are found in person Y. Therefore, person Y is of X group.

Duster goes on to suggest that the next iteration of this logic is as follows: Most of the time, group X's members share SNPs A–C, and group Y's members share SNPs B–D. Therefore, group X is genetically different from group Y. Reminiscent of the infamous syphilis experiment of Tuskegee,[43] of the U.S. government's establishment of Indian blood quantum authentication measures and the genocide it represents,[44] and of the invasiveness of forensic sampling on an already ethnically predetermined population of people, Duster alerts us to a science that can be used to discriminate between individuals based upon the purported biological differences between ethnic groups. The effort to find the genetic contribution to diabetes concerns us here for its potential to discriminate between Mexicanas/os and non-Mexicanas/os based upon the genetic differences purportedly discovered by the scientists within the diabetes research enterprise.

GOOD ENOUGH FOR MEDICINE AND FORENSICS: AIMS, ALUS, SNPS

Part of the conundrum of race in the genomic era is that the same genetic methodologies used in medical research are used in forensic science. Two campus visitors with whom Nora made appointments are worth noting. The first worked in a lab in the U.S. South that specialized in admixture estimates using Alus, which are mobile chunks of common genetic elements with particular recombination patterns. The researcher worked in a lab that had funding from the CIA for forensics research. The second was a computational theorist from an internationally known computer firm who met with Nora to discuss his computational network theories. He noted that his theories were being developed for forensics as well as medical applications. Nora was interested in meeting with them because both Alus and computational network theories might aid in her admixture estimates and other methodological challenges. The year was 1999, and the scientific defense about the usefulness of race, racial admixture, and even American racial taxa had not yet surfaced.[45] Researchers were still simply reporting specific markers or other statistically significant loci at conferences and in the literature.[46]

Recent ethnographic work with scientists using AIMs, which scientists claim can identify the ancestry of the DNA donor, reveals how these specific genetic markers are now used to configure racial groups. Detailing the use of ethnoracial populations that circulate through a San Francisco genetics lab, Fullwiley illustrates that AIMs configure biologistical ancestral groups that parallel old forms of racial thinking.[47] Fullwiley shows how AIMs are a technoscientific model of human variation that meets specific historical, financial, and medical purposes—to wit, to find old racial groups often corresponding to the five races of man. Following a pattern of tautological reasoning and other data-framing techniques, AIMs researchers select those markers and loci that are most likely to fit North American ideas about racial groups. As Bolnick, Duster, and others have observed, scientists reify race as a biological phenomenon because the genetic technology they use finds those groups they set out to find.[48] As Fullwiley notes of the alleles chosen for a given AIM, "The very continents and peoples chosen for this product were selected due to their perceived proximity to what we in North America imagine race to be."[49] For those researchers with whom Fullwiley worked, "making race" was not only acceptable, it was the point of their work.

Forensic anthropology contains its own racial logics. Surveying the field of forensic anthropology, Smay and Armelagos argue that race is used along a continuum from natural category to unsupportable by biologic observation.[50] In the race-as-a-natural-category camp, researchers uncritically use race as "clear cut biological categories."[51] Researchers such as Rhine, for example, use the race concept as a valid way to biologically parse human populations.[52] It does not seem to matter to those who fall into this category that their work is outside the debates about biological race.

The second school of thought Smay and Armelagos identify is the race-as-Newtonian-physics position. Scientists who fit into this category, they argue, understand that while it may not be precise, delineating humans by racial typology is close enough for applied work.[53] As the category's name suggests, Smay and Armelagos compare this race usage to Newtonian physics, which, though inaccurate in light of the theories of relativity, still can be used to explain a particular class of events that affect human day-to-day affairs.

The third school of thought, observe Smay and Armelagos, is the race-as-a-necessary-evil position. Forensic anthropologists who adhere to this position are stuck in a professional hard place.[54] While bearing questionable scientific merit, racial typing of forensic evidence is required by the medical-legal exigencies of their profession. For these anthropologists, it is important to accurately label, not question the validity of the label. In other words, the forensic anthropologists' role is to make an educated determination as to "how the person would have been identified in life"[55] to help identify human remains, find missing persons, and be used for other forensic purposes.

Finally, Smay and Armelagos discuss the group of researchers who argue for the nonexistence and nonutility of race.[56] These researchers argue that forensic anthropologists—from whatever camp—or any other scientists, for that matter, who use folk taxonomies are irresponsible. Their position is that scientists who use racially identified populations for research support the false lay assumption that race is biological and thus perpetuate racism.[57] "Nothing is to be gained by using a model that we not only know is unsupported by data, but also to be potentially socially destructive," the authors write.[58] Smay and Armelagos conclude that the public is not ready to do away with race, and hence those scholars who argue against it fight against the social tide even though their position is supported by the evidence.[59]

So where do Nora and her collaborators fit within these racialization rubrics? One day over lunch, I mentioned to Nora that I would be gone for a few days attending the American Anthropological Association meetings. I remarked that I would be giving a paper titled "Social Prescriptions: Race, drugs, and the making of diabetes-gene-carrier-populations." Nora protested, "We didn't make these [populations]; we inherit the population descriptions from [those who collect the samples]." For her, disease-gene-carrier populations were not made at all. They were, in fact, already in existence prior to her involvement. This inherited factor does not mean that Nora and colleagues think that race is real. For Nora, the Mexican American taxonomy in her publication is, like the necessary evil group evaluated by Smay and Armelagos, good enough for her purposes. The labels are not accurate, but they work for their research.

My interlocutors argue that the SNPs that comprise the at-risk haplotype for diabetes do not code for race as a biological or social category. Rather, they are simply allelic variations found in Mexican Americans, Finns, Germans, and Zapotec Indians but in different frequencies. In fact, Nora and Gary publicly object to the presumption that their work pertains to specific ethnic or racial populations. "We're trying to understand the molecular basis for the disease," explains Gary.[60] The goals of Nora's work are to understand the biological contributions to disease susceptibility that can be applied to all humans. This proposition is one that forensic sciences cannot as easily claim. "We are [universal] human geneticists," Nora's mentor, Gary, said, angrily decrying *Nature Genetics'* insistence on a Mexican American label for the title of one of their publications.

Gary's point is that the consequences of diabetes genetics research—a better understanding of the molecular basis for the biological contribution to a complex disease—affects us all. In other words, what affects Mexican Americans affects us all. However, the robust usage of population genetics requires continual vigilance against inaccurate assumptions about the meaning of admixture. For example, Nora wondered out loud while reading a paper if the notion that Asians are more homogeneous is biased. "Most of the admixture studies are between black and white (populations)" she remarked. And when I asked about the accuracy of the admixture estimates of the Mexican data set, she replied: "We've got one haplotype for Caucasians and one for Native Americans. We assume a homogeneous Mexican American population randomly mating. But that's not the case, really. Some of our families could be first-generation admixtures and some old longtime admixed. Without knowing this, my evidence for linkage is compromised." Polygenes and SNPs, they argue, are universally distributed genetic material that occur at different frequencies. Getting those frequencies right is the aim of Nora's work. Thus, while SNPs are being used for analyses of genomewide significance, they are not used to identify genes specific to any one group. Nora and Gary would like to know the genetics of populations because they want to understand the biology of the disease, not the biology of the group.

In other words, Gary and Nora work as *genetic* epidemiologists who borrow existing taxonomies as a means to a scientific end. Recall the labels on the Styrofoam boxes Pedro handled in the walk in cooler; boxes that were labeled by dozens of lab or field office workers over decades of research. These labels were obviously inherited from the census and other sociopolitics of identity at work during the era in which they were collected. It is difficult thus to claim that Nora and Gary are reiterating biological race even though they use racially and ethnically labeled DNA. The population identifiers simply denote the ethnoracial identity of the donors as understood and practiced by scientists at the time and place of DNA donation. I am not saying that the racial discourse of Gary and Nora are exceptions to the productive capacities of discursive formation. Rather, I am saying that the reiterations, if they exist, do not originate in the laboratory. To resolve this puzzle first requires that we look again at the no-race critique.

BIOLOGICAL OR SOCIAL

An examination of the arguments in the no-race debate reveals the complexity of racial discourse in and out of the diabetes enterprise. To make his argument, Duster cites the principle that "physical variation in the human species have no meaning except the social ones that humans put on them," which is taken from the American Anthropological Association's Statement on race.[61] Duster argues that the association's statement gives the impression that the biological meanings that scientists attribute to race are biological facts, while the social meanings that lay persons give to race are either (1) errors or mere artificial constructions, or (2) ideas incapable of feedback loops into the biochemical, neurophysiological, and cellular aspects of our bodies.[62]

Although correct in his critique, it is ironic that in interpreting the AAA statement as a misunderstanding of the social construction of race, Duster—not the statement—constructs the separation between biological facts and social ones. It must be remembered that scientists place social meanings onto the physical variations they construct.

A conversation with Sally, a quantitative geneticist who works in Nora's dry lab, illustrates a related example of how the social is always already part and parcel of genetic analysis. While explaining the ways she incorporates multiple variables into her algorithms, she noted:

> The nature of our health care system makes age of onset not a good indicator because people don't go to the doctor when symptoms appear . . . and the poorer a person is, the longer they have lived with the disease. In France and the UK, where there exists state-sponsored health care, age of onset is a good variable to work with.

Here we see how the health care system of the United States affects the algorithms used by computational scientists. This is far from a knowledge-making practice isolated from the social world by method or statistics. This is the norm. As I will show in subsequent chapters, the social, historical, political, and economic conditions that make populations intelligible are always already part and parcel of DNA research. After all, without bodies (however labeled, classified, and segregated) there could be no genetic knowledge.

Of course SNPs will be used to discriminate between individuals and populations. That is their function. But the population groupings are already established. There is nothing arbitrary about the geographic, linguistic, and other means by which we identify and are identified by others. SNP-based research that is used to ethnically classify people reiterates an old taxonomic system that has been shown to be profoundly social. However, they—or DNA more generally—can also be used to exonerate death row inmates or to better understand the biology of disease. To denounce SNP-based research as having "some not-so-hidden potential to be used for a variety of forensic purposes in the development and 'authentication' of typologies of human ethnicity and race"[63] is to overly emphasize the technology at the expense of the context and conditions for its production and use. Thus, an understanding of the coconfiguration of populations and discriminating medical-genetic technologies is obscured rather than clarified.

I share the call for empirically grounded characterizations of the ways race becomes biological, but not that for summary dismissals.[64] My concern with a no-race critique is not with the conclusions. Rather, my concern is with any argument that dismisses out of hand any instance where race seemingly appears in science. Even in Duster's account, the slippage between the biological and the social that his argument constructs seems objectionable. Calling attention to the potential of new genetic technologies to be used to bolster knowledge that has been shown to support prejudice, discrimination, and genocide is an important contribution. However, equal vigilance must be paid to the complicated ways social analysts of technoscience reiterate the false binaries of society/science and of scientist and laity. As Marks notes, "Merely calling racial issues 'racial' may serve to load the discussion with reified patterns of biological variation and to focus on biology rather than on the social inequalities at the heart of the problem."[65] In this regard, my task here is to unpack race in practice (as subspecies, subtype, and social category) to tease out the cultural processes and sociological consequences of deploying race and ethnic categories in the genomic milieu.[66]

CONCLUSION

While we must be vigilant about the varied uses of SNPs in science, we must also strive to document the conditions that make SNP research possible and productive. This means detailing the political, economic, social, *and* scientific exigencies of SNP-based research practices. In this chapter, I have focused on the latter. To be sure, SNPs or, more precisely, the population-specific haplotype groups that are constructed out of them, are textual representations of a priori classifications of groups. These representations are neither arbitrary nor inconsequential.

Drawing upon Bakhtin, linguist Fairclough notes that a text at times can be both repetitive or creative.[67] That is, the use of a text (or label, in this instance) can reproduce social conditions by drawing upon historically particular discursive practices. "Texts negotiate the sociocultural contradictions and more loosely 'differences' which are thrown up in social situations, indeed they constitute a form in which social struggles are acted out."[68] Yet, as the use of ethnic and group labels within the diabetes enterprise illustrates, the productive power of texts is only discernable within specific procedures of meaning making. Neither the scientific nor the sociological should ever be made to appear as standing alone.

To press the point further: the social conditions that underlay the use of DNA and the written, printed, computational or visual texts or utterances of ethnoracial taxa that name this genetic material remain to be explained if consequences are to be discerned, prevented, or enabled. Neither the labels alone nor the means of their acquisition are sufficient. My interests are the conditions that make such problems themselves imaginable. This is not for the sake of our imagination alone, but rather so that we can appreciate our contemporary predicament in transformatively productive ways. And to do that well, we should trouble the borders and bodies crafted of the natures/cultures of race, science, and disease.[69] To merely pronounce, even after carefully presented ethnographic evidence, that race is biological here or social there profoundly misses the most interesting and important part of this story. To wit, the impulse to make race one or the other, social or biological, drives the material and semiotic interplay within chronic disease genetics. Just as the normal and pathological were made manifest by the physiologists' and physicians' work to separate the two,[70] the undisciplined (social, biological, humanist, juridical) pursuit of the causes and consequences of disease and race by a heterogeneously preoccupied and interested host of corporate, state, and academic scientific actors is itself bringing the "apparatus of naturalcultural production," into being.[71] This is the cultural phenomena that captures our attention. It is the impossible and unbearable predicament of attending to an instance of biosocial negotiation haunted by eugenics and the future perils of disease epidemics among socially, economically, and otherwise marginalized peoples. It is this predicament of culture that has vexed anthropology since Franz Boas's attempts to demonstrate the inadequacies of craniometry or Montague's critique of physical anthropology.[72] That is, how to account for human variation without reiterating the "apparatus of naturalcultural production," which presumes that human variation can ever be explained as either social or biological.

We see that the labels that Nora and Gary use are inherited from outside the lab. Further, Gary and Nora are not interested in SNPs in order to produce genetic differences between populations. Do Gary and Nora rebiologize the populations by using them in their research? What

I have found in diabetes research is not the constructing of biological race as a human evolutionary subspecies or even human types.[73] Duster's point, however, is that race is real if people believe it is. For Duster, SNP research supports this belief because SNPs make biological differences between racially labeled people imaginable.

Fullwiley's direct queries to pharmacogenomic scientists about their concepts of race and Kahn's interrogation of the consequences and economic motives behind an "ethnic drug" BiDil are instructive here.[74] Allelic variation and the computer simulations it inspires provide analytical tools with which diabetes researchers hunt for genetic contributions to diabetes. What concerns us here in assessing the diabetes enterprise are those categories that make and are made from scientific knowledge and the local sites of origin of those categories. I ask the reader to withhold full determination of the productive capacity to make biological race through SNP technology deployed within diabetes genetic epidemiology until beliefs about racial difference are shown to accompany material consequences of those beliefs—in other words, until racial discourse within the diabetes enterprise has been fully characterized.

Diabetes scientists I worked with do not make evolutionary arguments about race per se. They instead make strategic use of racially labeled data sets because those are what are available. Therefore, it would be inaccurate to argue that the content of diabetes discourse relies upon subspecies arguments even though their labels suggest it. To conclude at this stage—as some critics would— that Gary and Nora are racists simply because they use population-based genetics for diabetes research ends the discussion precisely where it should begin. This is not to say that a present practice should not be assessed for its consequences. In this chapter I have intentionally maintained a presentist pretense to disentangle the specific procedures that make racial discursive formation productive of social relations of inequality based upon presumptions of essential difference.[75] That is, I have not analytically linked Gary's and Nora's use of ethnoracially labeled DNA to historical abuses of science. To fully appreciate the downstream consequences of the present-day practices of genetic epidemiology, it is far better to begin with an ethnographic characterization of the co-configuration of biology and society.

Returning to the rhetorical question posed earlier in this chapter: If there is no genetic basis for racial classification, why does it persist? The conundrum for human genetics in all its expressions (genomics, medicine, forensics, anthropology) lies in the social underpinnings of race. That is, it is important to recognize that race, while not a biologically based phenomenon, is a social one that appears in biomedical milieu just as it appears in the popular imagination. Because the distinction between the biomedical and popular imaginations is artificial, the no-race school of thought warrants our attention. For it cannot be argued that race has no consequence in the legal, corporate, educational, and workaday world of American towns and cities, as even a superficial interrogation of the U.S. judicial system demonstrates.

This book begins with the race/no-race conundrum precisely because it is the aim of this project to offer ethnographic evidence to the no-race school of thought. I do not pretend neutrality. Drawing upon Omi and Winant, I suggest that race be thought of as "a concept which signifies and symbolizes social conflicts and interests by referring to different types of human bodies."[76] The differences in human bodies are not, as Duster and Omi and Winant imply, arbitrary.[77] They are derived from a complicated interplay of the processes of scientific knowledge production and contemporary political exigencies, processes this book seeks to productively explode.

In this chapter, I have argued that (1) words that describe groups are inherited from outside the labs, and (2) population taxonomies used in Nora's and Gary's lab are entirely social. I have also shown that in misrecognizing that science and society are inseparable, critics of race in medicine make present-day predictions of future social consequences based upon past abuses of race in science and medicine. Thus, the critiques of race in science on the grounds that it rebiologizes race imputes a power to "science" it does not have. The racialization and the pernicious effects of claiming that groups are biologically different are a function of racial discursive formation. These discursive formations are crafted of procedures "whose role is to avert its powers and its dangers, to cope with chance events, to evade its ponderous, awesome, materiality."[78] It is a materiality that will be more evident as we analytically detail other phases of knowledge production within the diabetes enterprise.

In the next chapter, I will detail the process of data gathering along the border between the United States and Mexico. This will initiate a narrative device that will follow DNA samples from their point of origin to the production and consumption of diabetes knowledges. Beginning on the border, where the diabetes enterprise first acquires data derived from Mexicanas/os, will enable an understanding of the workings of racial formation wherein the "different types of human bodies forged out of specific social conflicts and interests" will be made explicit. Thus echoing Omi's and Winant's concept of racial formation, Visweswaran asserts, "Races certainly exist, but they have no biological meaning outside the social significance we attach to biological explanation itself."[79] Such explanation is far from arbitrary. Failure to recognize that race is different from social and political difference is to forget that "the category of nature (or biology) is itself founded on the cultural distinction between nature and culture."[80] Thus Visweswaran writes:

> The middle passage, slavery, and the experience of racial terror produce a race of African Americans out of subjects drawn from different cultures.[81] Genocide, forced removal to reservations, and the experience of racial terror make Native Americans subjects drawn from different linguistic and tribal affiliations: a race. War relocation camps, legal exclusion, and the experience of discrimination make Asian American subjects drawn from different cultural and linguistic backgrounds: a race. The process of forming the southwestern states of the United States through conquest and subjugation and the continued subordination of Puerto Rico constitute Chicanos and Puerto Ricans as races.[82]

The question is not whether race is biological and whether its use in genetic sciences necessarily leads to harm. Rather the question is; Can genetics researchers looking into an important medical condition afford to misrecognize the fundamentally social meaning of race in understanding patterns of disease and health? That is, can researchers interested in the etiology of disease ignore the impact of discriminatory experiences and social inequality on marriage, diet, educational and occupational attainment, access to health care, healthy living and working environments? More important, if they can, why?

CHAPTER 2

Genes and Disease on the U.S.-Mexico Border

The Science of State Formation in Diabetes Research

Anchored at the hub of the consortium at the University of Chicago, I followed the use of DNA data through the pathways of collaborative research. I learned from Nora and other consortium members that the main data set that Nora had been working on came from a Texas researcher who had been gathering DNA and anthropometric data from Mexicana/o families for decades. There were more than ten thousand individuals in this data set, all of whom came from one South Texas area and its northern Mexican counterparts. At Nora's suggestion, I contacted the researcher and scheduled the first of many visits to his field office and the surrounding community.

I arrived on a clear but hot May morning and met Carl, the principal investigator, at the airport. Carl coordinated my visit with one of his own: his labs are based in a large urban research university. As a gesture of thanks for introducing me to his field office, I offered to drive from the airport to the field office an hour away. We drove along the Rio Grande to "Sun County," the (fictitious) jurisdictional name[1] of the Texas side of the area he has sampled for nearly three decades. During the drive, I queried Carl about the sampling operation, about the community, and about the consortium. Before we arrived at his field office, we took one detour to view a place along the river where for centuries people, goods, and livestock had crossed the Rio Grande. Veering off the freeway, we followed a two-lane road for several minutes, then pulled onto a remote dirt road. Carl recounted how drug traffickers and coyotes (smugglers of humans) use flotation devices, boats, ferries, and paid swimmers to cross their chemical and human payloads.

As we pulled up to a clearing along the banks, two Immigration and Naturalization vehicles were parked window to window in opposite directions about 20 yards from where we stopped. The glare of the sun and tinted windows of the Ford Rangers made it impossible to see the agents. The full-size four-door sedan I had rented made for an awkward moment as I imagined being interpellated by la Migra as a chauffeur with his patron surveying a favored commercial artery. The river was down a 15-foot embankment and was approximately 40 yards wide. We didn't stay long. After Carl recounted a bit of the history of this particular crossing, pointing to an old cable that had once been part of a crossing apparatus, we left.

We arrived at the field office in time for Carl to treat the staff and me to lunch. I was not expecting the equivalent of a red carpet, but generosity is a defining feature of the sampling field office and staff. I gave a short introduction, and then each staffer explained a little about his or her particular job at the center. I would stay for several days, I told them, and Carl issued a blanket edict that I should be treated well. Carl had a 7 P.M. flight, so about three hours after we arrived, I drove him back to the airport. I exchanged rental cars for a nondescript smaller one and returned to Sun County.

The movement of people, blood samples, and data is a central feature of the diabetes enterprise. Carl's operation, like the rest of Sun County, does not distinguish between Mexicanos who live in Texas and those who live across the river. Up and down the border, inland a few miles to Carl's lab, across the four bridges that Carl's team uses to cross into Mexico, round trips, or "vueltas," are routine for this sampling effort. Samples are taken from Mexicanas/os in the entire region. Nearly 60 percent of field office time, is spent on vueltas of one sort or another. My life of vueltas would begin the next day.

The field office, in El Camino, is the hub of the field research practices. It is a nondescript one-story converted house in a residential area about four blocks from the highway. A routine day at the field office begins around 7 A.M. My first day there, I meet the center office manager, Judi, and two staff members, Rosa and Virginia. We board a late-model mini-van emblazoned with the university logo and drive north 20 miles to the next town. Once in town we turn left at the second stoplight, one of four on this highway. Five hundred feet later we enter the point of no

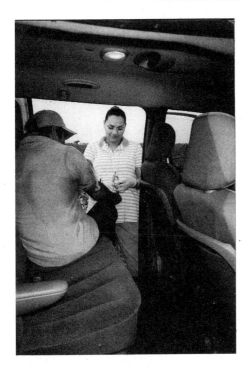

FIGURE 4. Field office staff collecting blood samples from a field worker. Photo by the author.

return before crossing the U.S.-Mexico border. Judi and Virginia fumble for the spare change they keep in a urine specimen cup in the utility compartment of the van. "I hope that is not recycled," I chide. Chuckling, Judi hands the 75 cents to the border official who glances at the van's passengers, exchanges morning greetings, and waves us across the bridge. As in all bottlenecks, our early-morning passage prevented much delay.

We proceed through the pueblo toward addresses Judi and Virginia know almost by heart. We stop to ask for directions and eventually retrieve Señor Zambrano and, after about an hour of driving, we collect Señoras Lopez and Espinoza from their respective homes. In the preceding vuelta or loop, we had doubled back through the rural Mexican back roads toward the pueblo directly across the border from El Camino. Judi and Virginia chat with their passengers as we approach the Mexican border guard kiosk. Now at the home crossing Virginia takes the lead this time in engaging the guard in conversation. Knowing the guard since high school, she chats about common friends, then parenthetically explains that we are with the university and that we are taking people in for health examinations for a research project. Fifty yards farther, on the U.S. side of the bridge, Judi pays the attendant, identifies us as employees of the university research center, and we are given the customary nod, smile, and minimalist hand gesture. "Bueno, have a nice day ladies," the guard says, and we proceed to the office, which is about eight blocks from the Rio Grande.

We return around 10 A.M. Parking next to the other five minivans, we disembark. Judi and Virginia lead the research participants into the building, which is now bustling with activity. The one-story office building is three blocks off the highway near the old center of town. It is on a street with other social service offices, small older homes, and several boarded-up businesses. Like the highway and most built structures in El Camino, the bulk of the approximately 1,100-square-foot office building runs parallel to the river.

Once inside, the passengers are led to their respective stations. The L-shaped office layout is divided into 11 semiprivate work areas, each designed for a specific task. Every square foot of the office is used for something. Even the walls serve as reference points for maps, forms, inspirational posters, work schedules, or photo galleries. As one enters, there is an intake cubicle made of 2-by-4 lumber and a recycled Formica counter where newcomers are first screened. Beyond the intake area is a cubicle with a scale, calipers, and tape measure for anthropometrical measurements and a waiting area that doubles as a meeting and consultation space. Directly opposite the main entrance is the retinopathy examination room. Inside the room are a desk and two eye exam stations. Here, full eye exams are given, and retinographic images are taken in accordance with strict research protocols.

To the right of the retinography area is the main section of the office. On the north side[2] is an area for the major blood draws[3] performed by the staff nurse. This cramped multiuse area includes the nurse's desk, a blood draw-chair with supplies at the ready, an empty table and chair used for one-to-one educational sessions, a TV, and another desk used for conducting the extensive medical histories that various research protocols require. Next to the blood-draw area is another bay of similar size that contains the storage freezer and a kitchen. Beyond the kitchen, a central hallway divides the office. On the north side is the lab, a restroom, and two small partitioned rooms for taking echocardiograms (echos) and electrocardiograms (EKGs), respectively. On the south side is a room with seven staff cubicles and one shared computer station. Judi's office, the only one with a door, is situated opposite the kitchen.

BORDER CROSSINGS

The filial, economic, and social ties between people along the river make crossing the official border necessary and commonplace. Though border patrol agents outnumber police 5 to 1, for locals the checkpoints are occasions to inquire about an agent's family—if familiar—or perform the minimal amount of deference required to get the go-ahead from a new agent. The data set comprises information on siblings who are both diabetic as well as on their other relatives with diabetes that the staff can enroll. Because family ties do not adhere to the imposed frontera/frontier, blood samples are regularly collected from Mexico. As Judi once remarked,

> One time an agent gave us a hard time for bringing blood samples back over the border. He had good questions and was probably following the letter of the law . . . but he didn't understand how things work around here. He's been reassigned. But we carry the Customs book's *Biological Use of Blood Sections* just in case another agent needs educating.

Though the river separates the land into two nation-states, for locals it is an inconvenience and a formality that punctuates the seamless ties between here and there, *entre aqui y alla*.

For some, the border is a reminder of the political history of their community. "At one time, this land was stolen from the Mexicans," one center staffer notes as we pass the mansion of a corrupt judge. The judge, like so many landowners before him, defrauded the unsuspecting by selling the same plot of land several times over. Land disputes, corruption, and violence are the subject of many conversations between the center workers and their research participants. Other common topics are jobs (or the lack thereof), migration, crops, drug lords, and of course family and health.

"Sun County," the (fictitious) jurisdictional name of the Texas side of this area, is one of the poorest regions in the United States and is known as one of the roughest drug portals on the U.S.-Mexico border. It is also known for its close multigenerational families and indifference to the formalities of border crossings, reflecting the persistent tenuousness of the symbolic and material dominance of the U.S. nation-state along the border and elsewhere.[4] Sun County comprises a series of Mexican pueblos and their South Texas counterparts along the Rio Grande. Like most of South Texas, Sun County boasts agricultural production (grapefruit, onion, sugarcane, sorghum), cattle ranching, and mining and other extractive enterprises as its dominant industries. U.S. Census figures from 2007 estimate that 32 percent of Sun County's total population lives in poverty and that this includes up to 45 percent of the county's children. Per capita income is a third of the state average, and nearly 20 percent of Sun County residents are registered as unemployed. High school graduation rates are less than 40 percent. Fewer than one in four residents have health insurance.[5] There is less than one direct care physician for every thirty-four hundred people (the state ratio is 1:661), so being seen by a doctor when ill is a luxury for most. Women must leave the county to find an obstetrician or gynecologist.

The region has a well-documented historical and ethnographic record. In his ethnographic examination of the cultural poetics of the region, Limón summons the earliest ethnographic and historical records of the area to highlight that the "lowest socio-economic class sector has historically waged the most intense warfare and suffered the most intense defeats, including, now, the imposition of . . . a racial and class-inflected postmodernity."[6] Scholars characterize the persistence of inequality along the U.S.-Mexico border as a continuation of the region's social history.[7] Born of the atrocities of a land-hungry state, the South Texas region is the site of countless battles between Mexicanas/os and Anglos. A half-dozen military forts stand as structural monuments, if not museums, of the seizure of land that was Mexico's and the incorporation by fiat of Mexicana/o residents into U.S. jurisdiction. The quickly forsaken 1848 Treaty of Guadalupe Hidalgo was but one event in many since, which Mexicanas/os did not quietly accept. Texas Ranger atrocities ensured generations of enmity expressed in heroic Mexicana/o folklore. Through it all, decade upon decade, Mexicanas/os, banditos, and rancheros are subjected to a common description in the Anglo imagination. As one historian says, "Half Indian and half Spanish, gaunt, dark, and of swarthy visage, with ferocious-looking brows and menacing mustaches, they were the 'Arabs of the American continent.' Feared by their own people as much as by the Americans, they exhibited 'but little advance in civilization.' "[8] One need only search contemporary nativist sources to read similar sentiments of contemporary disdain for Mexicana/o peoples, especially immigrants.

Scholars of the region have amply demonstrated that the transformation of the border region has fueled and been fueled by the political and economic "wars of maneuver" for more than 150 years.[9] A zone of often violent conflict, the region has endured two wars (three if the fallout from the U.S. Civil War is included) and a long history of Anglo domination of purportedly inferior Mexicano/a peoples.[10] In a poignant depiction that brings us to the present, Limón summarizes the transformation of the political economy of Texas thusly:

> [Anglo] Americans came to a new environment to create a new politically and militarily sanctioned culture and economy. The latter would be based on commercializing south Texas into a major agribusiness sector responsive to the demand for food in industrializing America. Based on the "appropriation" of Mexicano land, more often by foul than fair means, this impoverishing social imposition on Mexicano society continued to be ideologically sanctioned by the same continuing racism, religious prejudice, and linguistic xenophobia that had been introduced with the [Mexican American] war.[11]

The contextualization of the border as a war zone, an analysis supported by numerous historical and contemporary events, is highly instructive for this present account of diabetes research in Sun County: Limón's field site, the rural areas upriver from "McBurg," overlaps with the diabetes DNA sampling project of interest here.

Sun County, unlike McBurg and other more urban areas, never attracted many Anglo settlers. It was and remains, a predominantly Mexicano region. Its doctors, lawyers, judges, teachers, and business owners are predominantly Mexicano as are the ranchers, agricultural workers, and those involved in illegal trade. The economic transformations have largely been influenced by changes in agribusiness and in the ebbs and flows of drugs and people between Mexico and the United States. Between the 1960s and 1970s, charter buses provided by processors, packing plants, and growers would line Main Street to carry workers to inland Texas and beyond. Today, such courtesy has been replaced by vanloads of workers stacked six rows high who travel at night on well-worn, well-known passages. Paying between $500 and $2,000 for the promise of delivery past the Texas inland checkpoints, many are dumped just across the boarder. Locals tell me that most do not stay. Their contacts find ways to get them through, or they return to try again later with another coyote.

Sun County's remoteness enables clandestine crossings, the sheer volume of which captures the surveillance and enforcement agents' attention. The locals, long term or migrant, are resigned to the political and economic forces that shape their community. As one middle-aged woman recounted, "Everyone knows who is involved in las drogas y otras cosas, Miguel [. . . drugs and other things, Michael]. Y tambien, that those [elected] guys in Austin have their hands in it too. It's a small town. We all know which ones have their 'side business' here in Sun County." Coupled with such resignation is pride and dedication to the community. One vice principal boasted that the test scores and graduation rates of El Camino's schools rival many from the Texas inner city. Murals celebrate local generals, picturesque landscape, and agribusiness breakthroughs. Local humor, folk songs, and church and civic groups all celebrate the region, its river, and its people.

It is in this historical space, under these political and economic circumstances, that Mexicana/o DNA donation must be understood. In this chapter I will characterize the complex data-gathering research practices in El Camino and examine the meaning systems that Carl and his field staff use to explain their work. This ethnographic material will be analyzed within the broad political and social context of the area. My assessment is intended to produce a cultural critique that will demonstrate that the scientific frontiers of diabetes epidemiology are configured by the political and economic exigencies of the national frontier.[12] It will be shown that the context of DNA sampling enables scientists to both exploit and construct stratified categories of difference founded upon the region's Mexicana/o residents' material conditions.

The second aim of this chapter, thus, is to illustrate the cultural consequences of diabetes science on the border. It will be shown that research protocols genetically diagnose Mexicana/o bodies, which aligns the scientific enterprise with the state enterprise of continued capital accommodation and expansion in the region. I will argue that the social relations of DNA sampling along the border discursively configure Mexican American bodies as biologically predisposed to diabetes. Further, I will show the ways Mexicana/o and Anglo alike are rendered hybrid subjects whose ethnicity is flexibly affixed to meet the scientific requirements of the enterprise and the sociopolitical patterns of identity in Sun County. As I argued in chapter 1, this pseudo-reiteration of race is not possible without the particular sets of social relations of DNA sampling, to which we now return.

MAKING HISTORY, MAKING RACE

Mexicanos/as in South Texas are making biomedical history. A search of the National Library of Medicine for Carl's publications produce nearly 90 publications appearing in numerous journals. In 2000, Sun County made international news headlines with articles reporting the "discovery" of a combination of genes that confer susceptibility to type

2 diabetes. These polygenes, discovered by analyzing the genetics of Sun County Mexican Americans, were announced in the journal *Nature Genetics*. The significance of this recent finding should not be understated. Finding genetic associations for type 2 diabetes, long viewed as a disease of environment and behavior, is what a *Nature Genetics* press release for the discovery calls "the holy grail of genetics." It launches a new era of medical genetics research because the methods and theories deployed in the diabetes research on Sun County Mexicanos/as can be applied to conditions like heart disease, obesity, hypertension, asthma, and a host of other conditions once thought of as predominantly environmental.[13]

LOCAL KNOWLEDGE AND EXPERTISE

Carl has a staff of nine public health outreach workers, all local women, who work to recruit, screen, monitor, and sample Mexicanos/as for his research. Without these local Mexicanas—the staff and the participants— Carl, the consortium, and the wide world of complex disease gene research would not enjoy the attention it currently receives in the press and in scientific journals and on Wall Street.[14] Success in acquiring DNA from Sun County and the border towns of the northern Mexican frontier requires a unique blend of social, political, and investigative expertise.

The research office is managed by Judi, a Mexicana in her mid-fifties, who has worked for Carl for more than 20 years. Judi translates Carl's paternal—and exacting—managerial style into a professional, yet down-to-earth, practice of data gathering. Throughout the center, used furniture and handmade curtains starkly contrast with the crisp white coats and scrubs many of the staff wear. The atmosphere is professional yet disarming. "It's about being low key so people feel comfortable," Judi explained in the customary English-Spanish code switching of the region. "Some people don't understand that we can't just treat people like, well, *tu sabes* [you know]. . . . People have to have *confianza* [trust]."

The ability to make people feel comfortable in a professional medical setting is the result of the dedication and understanding that the office staff bring to their work. Judi's professional ethos is one of caring and service to her community. "If I can help just one person feel good today, I have accomplished something," she remarked. Similarly, while driving through a field toward a group of field workers weeding small cotton plants, Lena recounted how as a child she and her siblings would accompany her mother to the fields. She recalled: "My mother would make a lunch for all of us, and we would eat between the rows. I know what they are going through, Miguel. I remember my mother would give us Kool-Aid if we helped her pick the cotton. Our hands were all cut up, but my mother's were worse." When we arrived to take the blood sample from "Chucho," one of the workers, Lena's ability to engender *confianza* was evident in her detailed small talk about the field, about cotton, and about working so hard when you are fasting, or in Lena's case a hungry child accompanying her mother to work.

This *confianza* is one aspect of the work that cannot be understated. It is more important to recruit and keep participants involved in the research year after year than knowing the precise thresholds for Hemoglobin1AC, than seeing more people in less time, than remembering when the blood samples get shipped, than washing the vans that shuttle participants, or even answering the intake form questions exactly—all items of great scientific import about which Carl might badger staff at a meeting. Without the *confianza*, however, people will not participate in the research.[15]

Judi and her staff deploy local knowledge and expertise in the recruitment and retention of research participants. I refer to local knowledge as the robust contextual, experiential, place-specific community understanding of what people in Sun County experience every day.[16] What Judi and her colleagues refer to as *confianza* is the net result of years of experiences with diabetes and diabetics, but more important, with the experiences of living and working in Sun County. Moreover, without Judi, her staff and the community of DNA donors, Carl's research could not be produced.[17] As one consortium member from Glaxo explained, "Without DNA, we can't do research." Or as Nora remarked, "You can't clone someone's gene if you don't have their DNA samples." This is a contribution to making scientific knowledge for which there is little recognition and, because Judi's and her staff's work does not fit the dominant models for Mexicana identity and social position, even less ethnographic analyses.[18]

This is more than a democratic pronouncement about the way scientific knowledge gets produced. Like engaged applied anthropology, community-based health research, and community-based participatory research in environmental justice movements, this local knowledge is a constituent element of the way diabetes genetic knowledge is produced.[19] The polygene finding and all others that relied upon Sun County DNA are literally coproduced by Judi and the center staff.[20]

Carl's relation to local knowledge makers who are responsible for participant recruitment is a complex one. There are deep, caring connections between Carl and his staff and between participants and the center staff. Many have participated and thus known each other for decades. "Carl drops everything when I need him to," Judi remarked as we were unloading shipping boxes one afternoon. When there is a problem with staffing, personalities, a participant, a community professional, or data collection, he comes. "He tells [staff] the big picture . . . the importance of the project and all that we have accomplished. It really makes a difference, and I appreciate that," Judi remarked. Pictures on the wall display more than 20 years of history at the center. Like a family photo wall, ages and surroundings progress through time.

Another feature of local knowledge is that it often entails oppositional discourses that reveal, rather than occlude, structured inequalities that are embedded in the knowledge.[21] In spite of the care with which Judi, center staff, and Carl treat one another and their community, there exists an internal critique. For example, Judi filled the confessional space that my presence created with stories of how Carl does not understand what it takes to manage eight outreach workers and maintain the *confianza* so essential to the center's success. "Our official titles according to the University System are clerk 1, 2, or 3 and administrative assistant 3 or something," she explained, looking for my validation. "They pay us a going wage for El Camino, then find the classification that matches the wage. We are all hourly." Given Judi's managerial duties—and hence unclassified/exempt status eligibility—I was sympathetic and agreed with the implicit critique. I tried to explain to Judi that perhaps Carl's business sense was how he kept the center funded, and her employed, for all these years.

Yet more than the wage inequities, uncertainties about the role of the center is an issue. Imelda, a recruiter who has worked on and off for Judi and Carl over the years, told the story of one participant, a man by the name of Fernandez. "Miguel, it is just awful. Poor Señor Fernandez, a U.S. citizen, had TB [tuberculosis], but because he hadn't had continuous employment in the fields he didn't qualify for SSI [supplemental security income] or Medicare. He moved back to Mexico to get care even though he's worked here all his life. Can you imagine that!" She volunteered the story after I commented on the large number of abandoned houses in town and in the *colonias* (subdivisions, colonies, settlements).

More pointedly, one health professional familiar with the center remarked that participants are never offered treatment. When I ask why, she answers, "Naci de noche pero no anoche" [I was born at night but not last night]. The explicit critique is that treatment would threaten the (un)natural experiment of sampling families and monitoring their progress toward complications. As one Web site says, the study "has completed sampling and extensive genetic typing on more than 5,000 individuals. . . . At this time, the main recruitment effort is to re-evaluate previous study participants to measure changes in their health over time and to perform a more extensive study of the hearts of the subjects, most of whom have high blood pressure."

Collecting DNA to study the genetics of susceptibility to high blood pressure and numerous complications of diabetes are also part of the center's activity. In fact, participants can be screened for retinopathies with a series of state-of-the-art retinal cameras, heart conditions with echocardiograms, as well as blood tests for lipids, glucose, and measures of blood pressure and obesity. While no treatment has ever been offered, Carl hounds his staff to follow up referrals to physicians whenever any clinical condition is found or even suspected.

Carl's hands are tied in his ability to provide treatment to participants. There are numerous prohibitions against providing health care as a form of de facto payment for participation in research. However the critique that no treatment is provided reflects the local frustration that health care is so hard to secure in Sun County. No one feels this more than local doctors. As one local medical official recounted, "I told the [federal] commission on border health that I am tired of surveillance. We know we have diabetes. We must fund solutions now to this epidemic." Another noted, "For clinicians, genes are important for us to know about. But for lay people, it can be used as an excuse to not do anything [about preventing diabetes]." Everyone, health professionals and lay people alike, remarks that fast-food chains bombard the community with advertising. One local educator wondered aloud if the advent of school breakfasts and lunches with highly Americanized and processed foods might account for the upward trend in diabetes among school-age children since 95 percent of kids in his school get both.

Those who expressed doubts were those intimately familiar with the work of the center.[22] This double consciousness weighs heavily upon my El Camino interlocutors.[23] It is important to note that the only time I received instruction for "off the record" statements was during these moments of critical doubt. The oppositional discourse is acute in its reference to broader patterns of inequality in the region. The critique of the federal spending on surveillance, the doubts about the effect of federal food programs, the lack of treatment in the midst of a shortage of physicians, the elected officials who have financial interests in Sun County contraband, and the exploitation of *confianza* to persuade people to participate in studies were all noted, resignedly, as among the externally imposed burdens the community must bear.

"It's our Valley culture to help one another," notes one health worker. Working for the center is a kind of activism born of the contradictions of finding work while building community. The ever-present critique just as often gets expressed as a joke, a saying, or a story. I interpret such expressions as cracks in the dominant discourse about South Texas, but also about its people. The critique, thus, reflects the spirit of South Texas, perennially critical, expressive, and nuanced.[24] In this way, the center reflects the community because it is created from within it, contradictions and all. The burdens of those contradictions and the responses to them are far from victimological. In Ruiz's words, "Struggles for social justice cannot be reduced down to a dialectic of accommodation and resistance, but should be placed within the centrifuge of negotiation, subversion, and consciousness."[25] They also reflect the social, political, and economic impositions of structural and symbolic violences upon a multiply marginalized rural area. These critical sensibilities oppose the fixed notions of a weak and impoverished community by revealing an awareness and discourse of these structural contradictions. As such, they resonate completely with the counternarratives for which the region is well known.[26]

IDEOLOGY OF PARTICIPATION AND
HUMANIST SUBJECTIFICATION

The stated objectives of the center's activities are summarized in the consent form for a genetics of retinopathy study. It reads:

> The purpose of this research is to learn why diabetes complications develop. I understand that this study is an extension of studies on the genetics of diabetes that I have already participated in. I realize that my participation may lead to no immediate benefit to me or my family, but may enable scientists to understand better how genes contribute to the eye and other complications of diabetes and thereby to help others.[27]

Each work station in the center has been meticulously designed around research protocols for numerous concurrent projects. Staff members keep track of their visitors with color-coded chips because at any given moment there could be a dozen people juggled between more than one research project: as one protocol is finished, a yellow chip is exchanged for a red. The most extensive protocol requires 36 different samples including blood, urine, and plasma as well as EKG, echocardiographic, and retinographic images. Though many jobs are shared, including routine office upkeep and administration, staff members specialize for particular research projects.

Judi and her staff often lead hectic work lives. Every square foot of the office is in use for much of the day. The staff, all high school graduates, are certified phlebotomists and certified lab technicians. One is a certified retinographer, and one staff member traveled to New York to become certified in echocardiography. Their commitment to *confianza*, however, does not stop them from referring to participants in a local vernacular that is coded into the endless paperwork they must keep for each one. "We have 'schedules' to pick up at 6:30, 'GRs' [genetics of retinopathy] and 'walk-ins' tomorrow, we need 600 'controls' by May," Judi directs the staff. Participants may arrive with names and addresses, but they are quickly transformed into schedules, GRs, walk-ins, and controls whose blood serum, red and white blood cells get separated and shipped to Carl and his collaborators for numerous genetic research projects.

The complexity of the work at the center—the blood work, retinography, echos, EKGs, glucose, body mass measurements, and more—are designed to capture biological data on Mexicana/o bodies along the border. As each new research subject is enrolled, the consent forms are read and discussed. An intake can take 45 minutes or longer. This intake process initiates the transformation of Mexicanas/os into research participants for the diabetes enterprise.

The staff calls them "participants," not patients, given that "we don't do any treatment." And participate they do. Thousands of individuals have participated over the years. Carl's emphasis on "participation" marks his vigilance against the Human Subjects protections about making false promises of benefit but also frames the relationship of DNA donation in the language of humanitarian egalitarianism. As opposed to the labels "patient," "subject," "donor" or "volunteer," "participant" ideology is frequently referred to in Judi's and Carl's recruitment pep talks. "By participating in this study, you will be helping your children" is one such participant recruitment phrase.

Carl's insistence on the label "participant" is a gesture toward the egalitarian participatory research practices of action research within public health and popular education.[28] It would be inaccurate to write this naming practice off as merely a means to distance research participants from patients to reduce the ethical quandaries associated with the confusion that might result should a participant think some treatment for diabetes was possible through his or her involvement. The field station does have the look and feel of a community clinic. Staff members wear nurses clothing, vitals and biometrics are taken when the person arrives, and back rooms contain complicated biomedical surveillance apparatuses. However, for Carl and field office staff, participation is a philosophical, rather than ethicolegal, orientation.

Carl recognizes that his success depends on community buy-in which in turn depends on the buy-in of his office manager, clinical director, and other staff: All have been members of the local community for generations. More important, Carl's and Judi's careers matured together in this field office. Thus, his connection to the community is palpably filial. Judi and the Sun County participants are like family. However, unlike the inductive epistemological commitments of my use of the term "participant-collaboration," Carl's "use of participants" in his study is just that: *their* use in *his* study. That is, Carl has defined the questions, the problems, the methods, the acceptable findings and has enrolled participants into his epistemologically reductionistic enterprise. This assessment is not meant to privilege inductive methods over deductive ones, nor ethnography over genetics. Rather, to fully understand the global apparatuses of DNA collection, circulation, and production requires an appreciation of the contours of its acquisition.

Participants in this respect are more like donors of time, energy, embodied knowledge of their diabetes, and, of course, blood. Taking participation beyond a gesture toward egalitarianism would require the DNA field office to include research questions and courses of action that are thematically generated by participants. Hence, the defining characteristic between Carl's participation and participatory research and action is that Carl's participants remain squarely the objects of study and not subjects of inquiry and action.[29]

Consent forms like the one used at the field office and Judi's dedication to helping the community call upon the ideology of participation and of volunteerism to create the conditions for DNA donation. Examining the creation of biobanks in Europe, scholars have noted that this type of participation is a set of social relations.[30] Whether blood, tissue, or genetic material, each transfer of biologic material is intimately part of the local discourse of exchange within each sampling effort. The genetics of chronic diseases presents unique challenges to these relationships because the long-term nature of the sampling efforts are tied directly to the community rates of these diseases. More than simple genetic reductionism in which the genome is treated as the dominant force in all things, the semiotic duty of a participant's DNA conjures a double ideological message:[31] first, that genes drive diabetes; and second, that individual genes can inform groupwide patterns of disease. Unlike biobanks in England, Iceland, or Sweden, where material is taken with unspecified and often blanket research interests, the Sun County sampling effort enrolls participants "as if" the community rates of diabetes were going to be reflected in the individual participant's DNA. On my first visit to the field office, for example, I asked Judi why there were so many diabetics in her community. She replied matter-of-factly, "It's in our blood." Judi's answering of the hail of biological determinism is not surprising given her responsibility for collecting DNA samples from Mexicanas/os in El Camino.[32] However, the essentialist notions of ethnicity in the phrase "our blood" warrants further scrutiny.

The sampling of DNA enacts a worldview that diabetes is a biological phenomenon alone and that the disease rates are the result of the differences within the participants' bodies. This is an ideological proposition. Ideology, writes Althusser, is a dynamic construction of a "system of ideas and representations which dominate the mind of a man or a social group."[33] This construct is an imaginary representation of one's real conditions of existence, which for Althusser was fundamentally based on the material relations of inequality between persons within class societies. "What is represented in ideology is therefore not the system of the real relations which govern the existence of individuals, but the imaginary relation of those individuals to the real relations in which they live."[34] In other words, an ideology is a symbolic explanation that we use to describe the world we inhabit.

For instance, targeting the bodies of Sun County individuals maps seamlessly onto the system of ideas that blames the poor for their poverty and the sick for their disease. The blame-the-victim ideology is the idea that if people worked harder, stayed in school, dieted or otherwise changed their behavior, they would not be poor or infirm.[35] Participating in research that targets individual bodies without reference to the pronounced structural inequalities that have shaped the region and lives of its inhabitants actively creates the "as if" worldview or ideology that diabetes is a biological—not social—condition. More important, the reduction of diabetes to an individual biogenetic condition that occurs through targeting individuals divorced from their contexts is a contradictory imaginary. That is, the ideological maneuver is not simply the reductionistic one that places individuals as the locus of the disease. Rather, in so doing, the configuration of diabetes as a biogenetic condition keeps the individuals in the crosshairs of blame—except in this instance, their behavioral inadequacies trigger their genetic ones. This is the double edge of the gene environment narrative when social variables are ignored.

RECRUITMENTOLOGY 101

In his astute assessment of the U.S. policy of research inclusion, sociologist Steven Epstein details the ways the civil rights movement made necessary the inclusion of women and minorities in clinical research.[36] Since women and minorities had been either excluded or abused in previous decades, medical research findings were skewed to reflect clinical universals based upon small nonrepresentative samples (e.g., white college students, white men, soldiers, etc.), or, worse, research was conducted in ways designed to reinforce folk ideas about social difference. The national policy imperative to include women, children, and minorities of color as research subjects and researchers spawned a new science of recruitment, which Epstein calls "recruitmentology." Recruitmentology draws upon the ethos that underrepresented people should be included and that their difference should be an object of study.[37]

Carl's field office might be considered as one of the ground zero sites of recruitmentology. The Sun County sampling efforts began at the same historical moment as the inclusion-and-difference paradigm that Epstein's work so thoroughly details. The reported motives for sampling were and are to improve the lives of Sun County Mexicanos. There is no question that Judi, Carl, and most of the field staff feel that their work rights a wrong and that theirs is a labor of love. The use of community workers, the narratives of trust, and the community service ethos that permeates the field office culture exemplify the best ways to recruit participants from hard-to-reach areas and populations. Though Carl's papers rarely speak of his recruitment apparatus and thus may not be formally part of the science of recruitment, I concur with Epstein's observation that the "theory and practice of recruitmentology have promoted new fusions of biological and cultural knowledge about the medically 'other.' "[38] For it is through scientific explanations being crafted from Sun County DNA sampling that sociological explanations of the conditions of life along the border are imagined in ways that conceal the sociocultural while foregrounding the biological.

Sun County Mexicana/o participants are recruited into a transnational diabetes research enterprise and thereby accept the hail of the historical and contemporary formations of Anglo and Mexicano relations. Althusser writes, "Ideology 'acts' or 'functions' in such a way that it 'recruits' subjects among individuals, or 'transforms' the individuals into subjects by . . . interpellating or hailing."[39] That is, by participating in this research apparatus, Mexicanas are further subjected to the logics of Anglo dominance, which is manifest in high poverty rates and pervasive medical neglect, both of which are causally implicated in diabetes. The humanist impulse to help the community only works as a response to the interpellating power of these ideological premises within the sampling enterprise. I draw upon Althusser because the hail occurs within a regime of historical inequality and violence akin to coercive apparatuses: police forces, military presence, the Immigration and Naturalization Service, the Texas Rangers, and so on.[40] That is, accepting the call to participate is a particular social relation between a state apparatus and a community. Unlike Althusser's configuration, however, the state apparatus imposes its contemporary threat through the structural violence of gross neglect and social inequality and is manifest in the targeting of the Sun County Mexicana/o community for sampling.[41]

The social relations configured in diabetes research recruitment and participation are, like Epstein's inclusion-and-difference, a biopolitical paradigm. To wit, recruitment and participation in the diabetes research apparatus are "an example of how biomedicine (for better or worse) gets politicized . . . and governing gets "biomedicalized,"[42] Further, Schneider and Ingram have observed that target populations are configured to fit the instrumental needs of policy makers.[43] They also demonstrate that the benefits and efficacy of a given policy often are prefigured by the type of target population the policy constructs. I argue that populations targeted for DNA sampling also are prefigured, as in public policy. In the case of Sun County community members, converting someone into a participant includes constructing him or her as a humanist, as a genetic carrier who represents the broader community, and as a passive, docile body upon which a benevolent bioscientific interlocutor can work for a greater good, one that is greater than the immediate needs of the individual, the individual's family, or the community.

In spite of the oppositional discourse, the hushed tones of critique never emerge into an appeal or movement for treatment or prevention. "Only more research," notes a health professional familiar with the DNA collection operation. Contrasted with movements to clean up toxic waste dumps, to improve the health of IV drug users, to screen people for diseases, the complete interpellation as humanitarian and politically docile "participant" is striking.[44] To imagine a genetic sampling field office that spent as much time and resources on prevention, community development, and disease management as is spent on surveillance and genetic sampling would require a very different kind of participant and participation. It would require a program in which a donation of biological data also required a donation of time to organizing walking groups, menu surveillance at the schools, health promotion at workplaces, to help those on diets manage caloric ledgers, and the provision of safety nets for housing, health care, food, and other services.

CONCLUSION: ANTIPOLITICS AND THE EPIDEMIO-LOGICS OF DISEASE

In chapter 1, I presented the rationale for the use of genetics in searching for diabetes cures. As I said there, geneticists use populations to understand the genetics of disease, whereas epidemiologists use genetics to understand disease in populations. However, the study of type 2 diabetes as a biogenetic condition runs counter to the social epidemiologics of disease. Further, treating diabetes as a genetic condition, as researcher, clinician, or patient, obscures the cultural epidemiology of the disease.[45] By examining the social explanations of disease as an alternative to the biogenetic epidemiologics, the cultural consequences of DNA sampling will become clearer.

The prominent use of Mexicanas/os on the border as a racialized population whose heredity confers susceptibility to type 2 diabetes is wholly consistent with the epistemological shift away from context and toward explanations of poor health that focus on and sometimes blame the individual.[46] An emphasis on risk factor research models has resulted in the erasure of the socioeconomic, historical, and political contexts of populations affected by disease. Life and ecological conditions have been replaced with a reductionistic emphasis on individual and molecular causes of disease. Pearce notes, "The decision not to study socioeconomic factors is itself a political decision to focus on what is politically acceptable" and scientifically imaginable.[47]

That Mexicanas/os have been targeted for such research is also not surprising. In fact, as the political history shows, the South Texas border region has always been part of state-sponsored or -sanctioned use of the Mexicano/a population. That Mexicanos/as are now used for genetic research, is, it would seem, an almost predictable progression from their use as cheap labor, as Other whose rights to own land or vote varied according to Anglo needs for land and political power, and as national enemy in the context of war and capitalist expansion along the border. Is it a coincidence that Carl's project began in Sun County at the moment—the 1970s—that the marginalization of Mexicanos/as had stabilized into what Limón argues is now a permanent status of political and economic stagnation? It is a moment now recognizable as keyed to the flexible accumulation characteristic of Harvey's "condition of postmodernity," in which labor and laborers are subjected to the whims of distant calculus of economic inputs and before this, Marx's "floating populations" as the social costs of industrializing agriculture.[48]

In spite of the convention of explaining the incidence and prevalence of health conditions through biological processes, the incidence of diabetes in the Mexicano/a populace constructed through Carl's research tells a different story when contextualized within the political and social history of the region. In this light, diabetes is strongly associated with the national political and economic transformations on the border over the last three decades, transformations that themselves reflect new regimes of labor control and the deployment of new technologies.

Beginning with the categories used in epidemiological research, Krieger and Fee trace the history of its use of gender, race, and class variables.[49] They demonstrate the ways scientific research configures health risks for populations in accordance with prejudices of the day. From the early nineteenth century to the present, they argue, the so-called biological factors used in biomedical research simply "confuse what is with what must be."[50] This confusion is done through several means. As we have seen from the review of American Diabetes Association abstracts, population categories identified within biomedical literature do not reference anything biologically meaningful but are presumed biological by virtue of their increasing frequency in diabetes research reports. As Krieger and Fee observe, race is presumed to be biological, affected populations are presumed to have biological reasons for their health condition, and physiological differences between populations are given near-magical deterministic powers for health outcomes.

The arguments against racial codes in epidemiology and those that fault epidemiology for the absence of class and socioeconomic status from analyses conclude that social-historical factors, not biological factors, more accurately predict and explain health conditions between and within certain populations.[51] Further, in a 2003 issue of the *American Journal of Public Health*, authors launched an explicit discussion about racism and racial-ethnic bias in health outcomes. Editors called for careful characterization of racial-ethnic prejudice and the physiological response to them.[52] Krieger proposes an ecosocial perspective that links racism, biology, and health and that includes economic and social hardships, toxic exposures, verbal and physical threats, unhealthy consumer messages, and substandard medical care: all areas known to affect health.[53] Nazroo, van Ryn and Fu, Harrell and colleagues, and Williams and colleagues in varying ways take up Krieger's call and offer evidence that economic deprivation, biased health care provision, the experience of racism, and community stressors all contribute to negative health outcomes.[54]

Earlier research by anthropologists argue that epidemiology and anthropology share vital epistemological similarities that, if brought together, would make a good corrective to the social blinders within conventional epidemiology that allow for arbitrary categories of race to persist.[55] Hahn's groundbreaking work importantly highlights the technical weaknesses of racial categories but stops short of assessing the basic assumptions embedded within the categories deployed by epidemiology and anthropology. Social epidemiologists (Krieger and Fee 1994a; Krieger 2005) argue that research that focuses on differences in health patterns between individuals from the same ethnic group would serve as a foil to the current research failures.[56] For example, one such failure is the decades-long quest to prove James Neel's thrifty genotype hypothesis, an effort that has been shown to be both technically flawed and theoretically unwarranted.[57]

These critiques, and the alternative etiological frameworks for chronic diseases they sustain, directly counter the reductionism of genetic epidemiology. They also call into question the veracity of the risk for diabetes for Mexicanos/as that the genetics approaches portray. Certainly a genetic susceptibility, inasmuch as it omits or minimizes the local biologies of diabetics, is nothing if not a biological reductionism. More than an epistemological critique, however, I have also tried to show that this reductionism is overly reliant upon research variables (population labels, biogenetic samples) whose foundations are empirically neither robust nor reliable.

For this discussion, the epidemiological patterns are important in their cultural implications. That is, I will leave to epidemiologists the risk estimates and the discernment of incidence and prevalence patterns of diabetes along the border. What interests me are the (anti)political implications of a genetics model that so squarely relies upon the ethnically admixed body of Sun County Mexicanos/as. That is, as Ferguson has demonstrated of failed economic development projects that conceal political circumstances, the genetics approach to diabetes is a kind of "anti-politics machine" that reinforces and expands forms of state power while depoliticizing the conditions in which people live.[58]

Chapter 1 dealt with the theoretical vexations of population differences and the debates surrounding the objectionable uses of racial categories in medicoscientific research. This chapter explored the ways the ideologies of participation, human service, *confianza*, and a biogenetic approach to diabetes enacts an "as if" proposition of the border that conceals social inequality. In the next chapter, I present the ways the historical, material, and semiotic inequities of Anglo-Mexicano relations co-configure diabetes genetic science through the search for and use of ethnic admixture. This aspect of the diabetes enterprise begins with the premise that the individual biologically represents the community, that DNA represents the individual, and thus that DNA is a proxy for the population of donors of Sun County. The "as if" required for this synecdoche works through a series of strategic conceptual substitutions that enclose and reframe DNA as the material manifestation of the unique biological composition of Mexicano/a participant donors. The notion that individuals can inform—statistically, conceptually, or literally—population-wide representative models (genetic, demographic, cultural) is not only an essentialism of the first order, it is a peculiar kind of epistemic and epistemological politics. The political implications of the ways in which one stands for many in this sociocultural milieu requires that we look more closely at the presumed ethnic composition of Sun County Mexicanas/os.

CHAPTER 3

Purity and Danger

When One Stands for Many

The Sun County community has been selected because of its ethnic composition, a composition that is explicitly racialized through a discourse of admixture. For example, Carl reports that the community was selected both for the high incidence of type 2 diabetes and for its presumed ethnic homogeneity. The early studies dealing with epidemiology and Mexican Americans paid considerable attention to estimating ethnic admixture. For these studies, admixture is operationalized as the percentage of genetic material derived from each branch of a person's ancestral line, in this instance narrated in ethnic terms. For example, one study published in 1986 proposed a method for estimating individual admixture probability and found that the admixture of Sun County Mexican Americans to be 65 percent Caucasian and 35 percent Amerindian. Two years earlier, the degree of Native American admixture was positively correlated with type 2 diabetes in Mexican American populations.[1] By 1991, the admixture estimates had been refined to 31 percent Native American, 61 percent Spanish, and 8 percent African. In 1993 another study compared polymorphic blood markers with self-reports of Mexican American grandparents with skin tone measurements. According to the study, the three methods for estimating admixture correlated poorly with one another, and none proved unique in the degree of positive association with any of three health outcomes of interest: diabetes, obesity, gallbladder disease. Still, the attention to admixture endured.

The attention to ethnic admixture, say scientists, is a means of adequately characterizing the genetic structure of the population of interest. The admixture estimates quantify the biological variation derived from a person's ethnicity. Ethnic homogeneity of the DNA donor population is important, say researchers, because it helps limit the amount of genotypic information through which scientists must sift and thus enables comparisons of established genetic admixture estimates with their newfound nucleotide patterns. In 1992, Carl's team attributed 99 percent of the total genetic diversity of Sun County Mexican Americans as individual variation within the population. They write, "The history of admixture is apparently old enough to have brought the entire Mexican American gene pool to a stable frequency of genotypes." Sun County Mexicanas/os thus were proclaimed genetically homogenous and useful for genetic and epidemiological studies.

ETHNIC HOMOGENEITY AND DIABETES SUSCEPTIBILITY

Let us return to the "discovery" in 2000 of a combination of single nucleotide polymorphisms (SNPs) that conferred a threefold risk for type 2 diabetes that Nora, Carl, and others published in *Nature Genetics*. In this piece, researchers concluded that 14 percent of the risk of diabetes for Mexican Americans and 4 percent of that for Europeans could be attributable to this SNP profile. Exploring this racialized susceptibility hypothesis and situating the admixture-susceptibility matrix within the context of Anglo-Mexicano relationships of the region where DNA donation occurs reveals disturbing sociocultural linkages between historical and contemporary nativist concerns about the Mexicana/o threat to Anglo well-being and scientific concerns about the susceptibility of Mexicanas/os to type 2 diabetes. Below, we will explain the admixture-susceptibility matrix and conclude with its resonance with contemporary and historical nativist impulses.

For this widely hailed finding, scientists compared the patterns of single nucleotides (A,G,T,C) of persons with and without diabetes and found that a combination that included two different versions of the same gene conferred the greatest risk. Scientists hypothesized that the heterogeneous pattern that conferred risk was higher in Mexican Americans as a result of their Native American ancestry, which is estimated to be 31 percent. The admixture-susceptibility hypothesis was not explicit, however. In fact, the principal authors of the publication took great pains to avoid a simple admixture explanation for the increased risk in Mexican Americans.[2] Instead, the authors explicitly reported that the haplotype (inherited SNP pattern) itself was not the result of admixture. It was not until a subsequent analysis published in 2002 that scientists directly attributed the increased frequency of the haplotype in Mexican Americans to the higher frequency of that haplotype found in Asian and Native American populations. While admixture does not create the haplotype, scientists use admixture to explain the frequency of the haplotype in Mexican Americans. In other words, admixture makes the haplotype appear more frequently in Mexican Americans than in other groups studied. This finding is entirely consistent, note researchers, with the established positive correlations between Native American admixture and type 2 diabetes among Mexican Americans.[3]

How can Mexican Americans simultaneously be an ethnically homogenous group and at higher risk for diabetes on account of genetic admixture? The answer relies on the definition of population homogeneity. Recall that the value of the Sun County donor group lies in part in their ethnic homogeneity. The community was chosen because it could be conveniently sampled, Carl explained, and was presumed to be 98 percent Mexican American. "The other 2 percent," Carl noted, "probably answered the Census wrong." Researchers report that comparing the expected haplotype frequencies with those found within the sampled group establishes that the data set is representative of the group as a whole. Homogeneity, then, refers to the degree to which Mexicana/o DNA data sets are homologous to and thus representative of Mexicanas/os in Sun County writ large. Interestingly, Finns and Germans are never described as admixed: Europeans, for the purposes of the genetic epidemiology of type 2 diabetes, are a homogeneous (not admixed) population.[4]

The rationale that researchers give for admixture estimates are that comparisons between specific data sets and the general Mexican American population data sets are needed to ensure that a finding was not simply an allele (bit of inherited nucleotides) characteristic of the sampled group. "We ignore allelic variation at our peril," remarked a genetic analyst involved in the project. In this way, Mexicana DNA is thus evaluated for its homogeneity, only in this instance it is the homogeneity of Mexicana *admixture* that is of concern for genetic researchers. In other words, this haplotype model is founded upon a notion of a standardized admixed Mexican body: simply put, a pure Mexican. However, in this case, the purity in question is the purity of the admixture, presumed to be a 31 percent blend of American Indian, 64 percent blend of European, and 5 percent blend of "other."

Beyond the rhetoric of the Human Genome Project, at its most formative moment, lies population sampling of which the Mexicanos/as of South Texas are but one instance. Initiated in the 1970s, the screening of Mexicanos/as for diabetes began as a statistical sampling of selected *colonias* in three Sun County towns. "The question was, How frequent was diabetes?" recalls Carl. "We went door to door. in randomly selected blocks in each of these three towns and enumerated everybody in the household [as] either diabetic or nondiabetic." From this initial survey, Carl's team invited every diabetic—the proband—and all of his or her relatives to the office for a complete physical exam. Carl recalled: "So we got these beautiful pedigrees based upon carefully collected blood samples. It was almost like a National Geographic expedition. We had a team of 10 to 15 individuals who would fly down on Friday, start seeing people at 6:30 and go until 5 on Saturday and again on Sunday morning." The team would then knock off around 11 A.M., "pack everything up, put the blood on ice, race to the airport and come home." From there, the samples would be further processed and shipped to collaborators around the country.

The essentialism evidenced in Carl's narrative of the beginning of the sampling effort fits with Nora's description of the need for accurate admixture estimates to do her analyses of the genotypes derived from the population. Carl relies upon Mexicana/o self-identity to construct population homogeneity. Recall that in chapter 1 I showed how Nora narrated admixture into the rationale for population sampling as a reasonable but imperfect way to limit extraneous genetic signals in the search for diabetes susceptibility genes. At the root of this rationale is the attempt to create samples that are, in effect, statistically Mexicana/o. In other words, the diabetes science requires a statistically robust population, a population that is as genotypically uniform as is possible and in which the variation is known. Recall how Nora explained her concerns for homogeneity in the population samples. Admixture estimates are important because, she said, "Even knowing where our families' grandparents were born tells me nothing about whether a family is pure Spanish or pure Native American." Carl's success in packaging the Sun County Mexicanos as an admixed population is evidenced by current admixture studies that rely upon his data set as source material for their admixture research.

For Mexicans, Puerto Ricans, and most other Caribbean peoples, a link between mixed-race status and disease was one among many made by nativists and physicians alike in the early part of the twentieth century.[5] Further, statements about race in fields as diverse as craniometry, anthropology, serology, and genetics dating to the formation of those fields in the mid-nineteenth century have also contributed to imagined difference-cum-inferiority of non-European peoples.[6]

Similar to Fullwiley's findings for Puerto Rican asthma genetics, individual admixture estimates have been made for the Sun County data set for studies dealing with hypertension.[7] For Tang and colleagues, Sun County Mexicanos are noted to be Native American (39 percent), European (57 percent), and African (4 percent). This is consistent, they note, with the admixture estimates of Mexicans from Mexico City but slightly inconsistent with Carl's original estimates from 1991 of 31 percent Native, 61 percent European, and 8 percent African. The specific techniques that Tang's team or Carl use to derive these estimates are less important than that they seek to derive admixture estimates in the first place. To do so requires a commitment to Old World notions of ancestral populations, but, more important, admixture estimates point their scientific imagination toward the bodies of Sun County Mexicanas and, consequently, away from social history and environment. A perfect example of this appears in this passage by Basu and colleagues.

> The recent history of Latin America, starting five centuries ago with the arrival of Christopher Columbus, has been one of large scale and widespread exchange between African, Native American and European genomes. These unprecedented events brought together genomes that had evolved independently on different continents for tens of thousands of years. . . . The various Latino populations of the United States represent [such] admixtures. . . . Populations separated by continental distances, whose genetic makeup was shaped through thousands of generations in distinct environments, were suddenly exposed to an entirely new world and unfamiliar environment.[8]

Note in this passage the ways the words "admixture," "exchange," and "suddenly exposed" are a neutral gloss for slavery, genocide, forced dispossession and relocation. And the unexamined premise underlying this quote is that gene flow (interbreeding) did not occur sufficiently to wreak havoc on the supposed independent lineages or genetic isolation by distance.[9] Further, the passage above perfectly illustrates a "biologistical construction of race" characterized by Fullwiley wherein precise molecular concepts of racial bodily difference somehow neutralize the often horrifying sociohistorical realities of interbreeding.[10]

MONGRELS, ZEBRAS, AND PURO MEXICANOS

The quest for scientific purity refracts earlier concerns with and about ethnic composition of Mexicanas/os. Scholars have amply documented that the racism that pervades the region is based upon the long-standing problem the Indian or indigenous ancestry of Mexicanos/as has presented for Anglo society. Menchaca's analysis of federal and state racial laws from the nineteenth to the mid-twentieth century showed that particular legal statuses and discriminatory treatments were congruent with the color coding of Mexicans based upon their Indian ancestors.[11] Analysis of earlier periods showed that little had changed between the colonial settlement era and the period leading up to the Mexican-American War. For example, De León showed how European settlers imported homologies of racial purity and Christian morality in the North American colonies.[12] Similarly, Horsman's analysis of the 1830s–1840s showed that beliefs in Anglo-Saxon superiority were used to explain Anglo successes in the northern Mexican territories.[13] Dispossession was justified on account of the inferiority of Mexicans as a weak race who, "like Indians, were unable to make proper use of the land . . . because they were a mixed, inferior race with considerable Indian and some black blood."[14] Similar sentiments were echoed by members of Congress to justify the Mexican-American War in 1846–1848.[15]

However, purity-cum-homogeneity is a highly problematic concept for other reasons. For example, I observed numerous people who "pass" for Anglo. When I asked Judi about these apparently Anglo participants included as Mexican American in the research data sets, she replied, "You mean the zebras? . . . Because of the [U.S. Army] forts, there are families here whose names are Hewlitt, DeForge, or Anderson, but they have diabetes, and we include them in our protocols." "What about a John Smith?" I asked, referring to a hypothetical participant *without* such a historical connection to Sun County. Judi said that a hypothetical John Smith could be screened for diabetes at the center, but his sample would not be used for research. The non-hypothetical Johns and Janes, whose surnames could be Spanish or English, were unquestionably categorized as Mexican American and included in the research samples.

Their connection to Sun County established their Mexicana/o identity for Judi. Similarly, two of the center staff, Alma and Lena, could pass for Anglo. Their light skin and hair and their English surnames blur any notions of homogeneity-cum-purity.

And yet, the ethnicity of Mexicanas/os in El Camino and of those who work for and donate to the diabetes enterprise is, as the political history of the region shows, a hierarchical one. Carl's '98 percent pure pedigrees' and his willingness to dismiss the other 2 percent illustrates the ways social group classification is not arbitrary. Of kinship and race, Brackette Williams writes, "When social classification meets hierarchy, their union is made possible by myths that fold social space back on itself to naturalize power differences that are legitimated in particular representations of the historicity of kin substance."[16] Mexicana/o purity is a myth. Many critical race theorists have shown that ethnicity is a malleable outcome of social and political processes. As, for instance, the changing status of Jewish and Irish immigrants demonstrate, "whiteness" is established through assimilation and class mobility.[17] The malleable labeling of Mexicanos from El Camino demonstrates that "Mexicanness" works in similar ways.

Moreover, in spite of their phenotype, Alma's and Lena's references to "us," "our community," and "our diet" indicate their ethnic self-identity as Mexicana. Judi's adherence to "our blood" and the inclusion of samples from "John Anderson" on the one hand supports, and on the other actively destroys, the alleged purity of the Mexicana/o DNA samples even as it reinforces the myth that Mexicana/o is somehow a meaningful biological construct. Hence Nora's concerns about purity, even as a purely homogenous admixed population linked through some magical biogenetic substance,[18] do not begin to address the profoundly social construction of Mexicanas/os in the genetic data sets.

Indian ancestry is a central ideological feature of the diabetes enterprise. Evidence of beliefs about blood-based heredity was easily elicited form field office staff when commenting upon the causes of diabetes. But so too were notions of social etiologies of diabetes. When explaining the causes of diabetes, staff members explain that genes and life conditions together explain diabetes. For example, on our way to an ice cream distributor to fetch dry ice for a Monday blood sample delivery, Maria remarks, "Genes are passed from one generation to another, but basically it's our way of eating." Being careful to explain the complexity of the diet hypothesis, Alma elaborated:

We see people whose parents have it, and now they have it. One woman [we know] makes a more balanced diet. Before she made BBQ, fajita, rice, beans, mashed potatoes, and a big glass of coke. Now just BBQ, rice, and beans only. Most folks don't go to [diet] classes because they think, "I'll take my pills so I can eat [or drink] whatever I want.' But just as bad or worse [for them], they don't have any options for screening [so they cannot really monitor themselves].

Lena explained diabetes as follows:

It's genetics, and [our] diet is terrible. . . . Anglos eat a lot of vegetables. We eat fruit when we could afford it, mostly melons, onions, tomatoes, and corn. When I was growing up we weren't introduced to vegetables or fruit really. Just beans, rice, meat, and tortilla. Also everyone walked, and no habia candy ni soda [there wasn't candy or soda].

Here we read how staff understands diabetes as a disease with both genetic and environmental etiology.

This split between genes and life conditions was further elaborated by Judi, whose unflinching acceptance of the biology of "Mexicanness" was complicated by her critique of public health discourse, which blames Mexicanas/os for their lifestyle failures. Complaining of the ignorance of health professionals, she notes, "Es que, people are always saying that we should exercise more. But where are we supposed to do that? The roads aren't safe to walk on, snakes and dogs are everywhere, and for much of the time it is too hot to be outside." We read in Judi's comments the simultaneous acceptance and rejection of an imposed biomedical discourse about Mexicana/o diabetics. On the one hand, Judi's first reply to the causes of diabetes is a blood-borne genetic one. On the other hand, she accepts that exercise would be a good idea but that blaming people for not exercising fails to acknowledge the local biology of an El Camino resident.[19] Judi recognizes the anthropological insight that bodily conditions must be understood as an interplay between biology and culture and the embodiment of the living conditions in the border region.[20] Thus, for field staff, the etiological frames of reference are split between genes and the life conditions of Sun County residents.[21]

Judi's affirmation of the hereditary etiology of diabetes and the blunt-edged identities assigned to some Sun County residents are necessary stages in the making of transnational protogenetic subjects out of research participants. Participants are not merely volunteering their time and DNA. Rather, through the diabetes enterprise configuration of their biological difference as that which confers susceptibility to diabetes, the participants, field staff, and researchers reiterate the subordination of Mexicanas/os based upon the naturalized differences between Indians and Anglos—a subordination that was upheld by the state institutions designed to dispossess Mexicanas/os from their land. Admixture so configured ideologically upholds social relations of inequality.

Elaborating on the processes of subjectification, Foucault argues that the "dividing practices" of an objectivizing science are essential to creating subjects.[22] He writes, "The subject is either divided inside himself or divided from others. This process objectivizes him. Examples are the mad and the sane, the sick and the healthy, the criminals and the 'good boys.'"[23] Echoing Althusser's notion of "the hail," Foucault sought to study "how men have learned to recognize themselves as subjects," in this case, as people whose ethnic group is interpellated as "diabetes prone."[24]

Therefore, "Mexicanness" for the diabetes enterprise is part taxonomy and part social identity bundled together in fictions of social and genetic homogeneity and purity. In this light, the diabetes sampling project is a "regime of representation" like that expounded by Escobar's analysis of development as a historically and culturally specific project.[25] Arguing that development discourse regulates populations through the use and creation of representations of peasants, women, and the environment, Escobar's analytic framework works for the representations of diabetics as well as it does for the "discourses through which people come to recognize themselves as developed or underdeveloped."[26] In fact, the resonance between the teleological ideology of development discourse and the biological fate of genetic predisposition constitutes subjects for research and subjects for development in similar ways.

By substituting "development" with "diabetic," we can see that naturalizing Mexicana/o ethnicity within an admixture discourse thus primes the production of scientific knowledge for the process of reinscribing Mexicanas/os into subordinate subjects of national and scientific objectives. And yet, as Yanagisako and Delaney observe, "inequality and hierarchy come already embedded in symbolic systems as well as elaborated through contextualizing material practices."[27] In this instance, "Mexican" is the symbol of blood-based ethnicity, which as we have seen, is shot through and through with hierarchical notions of inferiority. The DNA sampling efforts thus are the contextualizing material practices that elaborate upon the ethnic hierarchy of the region. At issue is what constitutes "Mexicana/o" ethnicity under these historical circumstances and within these sets of scientific practices. The wedding of identity and genotype in the racially stratified border zone of conflict shifts the nationalist enterprise of regional hegemony onto the meanings of "Mexicanness." By relying upon the ideology of admixture and hereditary disease etiology as the rationale for Mexicana/o sampling, researchers and field staff construct research participants as genetic carriers in a stratified social order that places a premium on genetic purity at the level of identity and genotype. The hereditary etiological framework for diabetes is consistent with the U.S. project to control the border through the surveillance and micropolitical control of the Mexicana/o peoples of the region. The ontology that results must be considered as part and parcel of the U.S. nationalist project of Mexicana/o subordination. In her analysis of the historical production and reproduction of racially defined substances, Williams writes, "[A] major objective of nationalist ideology has been to invent a unitary substance," in this case biogenetic, "and to link that substance to a sociopolitical unit and its economic structure."[28]

More than simply an imposed ontology, the Mexicano/a participant is a dynamic interlocutor in the construction of Mexicanness and non-Mexicanness, and of the individual, social, and political bodies to which the label refers. As Scheper-Hughes and Lock observed, the body is "simultaneously a physical and symbolic artifact, is both naturally and culturally produced, and is securely anchored in a particular historical moment."[29] More than overlapping analytical or epistemological approaches, the Mexicana/o body constructed in the diabetes enterprise is a site of the confluence of individual experiences of illness and of well-being, of the representation of the social history of the U.S.-Mexico border and Anglo–Mexicano–Native American relations, and the regulation and disciplining of Mexicanas/os individually and as a class of people. The dynamics of this process, its contours and the boundaries it crafts of bodies, geographies and identities, are seamlessly locatable as befitting the contemporary quest for biocapital.[30] That is, the Mexicano/a body is a fulcrum of biopolitics and governmentality upon which great investment and potentially profit (scientific, material, symbolic) teeters: profits, I will show in subsequent chapters, that require specific configurations of the Mexicano/a body, specific Mexicana/o subjects.

RISKS FOR A BIOSOCIAL GROUP

In his analysis of the Human Genome Project, Rabinow explores the alterations in the modern forms of power over and through the body as an object of discipline and the population as an object of analysis, control, and welfare, which surface in the relentless pursuit of the human genome.[31] Inspired by Foucault's concept of biopower, Rabinow analyzes the specific rationalities that emerge within practices and institutions designed to apply genomic knowledges to questions of life and labor.[32] Genetic epidemiological practices that attempt to understand the genetics of diabetes is one such institution and an ideal site through which to ethnographically flesh out Rabinow's insights into this phenomenon that he calls "biosociality."

To begin, we must consider diabetes as an illness that is thoroughly inflected with a rationality of risk. But this is not merely a statistical artifact of probabilities for the likelihood of the disease, though it is this to be sure. Diabetes in Mexicanas/os is a condition now attributed—14 percent of it at least—to a heritable pattern of nucleotides whose presence is explained as a result of ethnic admixture. As one scientist explained to me in an e-mail, the risk haplotype "appears to be found more often in Mexican Americans because they are found more often, on average, in Asian and Amerindian populations." In this light, the diabetes susceptibility haplotype produces a risk group whose social environment is relevant to its suffering only as an ontological necessity that defines the quantitative parameters of risk, 14 percent, and the typological purity of the ethnoracial subject, the Mexican American of Sun County, Texas.[33]

The diabetes susceptibility haplotype transforms the conventional epidemiological concern for predicting which persons will become ill to predicting who is an ill person. The creation of the Mexicana/o diabetes susceptibility haplotype is, in Rabinow's description of biosociality, an "identity term . . . around which and through which a truly new type of autoproduction" has emerged.[34] In this instance, "Mexican American," the social label, has been transformed via the practices of genetic epidemiology into a natural one. Though similar, this transformation is different from simply racializing Mexican American ethnicity. As Miles and Brown write that racialization "denote[s] a dialectical process by which meaning is attributed to particular biological features of human beings, as a result of which individuals may be assigned to a general category of persons that reproduces itself biologically."[35] Whereas racialization is the attribution of innate fixed biological differences between human groups labeled with ethnic-, cultural-, national-, political-, or geographical-based taxonomies, the emergent biosocial category of diabetes-susceptible persons are in fact a newly discovered natural class of human. In this new assemblage, carriers of the risk haplotype are made visible through the prism of heritability[36] within the new genetic technosciences. The simultaneous homo-heterogeneity conferred upon the Mexicana DNA data set affords a glimpse of the social conundrum presented by complex disease genetics.

In this case of genomic knowledge making, the enduring processes of social stratification *and* the technoscientific means through which these processes come to be normalized, even internalized, come into view. When Mexicana/o DNA is transformed into quantified admixed matrices of risk—in this case, 14 percent disease risk that is derived from 31 percent Native American admixture—the Mexicanas/os from whence the DNA comes now embody such risk simply by virtue of membership in the sampled group. What is more, the *social* conditions of Sun County Mexicanas/os become the *biogenetic* conditions of Sun County Mexicanas/os. The diabetes genetic research enterprise is thus an instance wherein the conditions of a donor's life, those events that shaped their physiological condition and the social and political history that attached itself to their lives in the form of an ethnic identity, are conscripted into the service of a biogenetic disease research enterprise.[37]

Central to my thinking of these ontological maneuvers are the polyvalence of race within the biologistics of admixture. The task at hand is determining how to account for and explain race or, as I prefer to call it, "ethnorace," which is simultaneously a taxonomic system, a social identity ascribed by others, a self-imposed identity, and a conceptual apparatus within the epistemic machinery of disease gene research.[38] In the latter instance, because it is reiterated again and again, each time with new technoscientific certainty and rhetorical force, it becomes "real biological human difference" because it is treated as such. By this I mean that, in its consequences, ethnorace within the diabetes enterprise and beyond enables ever more and expanding possibility for its own existence and demise.

By demise, I mean the scientific ruptures in which, as Fullwiley, Kahn, and others demonstrate, the truth claims figuratively and sometimes literally do not add up and thus require a reframing. I also mean the fundamental contradictions that are so often articulated with talk of matters of race. How is it that Mexicana/o admixture comes to be once again a dominant feature in the making of a social and biological problem such as type 2 diabetes? The rhetoric and ontological sleights of hand that conjure the antimiscegenation and degeneracy tropes of old do so in what Hall aptly describes as articulation.[39] That is, in a nonreductive way, structures of inequality and meaning systems converge in a historically specific conjuncture to reiterate difference—in this instance racialized—that is at once structural and ideological.

These iterations of difference need not be flat-footed one-to-one correspondences to what scientists say they are doing when they deploy admixture estimates: The explanations scientists give can vary from the sociohistorical significance when placed in a broader frame. Gary and Carl would shudder to be associated with nativist claims, although other scientists may take it in stride.[40] However, the homologies between the deployment of admixture estimates by researchers using Sun County Mexicana/o DNA and the social and political use of mixed blood by nativists and eugenicists in the United States are striking. Race, then as now, "works like a language,"[41] discernable only in context, to represent and compose a world of human creation.

Articulation is not causal, but it is not random either. When we account for the material and semiotic relationships embedded within claims about admixture or biogenetic human variation, the political implications come into view. Just as possessive individualism and the Protestant work ethic were and are building blocks of industrial capitalism, so too is bioethnic difference a response to threats and endangerment.[42] In this instance, the movement of (predominantly) Mexicanos across the border—as people have for five thousand years[43]—is perceived as a new threat under the conditions of huge demographic shifts in the United States and the chronic effects of deindustrialization and a failed, consumer-driven economic structure during the rise of neoliberal governance. In the case of the diabetes enterprise, bioethnic difference is now, as in past eras of mass migration and economic turmoil, a means through which threat and danger are expressed and managed.[44] As Chavez has compellingly demonstrated for the contemporary moment, the Latino threat narratives are perpetuated through the images of "anchor babies," the invasion of criminal border crossers, public proclamations against the darkening of Anglo-American people, or media accounts of the diseased immigrants (nonwhite and largely Mexican) who threaten the United States.[45] In the case of type 2 diabetes among Mexicanos, dangerous and endangered and threatened and threatening operate as two sides of the same coin.[46]

By deploying the ideology of admixture and hereditary disease etiology as the rationale for Mexicana/o sampling, researchers and DNA donation field staff construct research participants as genetic carriers in a stratified social order that places a premium on genetic purity. But more, the wedding of identity and haplotype in this racially stratified border zone of conflict shifts the long-standing U.S. nationalist enterprise of regional hegemony onto the meanings of "Mexicanness" itself. In other words, what might be characterized as a technoscientifically enacted ontological sleight of hand, the threat to the social order is not merely some external racialized Other menacing the borders of the nation-state. Rather, this making and breaking of boundaries and borders is being internalized through the contests of postgenomic specifics of genetic differences within the registers of diabetes haplotype science. In this manner, genetic epidemiology of type 2 diabetes naturalizes the Mexicana/o body as an admixed transnational protogenetic subject characterized as a biological and social problem in need of a solution.[47]

The risk of diabetes in this episteme is that as an epistemological artifact it serves as a means of subjectification. By accepting the biogenetic risk narrative, affected people cede the sociocultural risk factors so central to disease. Many have observed that risk derives its meaning from its social, cultural, and historical context.[48] In this vein, I argue that context of the U.S.-Mexico border is co-configured by the risk calculus derived by the diabetes enterprise. It is a bidirectional semiotic and material phenomenon. As subjects of analysis, Mexicanas/os serve as more than a population at risk. The essentialist notions of Mexicana/o ethnicity inherent in the etiologies of DNA sampling efforts construct Mexicana/o ethnicity as a risk in its own right. For example, the subtitle of a *Wall Street Journal* article reads, "In Rural Texas, Scientists Seek Genetic Cause for Diabetes in Mexican American Clan," and also references the standard Hispanic risk statistics, the homogeneity trope, and the heritability theories being redeveloped by Carl and colleagues.

This book follows Lupton's charge to bring empirical material to bear on the configuration of risk at a particular time, place, and for a particular set of people.[49] I do not seek to create an overdetermined analysis in which social and political etiological forces seem just as ineluctable as the biologisms appear in biomedicine. Rather, I intend here to offer a beginning point for ways to critically bridge the biological and the social, nature and culture, individual and society without succumbing to a naïve reductionism or summary dismissal of uncritical epidemiological analyses. Frankenberg, Williams and Collins, Cooper and David, and Krieger and Fee all try to coerce the epidemiological gaze outward to social history and social structure.[50] Similarly, cultural epidemiology, biocultural synthesis, embodiment theory, and a range of emergent models that control and account for contextual environments broadly defined offer promising visions of research approaches that are robust and capable of attending simultaneously to the biological and sociocultural complexity of human life.[51]

CONSEQUENCES OF CONTEXT

In this chapter, the DNA sampling practices have been placed in social and historical context. We have seen that the complex measurements and biological sample taking occur as a result of Mexicana/o participation as research subjects and field workers. Further, I argue that this voluntary participation is consistent with the nationalist enterprise of subjugating Mexicanas/os along the U.S.-Mexico border and thus is a racial project of the first order.[52] I have also compared the hereditary and social etiological frameworks for disease to assess the configuration of Mexicana/o ethnicity as a biological risk factor. Stepping back further from the empirical case, additional consequences of the DNA sampling for the diabetes enterprise can be discerned.

Tapper has shown how sickle-cell anemia first worked to construct African blackness, then how blackness was used to explain sickle-cell anemia.[53] He also shows how the public health campaigns dovetailed ideologically with the post–civil rights movement demand for full citizenship for African Americans, making full membership more conditional upon whether or not African Americans regulate their bodies (personal choice of partners, early testing, adoption) to control the spread of sickle-cell anemia. Tapper's "technique-of-self" thesis,[54] however, does not forge a bridge between epidemiological or biomedical claims and the social-historical causal claims because it does not address the legitimate ways biological approaches to sickle-cell disease can address social etiology or visa versa. To reiterate, the use of Mexicanas/os within the diabetes enterprise is not a waste of time. It is not that the incidence and prevalence of diabetes among Mexicana/os is uninformative. Rather, what this examination of the production of diabetes genetic epidemiological knowledge seeks to explain are the cultural meanings of the use of Mexicanas/os. In other words, the use of Mexicanas/os in diabetes research is informative, but informative of what?

The diabetes genetics research enterprise configures Mexicanos/as as diabetes prone by virtue of the bits of genetic information they carry. These bits of genes, SNPs, are the material and semiotic nodes conjured from the bodies of Mexicano/a research subjects.[55] It is a subjection that is based upon the racialization of Mexicana/o bodies and upon the relationships between the state-funded research enterprise, instantiated by the Human Genome Project and the sociopolitics of the U.S.-Mexico border. One very important aspect of the polygene discovery that is implied rather than stated in the *Nature Genetics* publication of this particular research is that the genetic material that confers susceptibility is allegedly acquired through admixture—one bit from European ancestors and another from Indian ancestors.[56] In spite of the evidence to the contrary, the boundaries of biological difference are being reworked within the sociopolitical space of the Sun County scientific enterprise.[57]

Devoid of the social and historical context of the border region, diabetes research hardly warrants a quarrel. Carl and his colleagues are respected professionals whose scientific projects are founded upon helping people with diabetes, solving public health problems, and making good use of federally funded data sets. Carl, for example, insists to his staff that any research subject with medical conditions identified in his or her screenings get immediate referrals. Nora remarked that complex disease research is the right thing to do with genomic data since so much public money was used to gather it. However, in context, the sampling of Mexicano/a DNA along the U.S.-Mexico border inserts into the very bodies of research subjects the governmental efforts to maintain the region under strict U.S. control. The recruitment of research subjects thus is the most recent form of a U.S. governmental project that transforms a dangerous zone of racially inflected conflict into a manageable population problem.[58] This form of "governmentality"[59] extends the control and surveillance of the population well beyond what the Immigration and Customs Enforcement, Census Bureau, Internal Revenue Service, or other agencies are able to do.

In the perpetual war along the frontier, the institutional mandates of state-funded public health research naturalize the continuing marginalization of Mexicano/as. As Yanagisako and Delaney observe of evolutionary origin stories, "The social was embedded in the natural, but in a particular version of it."[60] The same must be said of the origins of disease among Mexican Americans. What are we to make of the persistent configuration of Mexicanos/as as enemy, Other, labor source, and now public health burden?

Switching analytical vantage points brings the scientific enterprise of diabetes genetic epidemiology in line with the national enterprise of capital appropriation and accommodation in the region. Under these conditions, the border can be viewed as a social and historical creation that makes possible the specific DNA collection practices of the diabetes enterprise. A unique location, the border is a transnational and global space within which, as Gupta said, "cultural forms are imposed, invented, reworked and transformed."[61] The attention given in this chapter to the political and social history of the space of DNA collection locates the scientific enterprise in two senses—as a space of subjectification and as a set of social practices that naturalize difference.

In this first sense, this chapter argues that the acquisition of DNA samples for the type 2 diabetes enterprise transforms Mexicanas/os into racialized subjects consistent with the decadeslong wars of maneuver between Anglos and Mexicanas/os along the border. The subjectification of Mexicana/os is accomplished because the conditions of poverty and disadvantage are exploited to recruit DNA donors. Additionally, through the process of "donation," DNA donors are transformed into "participants," which, in true Althusserian terms, is the hail that interpellates them.

In the second sense, the geography of the border space, on the edges of two nation states, offers an "ethnoscape"[62] of persons whose embodiment of difference shapes and is shaped by the politics of the region and by extension the perpetual struggle between the United States and Mexico and between Anglos and Mexicanas/os more generally. The political context of DNA collection locates the border as a space of ontological contestations through which the identity and subjectivity of its inhabitants are reworked in particular ways. Now crafted of genomic material, this border zone becomes a DNA-scape that recomposes geographic and social topologies of inequality and differentiation in a postgenomic guise. This chapter demonstrates that while the ideology of diabetes science may interpellate Mexicanas/os into state subjects, it does so by naturalizing a particular social order.

Thus, the frontiers of science are being co-configured by the political and economic exigencies of the frontiers of nationhood. Mexicanos/as are conscripted as racialized research subjects by scientists desperate to appeal to the authority of objectivity. The use of ethnicity in this context transforms it into a taxonomic metacategory that fits easily within the discourse of biological science. Race, however, is not a biological concept. Yet, as I will show in chapter 6, this "bioethnic conscription" fuses the social history of Mexicanos/as with their purportedly biological essence. Not unlike the well-documented exemplar of biomedical constructions of women's bodies based upon concurrently prevalent social prejudices,[63] genetics researchers' use of a border population illuminates the manner in which Mexicano/a ethnic identification—and the social history through which it is forged—is taken up in biological knowledge. In this process, research participants become transnational protogenetic subjects irrespective of their national identities and allegiances.

Returning to the myriad ways Mexicana/o bodies are defined, located, surveyed, labeled, diagnosed, screened, genotyped, and analyzed, we see yet another important transformation of the social body into the biological body. Prior to participation in the research, Mexicanas/os with impairments in glucose metabolism are often undiagnosed. Participation ensures a diagnosis and a referral to a physician if needed. The diagnosis occurs within the epidemiologics of genetics and thus conscripts the participant into the essentialism inherent in the hereditary etiological model. Taussig points out that a diagnosis redefines a person "firmly within the epistemological and ontological groundwork from which the society's basic ideological premises arise."[64] It was shown above that for diabetes epidemiology, the "epistemological and ontological groundwork" inherent in the use of Mexicano/a bodies is predicated upon notions of "racial" admixture, the pseudo-biological consequence of conquest, and, additionally, the elision of the highly stratified structural context of Anglo-Mexicano relations in the region.

Thus, in the context of the persistent representation and treatment of Mexicanos/as as an enemy, an Other, an uncivilized brute, a squatter, a thief, a peasant, a half-breed, and now a carrier of susceptibility genes, Mexicanos/as on the border fulfill an embodied role as racialized objects of research. Further, that government agencies pay for most of this research is an important fact. For what was once a military and business practice—the making of controllable border subjects—is now also carried out by biomedical institutions with money from U.S. government agencies.

Another way to imagine this is as follows. If in the era of conquest and dispossession the half-breed mongrel race threatened the natural and thus social order, in the contemporary era of genetic admixture, the miscegenational metaphor reconstitutes the social order as a response to the epidemiological monster called type 2 diabetes in Mexicans and Mexican Americans. The monstrous person is no longer the one dimensional target of governmental concern. Instead the bodies (social/biological) of Mexicanos are marked as outside the genotypic norm by virtue of the risk carried in the Mexicano haplotype.[65]

I have striven to accentuate here that the local context of DNA acquisition matters in the assessment of the diabetes research enterprise. To understand the context makes a raft of troubles for the humanistic rhetoric of screening, treating, preventing, or curing type 2 diabetes, but mostly illuminates the conditions that make possible the diabetes genetic research enterprise. First, Mexicanos/as are not willing participants in research. This does not mean they are screened against their will, but rather that participation in research screening for a debilitating condition that occurs in a space of 150 years of political and economic subjection, when no viable alternate means of surveillance is available, is hardly voluntary. Who would *not* participate in a research project if it was the only way to gain lifesaving knowledge for oneself and one's family? In fact, one field office worker told me that people with insurance coverage are hard to recruit.

Second, I have tried to demonstrate that the bodies sampled for research make knowledge possible. Without DNA, research comes to a standstill. Yet, as the case of Sun County illustrates, acquisition is no simple affair. It involves multiple levels of administrative and interpersonal prowess. What is more, Mexicano/a DNA is valuable to the genetic economy of diabetes research. In the chapter that follows, I will show that the material and cultural capital generated by the processing of blood samples flows away from the donors.

In addition to the contextual and political economic critique I have offered here, particular attention must be paid to the body as a field through which biological and political discourses are construed. Up to this juncture, my quarrel has emphasized the place and use of particular bodies. The diabetes research enterprise is not unique in its elision of the political context of knowledge production, as the criticisms of Frankenberg, Williams and Collins, Cooper and David, and Krieger and Fee all demonstrate. It is, as so many have observed, impossible for context to creep into biomedical discourse because to do so would disrupt the frame of reference for the entire medical industrial complex.[66]

The body conjured by the diabetes research enterprise instantiates Lock's insight that bodily conditions must be understood as an interplay between biology, history, experiences, meanings, and social context.[67] Thus, the stakes for those whose ethnicity is conscripted for biological narratives of diabetes are costly. Simply put, the diabetes genetic research enterprise would lead us to conclude that Mexicanos/as are *biologically* predisposed to diabetes. That this assertion happens to fit a long-standing pattern of Mexicano/a subjugation, the elision of which requires ethnographic unpacking, demonstrates the extent to which science supports the state's production of racialized Others in such spaces of contestation as the U.S.-Mexico border. Recall Duster's critique of the empirical arbitrariness of racial typologies used in biomedicine.[68] The point argued here is that the populations are not arbitrary, empirically or otherwise. In fact, when the conditions and contexts of donors' lives are included in the epistemological framework of medical knowledge, Duster's warnings about biological racial profiling are more easily understood.

The diabetes enterprise thus illustrates how scientists like Carl and his colleagues are pressed into service of the U.S. nation-state's perpetual assertion of its social and political hegemony. This assemblage of state, academic, and corporate research is nothing new nor unique to the U.S.-Mexico political milieu. As Paul Rabinow has remarked of the alliance between France's state genomic laboratory and a patient group, "What is distinctive—and 'contemporary'—in this situation is not its radical newness but its assemblage of old and new elements."[69] Notwithstanding Judi's comments about public health workers blaming diabetics on the research subjects' sedentary lifestyle, the complete absence of patient advocacy voices within this specific assemblage endows this research enterprise with a preponderance of by now familiar biopolitical elements.[70] Hence, though not overdetermined, the scientific frontier of diabetes genetic epidemiology contains a double edge. One side is the humanist effort to prevent chronic disease, while the other is a "technique of power" aligned—historically, politically, and economically—with the nation-building efforts of the past century and a half on the U.S.-Mexico border.

CONCLUSION

For the purposes of this discussion, the racialization inherent in this practice is but a starting analytical point to understand the racial emplacement of Sun County Mexicanas/os. Racial emplacement occurs when group identities come to stand in for group biology. In this instance, Carl's biogenetic rationale for why Sun County Mexicanos/as are appropriate for genetic research reflects the formal logics of classification while simultaneously "torqueing" the way Mexicana/o is a label that references a specific group of people linked to a specific place and time, such as Sun County, Texas. What is of particular interest are the scientists' attempts to quantitatively characterize the ethnic homogeneity of the Mexicana/o population as a means of understanding the incidence and prevalence of diabetes. As Stefan Helmreich observes, "Individual biographies are twisted into tortured shapes that materialize in the negative space that opens up when powerful classification schemes do not line up in the local logics of everyday life."[71]

The practice of racial emplacement—that is, characterizing the population structure of an ethnic group like Mexican Americans—is not merely a simplistic typological exercise. Rather, it is an epistemological practice that works on the meaning-cum-location of diabetes itself, and thus is also an ontological cultural operation. Locating diabetes within Mexicana/o ethnoracial admixture cleaves both Mexicanness and the illness called diabetes from the social histories that produced the ethnic label and the socially embodied conditions that contribute to the disease. Racial emplacement is repeating itself for numerous ethnic groups for numerous diseases in attempts to gain empirical purchase on the biology of human variation.[72]

That diabetes scientists begin with a social label for their population of interest (Mexican American) and then characterize the ethnic group according to its percentage of genetic admixture from Native American, African, and Spanish inheritances, presents an interesting object lesson for the study of the coproduction of science and society.[73] On the one hand, the need for valid population constructs requires the most accurate characterization of the population structure possible. On the other hand, the history of Mexicanas/os in the Sun County region of the United States is bedeviled with conflict, often violent, that is itself rationalized by reference to the racial impurity of the Mexicana/o. Classification, genetic characterization, and political history are thus conflated.

CHAPTER 4

Collaboration and Power

Processing Cultures and Culturing Data

In her famous essay titled "Situated Knowledges," Donna Haraway writes, "Critics of the sciences and their claims or associated ideologies, have shied away from doctrines of scientific objectivity in part because of suspicion that an 'object' of knowledge is a passive and inert thing."[1] I am both haunted and vexed by Haraway's unrelenting insistence that we do better than simply point out the obvious power implications of a technoscientific find. Yet, there is a place, in the analytical practice of making a partial account,[2] through which the power of the knower must be accounted for. In this chapter, I examine the practices of collaborative data creation and sharing and assess them for the ways the bodies of DNA donors are made into objects for the research enterprise. Central to this objectification is the conversion of DNA into data sets, which requires a heterogeneous set of skills, technologies, and processes. Laying out these social and techno-logical practices demonstrates the ways Mexicana/o donor bodies are made to span texts and worlds, in the syntactical registers of statistical noise, pure data, and power. We begin by situating data collection and the conversion of blood samples into genotypes.

"Aren't you bored?" asked Alma. Having returned from a home visit where field staff retrieved blood samples, I had been watching her for nearly 20 minutes prepare the samples for storage in the freezer. Though everyone spends time in the lab processing samples from participants, Alma seems to be most at home there. The lab is located at the back of the building. One wall is covered in shelving and a 10-foot countertop that serves as a wet lab. Two freezers, a closet, and a bathroom are also part of the lab space. A small centrifuge, pipette equipment and shipping supplies are neatly arranged on the shelving and lab bench wall. After a blood draw, samples are placed in the centrifuge and spun down into plasma, buffy (white blood cells), and the reddish serum. Then they are separated, labeled, and stored for shipping. Alma prepares samples for Houston once a month. "Mayo [Clinic] goes out on Mondays," she explains. Other research projects necessitate samples of blood, lipids, urine, plasma, or images (echocardiographic and retinographic) to be sent to San Antonio, Madison, and Chicago. For each study, Carl's Houston staff sends carefully prepared shipping supplies to the field office. Zip-seal storage bags, pages of preprinted labels, shipping labels, and checklists arrive at predetermined intervals. Pages of labels printed with participant identification numbers, protocol codes, dates, and other information are placed on the 8.5 mL Vacutainer tubes color coded by research project. For each participant there are numerous labels corresponding to the various samples taken, which are coded further for each research project to which they have donated. Houston knows well in advance who will be sampled and when the samples are to be shipped.

When shipping samples off to collaborators, field staff can get a bit edgy with one another. "We need more ice!" Maria announced to her colleagues in anticipation. "Did we get those boxes yet? Who ordered them? *Ay*, come on you guys, someone call Airborne [Express] and tell them we need about 12 more," she cajoled. Later that afternoon, Airborne Express arrives with stacks of boxes, some empty. "We must open everything," Maria says, directing her more junior colleague. In addition to the empty shipping boxes, more forms and labels arrive. Consent forms, intake forms, and cardiac referral forms are quickly sorted, counted, and taken to the various places throughout the center where they will be ready for use. "If you need any supplies, I'm doing the order," Maria calls out loudly to her colleagues. It's after 5, and the last participant left about an hour earlier. "The woman [in Houston] who fills our supplies order is going on vacation, so we need to order this week," she explains. The mood around shipping is not one of *confianza*, but rather of ensuring that the samples get to collaborators in adherence with strict guidelines. A box that is improperly prepared could mean the loss of dozens of samples—a time-consuming setback.

Judi and her staff often spend time talking about quality-control issues. A mislabeled vial or improperly filled out form, once discovered, immediately requires a response. Before shipping, staffers exchange paperwork to check for any errors, missing information, or anything else that would incur a call from Houston. The work of the field staff is to make the samples conform to the specifications of the entire collaborative diabetes enterprise. Therefore, an error early on in the development of a data set wreaks havoc downstream in the research process.

Judi and her staff work to render the lived conditions of donors' lives accessible to researchers around the world. In this chapter, I will follow the blood samples from their point of acquisition on the border to the next node in the collaborative network, to Chicago at the labs of Nora and Gary. Examining the processes of data sharing between collaborators in the diabetes enterprise demonstrates that collaboration requires the regulation of ideas, practices, and populations. Converting bodies into data sets is a requirement for the production of knowledges based upon those bodies. Specifically, I argue that researchers develop, prepare, and narrate "good data sets," which require that researchers perform what I will call "articulation work." Articulation work occurs when researchers reconcile diverse frames of epistemological reference, just as an accountant reconciles a ledger.

The challenges to this reconciliation are that bodies, data sets, and technologies (and sometimes the behaviors of collaborating colleagues) are unruly things. This requires several moves on behalf of the scientist that convert the unruly, into workable objects for analysis. As Haraway writes, "It—the world—must, in short, be objectified as a thing, not as an agent; it must be matter for the self formation of the only social being in the productions of knowledge, the human knower."[3] We will see in this chapter that diabetes science collaboration across disciplines, geographies, and methodologies requires (1) a shift in scale, (2) an emphasis on a biology based on digitalized information, (3) the rhetoric of objectivity, and (4) data that no longer represent active donors' bodies but rather a passive and quiet compilation of quantitative information. As Haraway puts it, "The object both guarantees and refreshes the power of the knower, but any status as agent in the production of knowledge must be denied the object."[4] We begin with the human-computer interaction.

HUMAN-HUMAN-COMPUTER COLLABORATION

On the first Monday of the year 2000, I walk across campus toward the lab. Evidence of Saturday's revelry still litter the residential streets. Now recognized by security, I pass through the hospital security checkpoints, ostensibly as an employee who has forgotten his ID card. I make my way to Nora's and Gary's office; Nora's new lab is not complete. Nora had not yet arrived, so Gary and I chat about the New Year hoopla. The office is not large enough to accommodate two people in the customary space requirements of professionals, so my spot next to the door allows an intimate observation of Gary's and Nora's work.

Gary's and Nora's relationship over the years had shaped their workspace expectations. Theirs was a constant back-and-forth. They would share e-mails, analyses, shoptalk, gossip, politics, and no small number of jokes and personal jabs. Gary, as the senior researcher of the duo, was immensely appreciative of Nora and her work. He would remark to me as if on camera, "My miserable life here would be nothing were it not for Nora. She's the brains of the outfit. I'd be lost without her." Gary's and Nora's desks were so close that they could hand each other a paper without moving their chairs more than six inches. Gary was the neater of the two. He would throw up his hands in resignation when Nora fumbled through the mountains of paper scattered in seeming chaos on her desk.

If Nora's desktop was disordered, her virtual life was not. In fact, the multitasking she conducted *in silico* mirrors the fluidity of her desktop file system and the sociality that drives her work. Much of the time Nora was in her office was spent conducting analysis. Working on several databases at once, Nora would toggle back and forth from one to the other. There was a main hard drive and two others she drew from. Her postdocs and all her collaborators were also networked, and, if one was having difficulty, she would log over to their workstation to problem solve. In the midst of her database surfing, she would answer the phone, read mail, chat with Gary and me, read her e-mail, all the while picking away at her primary data set, which was usually the one closest to a deadline for publication or a meeting presentation.

Nora's labor is structured around the social networks she creates. Hers and Gary's face-to-face interaction mirrors the seamlessness of her collaborations with scientists from around the globe. Nora's collaborative network relationships are enduring forms of sociality through which the diabetes consortium membership produce knowledge. Dispersed through geographic distances and reliant upon digitized collaboration, Nora maintains dozens of active professional relationships through several networks of which the diabetes enterprise is only one. All of Nora's collaborators say their involvement was in part because of their relationship with Nora.

Scribbling notes on the back of whatever piece of paper is handy, Nora notes statistical likelihood scores, SNPs, or some other numbers of interest. There are hundreds of data sets that she draws from. Each data set is tied to a collaborative relationship within Nora's social-professional network. Each time a set of population samples is genotyped, it is placed in its own data set. Nora then tests, checks, evaluates, and conducts simulations on the data sets. Day after day, between meetings, remotely from home, while on the phone, she runs various tests using FORTRAN. Nora writes the routines and subroutines in a series of cascading if-then statements that often fold into one another. Embedded into the routines are other software programs, some she developed, some developed by colleagues: None is off the shelf. In at least one instance, when they needed an off-the-shelf program to run a specialized query, she used her network to contact the programmers, who sent her the code to alter it. The software programs read and test the genotypes of the data set of interest described in alleles. Over and over again, she checks them for errors in genotyping, for expected inheritance patterns using the long-established Hardy-Weinberg algorithm for determining homo and heterozygosity.

Nora's realizations come in bits and pieces. There is never a monumental moment when the computer finishes its computation and the data suddenly jump off the screen. For example, the realization that heterozygotes for one piece of a gene were at greater risk than homozygotes came during one of her analysis sessions. It was on that day that Nora caught an inkling that ethnic admixture might confer increased susceptibility to diabetes. Her realization occurred while toggling between windows on her screen comparing the heterozygotes with the homozygotes for each SNP. Nora uses SNPs as analytical categories by which to measure variation between siblings and populations. Instead of whole genetic variants, Nora is evaluating SNP variations and, thereby, isolating the susceptibility gene products within populations.

After programming her FORTRAN command routines, Nora examines the report generated by the queries she runs. On one occasion, she compared the values beneath each y-axis number and the corresponding homo- or heterozygosity pattern for each SNP. Across the x-axis were numerical names for the SNPs corresponding to their position relative to the marker used for genotyping. Genotyping is essentially a report of the presence or absence of a set of markers whose location and frequency had already been established.

I noticed during one of her analytical moments at her computer that Nora was comparing those patients who were homozygous for some

SNPs while hetero for others. She noted to Gary, "It's puzzling that there is no high risk with homozygotes. I put tables together, and if you take all polymorphisms across Calp-10 [a suspected risk molecule], there are four homozygous individuals who are controls for the high-risk allele, but there are none in the patients." Nora did the comparisons between patients and controls for Calp-10, made a list, and handed them to Gary, who dispassionately entered the results in his laptop. Gary was the chart maker. Nora then repeated the comparisons with the g protein coupled receptor, another suspected risk molecule. This data would later become the key finding to appear in the *Nature Genetics* article of 2000.

Nora's quantitatively oriented genetics work is the backbone of research collaboration into a complex disease like type 2 diabetes. Her genetics expertise is part statistical, part technological, and part social. "While I disliked it at the time, I am so glad that my advisor forced us to learn FORTRAN," she recalled. In terms of her collaborative involvement, Nora has leveraged her multiple talents well. She is overworked, however. At any given time collaborators from around the globe are waiting for something from her. Nora describes these as debts, "I owe 'Steve' something," she recently remarked of a British colleague. Her sense of responsibility to her work, to her colleagues and to the judicious use of resources is palpable. Even under the most stringent deadlines or uncollegial treatment by associates, Nora seldom gets flustered. "I'm too nice," she confessed during a bitter battle over lab space with some associates.[5]

Gary gives plaintive voice to the demands upon Nora. Everyone wants something from her. A talk, a consult, an interview (me), analysis of a data set, help with study design, supervision of a project, results from a simulation. Though uncompromisingly supportive of her talents and professional interests, his "support" is often delivered as complaints about work that is past due. They are complaints that mirror, if not co-create, Nora's debtor mentality. Important here is the way collaboration involves multiple exchanges of data, intellectual service, and computational time. The diabetes enterprise works as a collaborative venture because of the solidarities established through these exchanges. Almost everyone owes everyone something.

In true Maussian fashion, to belong to the consortium requires an initial transfer of data. I use the term "transfer" rather than "gift" because, as Maurer observed, Mauss's theory of the gift wavered between the pure gift and the commodity.[6] That is, on the one hand, a grand theoretical concept that defines social relations structurally in a series of solidarity-enhancing exchanges that operate seemingly outside of the calculated, adequated economic rationalities. And on the other, Carl is working with a wholly discernable calculus of value of the goods or services exchanged between rational interlocutors. Collaboration within the diabetes enterprise instantiates Mauss's qualification of his theory that gift giving is simultaneously calculated and not calculated. A gift is a gift, not a utilitarian contract for certain return. However, Mauss observed that gifts operate within a cultural logic of exchange such that giving creates structural solidarities between those involved. Referring to the Trobriand Islands, Mauss observes, "This notion is neither that of the free, purely gratuitous rendering of total services, nor that of production and exchange purely interested in what is useful. It is a hybrid that flourished."[7] Owing Steve work, thus, is Nora's externalization of the expected return of services for Steve's contribution of a data set. And yet the giving of the data set was itself an act of professional solidarity to a trusted colleague whose services can make of it more than it was before. What is created in this exchange is the networked sociality of the consortium with both the rights and obligations of solidarity to the enterprise that is membership via data set contribution, and the hoped for outcomes of scientific discovery. It is an exchange across time and space, occurring between humans and their computational media.

SCIENTIFIC MEETINGS: FACE-TO-FACE COLLABORATION

Perhaps the most public forum for collaboration occurs at scientific meetings. At least three times a year consortium scientists from far-flung laboratories meet to share and exchange research developments at scientific meetings. Since 1937 diabetes has enjoyed its own scientific conference. There are dozens of conferences, mini-conferences, symposia, international meetings, and other gatherings that are organized to enable the exchange of ideas.[8] Consortium meetings are scheduled to coincide with meetings that investigators already plan to attend.

Because I was interested in scientific collaboration, scientific conferences surfaced as important sites to document the ways that scientists from different disciplines and institutional contexts work together. Conferences are redolent with opportunities for ethnographic collaboration.[9] Aside from the formal presentations, numerous informal events occur. My interests were in a specific diabetes consortium, its members, their collaborators, and the work they produced collectively. I was also interested in the array of topics next to which diabetes genetic epidemiology is situated.

The 1999 conference of the American Diabetes Association had some eight thousand participants; of those, thirty-eight hundred were clinicians, fourteen hundred were research scientists, and another fourteen hundred were diabetes educators. To remain focused, I stratified my participant observation as follows. I first wanted to follow researchers and interview them if possible. I looked up their names in the abstract books, went to their sessions, and noted their collaborative partnerships. Next, I used the thematic index to find other sessions that directly dealt with type 2 diabetes, genetics, and populations. I deliberately avoided the diabetes education sessions because I was most interested in genetic epidemiology.[10] Occasionally, I would attend a session that was more general, something on physiology, diagnosis, or collaborative partnerships between, for example, Glaxo, Roche, or Millennium and the NIH. Because Francis Collins, then director of the NIH's Human Genome Project, was still making his promotional rounds, I attended a few sessions in which he was featured, if only to capture data on how the US-Human Genome Project was being intellectually positioned vis-à-vis diabetes genetic epidemiology.

The advantage to a scientific meeting is that often researchers would frame their work differently for a broader and perhaps more skeptical audience. Such alternative framing requires researchers to better articulate the discursive context of their contributions to the intellectual project and their specific research. It also aided in my general comprehension of the particular method or finding being discussed. The disadvantages to scientific meetings are that they are immense and researchers are busy. Consortium meetings were almost always connected to scientific meetings because, logistically, it was most efficient. Meetings are events that simultaneously illustrate the possibilities of overcoming geographical distance and time limits. Scientists come to share results of a few months' or years' worth of work with diverse audiences from the United States, western Europe, Japan, and elsewhere.[11]

My first American Diabetes Association meeting occurred when I was conducting prefield explorations. I had recently failed to secure permission to work at Glaxo and placed all my field site hopes on Nora at the University of Chicago. If Nora was not amenable to my sustained observations, I would be forced to begin my field site search anew.[12] After talking my registration fees down from $365 to $75, I prepared to meet with Nora and somehow persuade her to allow me to come spend time in her lab. It was the 1998 ADA meetings and Nora and I would meet in the registration area. The registration tables were situated in one corner of a huge sunroom/meeting hall of the San Diego Conference Center.

We walked over to a series of about 70 banquet tables that occupied the front third of the hall. The interview began with me asking her about the consortium. During our initial phone call, Nora had relayed her feelings about why the consortium was needed and the right thing to do.

> *Me:* What is your role in the consortium?
>
> *Nora:* Gary and I think it ought to be done, and it's the right thing to do. For one thing, you can't work in this too long without realizing it's gonna take big data sets, clever and hard molecular work. It's foolish not to make optimal use of the data sets. I mean, taxpayers paid for these data to be collected. It's a moral obligation to get the most out of it as you can.

I asked for any updates on the consortium work. How it was going? What were the setbacks, if any? Any results or publications? I then asked about biographical information. How long have you worked on diabetes? Where did you work before this? What did you work on before this? Next I described my project. I had a one-page abstract of my research that posed my research foci as follows: (1) scientific collaboration, (2) the use of ethnic populations in research, and (3) the shift from endocrinological to genetics-based approaches for a complex disease. Like a true teacher, Nora corrected the terminology a bit to make it clearer and more accurate. The exchange would be emblematic of many to follow.

After the interview, I set about describing my methods: participant-observation (i.e., purposeful hanging out and participation) at labs, meetings and field sites, and interviews. I asked if she would please ask the consortium if I could attend their meetings. At the end of our meeting, I thanked her and asked if she would consider having me conduct my fieldwork at her lab. She said that I would be welcome to visit her lab. When the interview concluded, I said that I would contact her again if I wanted to take her up on her offer. That afternoon, Nora had a steering committee meeting in which she asked if I could attend the full consortium gatherings. There were no objections, and I attended the consortium meeting the following morning.

The consortium meeting began at 7 A.M. Two years earlier the first such meeting also began early. What was planned as a one-and-a-half-hour meeting lasted six hours. "The interest was so high," remarked one member. "We just kept brainstorming." This meeting was more predictable, however. The business of the morning was to report on progress for chromosome 20 and clarify which chromosomes would be pursued next. The overall aims of the consortium were to conduct linkage analyses to search for susceptibility genes for diabetes. The task at hand was to construct a map that was based upon the genotyping work of consortium members. One statistician, whose nonprofit research institute offered the computer storage space for the immense data files, took the lead.

The statistician reported that he had just received some data sets, so no final Ch20 report was ready. He also reported that the files were so large that even without the new data, the software crashed. The data sets needed to be rescaled. Members discussed whether to alter the software, the data or the way the data was fed into the software. One researcher volunteered to call the software developer, who was not there, to ask about altering the software.

The second issue was how to fold in new data once the map was complete. The group decided that it would not redo the marker map but would add the collective markers to the new data set. The resolutions to the various issues were reached by dividing up the workload. One scientist would explore marker maps for the next chromosome. Another would scout the French reference database (CEPH), and one would evaluate the Marshfield clinic's 8,000 to 9,000 pre-mapped markers. There were no overt disagreements, and so the motions and seconds and votes were performed with perfunctory resignation. The meeting ended with the agreement that the analysis subcommittee would address the remaining issue of how long and how many markers to use for the map of Ch20.

This seemingly mundane description of the collaborative practices planned and carried out at a consortium business meeting conceal a host of anxieties and potential conflicts. During my second meeting, after having interviewed several of the members, visited them in their labs, and spent months with Nora, a conversation occurred that I could not quite understand. I was accustomed to asking Nora or someone else for a breakdown after a technical conversation, or looking something up in published sources when I did not quite follow the conversation. This instance was different. Consortium members were clumsily deliberating about which chromosome to map next. The debate seemed to center on a set of markers that would be used for one of the chromosomal maps.[13]

Nora later explained what the hemming and hawing was really about. A senior but not central contributor to the consortium had invested years in the development of several markers on a particular chromosome that most consortium members no longer used because a set of better markers had been developed by someone else. To include the senior colleague's genotypes would require the use of his markers. Consortium members were in a conundrum. They wanted the data from the colleague's samples but did not want his genotypes or markers. The senior colleague, who was not present, would not be keen to share his data if his markers were not used. The tension was palpable, with a few at the table arguing on behalf of the senior colleague. It was resolved by someone volunteering to contact the absent colleague to discuss the possibility of regenotyping his samples, at considerable cost of time and money, as a way to validate his markers while at the same time enabling a standard set of markers to be applied to his DNA samples.

WHAT IS A DIABETIC: STANDARD VALUES, PURE AND POWERFUL DATA

Though Nora was trained as a geneticist, her expertise draws upon quantitative analysis and computational tools. Biostatisticians, bioinformaticians, and quantitatively minded geneticists like Nora, are all central to the collaborative efforts of the consortium and the representation of their collective efforts. For this discussion, I will refer to such researchers as statistical analysts. These are the power brokers of the consortium. Their role in diabetes research is to search for and create pure and powerful data.

For a genetic finding of a complex disease like diabetes to be taken seriously, the data sets must be powerful. This means that at each stage of research, from the selection and screening of populations to the genotyping of the DNA to the analyses of each data set produced by each collaborator, each data set must adhere to strict rules. Nora's job is largely to make the disparate data sets articulate with one another. The case for standardized data sets is narrated in terms of degrees of power and noise.

Much of Nora's collaborative efforts involves "cleaning up" data sets to make the results more powerful. That is, getting one person's genotyping information into useful, informative shape so that the data could be merged with a larger set or sorting through an old marker map with a newer one to make the case for one set of markers over another.

The standard test of the power of a finding is expressed in its logarithm of the odds (LOD) score. A LOD score is a way to quantitatively analyze a data set to determine if a marker (a bit of genetic material) is linked (inherited together) with another. If so, then scientists can compare a known marker with unknown others to infer an association that may lead to a putative inherited disease marker. Conflicting findings between one researcher's results and another's, is often described as "noise." Results of data deemed questionable figure prominently in discussions of data sharing and analysis. One consortium member puts it this way:

> There's a long list of reasons why studies might fail to replicate. The most discouraging of which is that it's all noise. And I think a lot of it is noise. The separating signal for noise is the problem here, because I think a lot of these wiggles that you saw on these graphs are LOD scores going up and down, and a high LOD score is supposedly a signal. But I think a lot of that is noise, and teasing out. . . . I mean, the diabetes genes are there somewhere. . . . And teasing out the real signals, where there actually is a susceptibility gene from the noise is a challenge. Part of the reason there's so little replication is because a lot of what we're looking at is, in fact, noise. That is a challenge.

Pure and powerful data also requires that at each stage in data set construction, for each population and each experiment, "robust" standardization and sheer volume must be created. One statistician explains it in terms of the number of members from one family who participate in a given study. He notes:

> If you want to get a genetic study funded, you need to say something about power. Reviewers always ask what is your response rate. Usually what lousy response rates will mean is that your families are going to be smaller if people don't participate. Because they're smaller, you're going to get fewer relative pairs. Because you have fewer relative pairs, you have a loss of power.

Statistical analysts speak with an almost evangelical undertone in their desperate attempt to raise the standards of research. High response rates are one such standard. Others, which will be discussed below, include good genotyping, informative and current markers, and a well-ascertained population.

The collaboration is made problematic because each researcher is trying to leverage his or her labor for multiple ends. The specific goals of collaboration are only one demand placed upon their research. There are conflicts. In one instance, Nora was struggling with a researcher who had made a map of a chromosome with markers that were no longer informative. "You want to use everyone's markers because they have a lot at stake in those markers being informative. But Ned's markers are not dense enough and actually detract from the statistical likelihood [LOD] scores we see when we use more recently developed markers." Some researchers are loath to give up their markers for the greater good of the consortium, and Nora must carefully negotiate each member's professional and scientific needs.

The pressures for powerful data are immense. Attention to statistical power must begin with the very first piece of data collected for a project. Statistical analysts often deploy a proselytizing tone simultaneously convincing and recruiting scientists to their kind of robust data collection. At one ADA meeting, two consortium members, one from industry, the other a nonprofit research institute, gave an introductory talk on powerful linkage analyses. In this instance, power is defined as the number of times statistical simulations produce significant LOD scores—those 3.0 or higher, which means the likelihood of the observed inheritance patterning occurring randomly is less than 3 in 1,000. Responding to a question about small effects of some allelic variants, Nora remarks:

> [It] is a hit-or-miss enterprise in terms of what you expect to find with any particular variants. There is a challenge, though, even if you have variants in front of you, you need a lot of DNA samples if you're going to have sufficient power to detect a weak effect, and we all would like to see those weak effects because each one of them tells us about a pathway that may be involved. Even if it only accounts for a small fraction of the heritability for diabetes, you wouldn't want to miss it.

Failure to conform to standard practices, use common diagnostic criteria, similar markers, common labels, and standard population selection protocols will also jeopardize the individual data set, which, when pooled with multiple data sets, then diminishes the power of the entire collaborative venture.

A senior biostatistician in the consortium, Franklin Akindes, addressed quality data as an issue of population selection and diagnostic criterion. In a talk titled "Simple versus Gold Standard Measures of Diabetes/Glucose Intolerance," Dr. Akindes argued to the approximately four hundred who had come to his talk that getting to the bottom of phenotypes is of utmost importance. Diabetes science would be greatly improved, he argued, by evaluating studies by the phenotypic screen each study used. There are different tests for insulin resistance, among them fasting glucose tolerance versus the homeostasis index for fasting blood glucose. If research subjects are selected by different tests, or different cutoff points for the same test, then when the data are combined, the aggregated data set is compromised.

Akindes' concerns strike at the epistemological foundation of the collaborative venture to find the genetic contributions to complex diseases. To wit, the presumption that genotype drives phenotype. Akindes was peering around the corner of the limits of genetic epidemiology echoing the growing scientific appreciation for the complex relationships between proteins and their environments. Genotypes are likely poor predictors of health outcomes. Even under strict experimental conditions, plant geneticists know, plants with identical genotypes will develop differently according to subtle changes in temperature, wind, soil, and a host of mostly unexplainable factors.[14] The gene, or the expression of a protein as a result of a genotype, is increasingly understood as an interplay of natural and social environments, extracellular matrices, interactions between and among molecules, and overlapping functional molecules that get expressed as a phenotype in networks of context dependency.[15]

Franklin Akindes' arguments stop short of calling the gene, as a determinative force for health, flat-out misguided. However, Akindes and his colleagues on the ADA panel did argue that attention to phenotype differences of all kinds were vitally important to advance the understanding of diabetes genetics. Panelists specifically mentioned that ethnicity, like other variables of interest to genetic scientists, should be interrogated. Akindes' message at the time was that researchers needed to pay more careful attention to phenotype to fine-tune linkage analyses results. He argued that phenotypic subsets must be created by breaking out, layering, and comparing multiple phenotypes with multiple markers. This would, he argued, enable a better understanding of locus-phenotype-trait interactions. Akindes underscores the complexity of collaboration. But, additionally, his arguments, which were repeated at multiple conferences, are emblematic of the consistent reminders to diabetes researchers that ethnicity is a highly problematic variable. His calls for scrutiny of population identifiers reminds the diabetes scientific community that ethnicity is a poor shorthand for phenotype.

Akindes' panel was only one of many that conveyed the seriousness with which diabetes scientist take their work. The ADA conference contained panels and papers on the best practices for taking blood, for sending blood, for processing genetic material, for determining which markers to use, for deciding which reagents to use, and for calculating how dense a map to make when attempting to genotype a particular chromosome. During the consortium meeting, some time was spent discussing which chromosome to map. Nora explained later that the next steps in such collaborations are complex and involve balancing the competing needs of individual researchers and their need to collaborate. For example, sometimes a collaborator's genotyping is fraught with errors, or in the case described earlier, is good genotyping but the markers used are outdated. Nora and her biostatistician colleagues have the unrewarding task of evaluating data sets for any number of common or idiosyncratic deficiencies. There are countless things that could go wrong, and it is usually not determined until the genotypic information can be tested to see if it conforms to the inheritance patterns expected of the data set. The work to create powerful data sets is a constant negotiation between individual interests and group interests. Nora's work illustrates how scientists and scientific practices occur across many institutional and social contexts, and thus researchers must routinely bring boundary objects such as categories of persons and genotypic patterns with them as a condition of collaboration.[16]

Scientists bring other things to the collaborative table. They bring their social relationships with other researchers and families, their competitive and other personality quirks, and, at least in one case, they bring an aversion to philosophy, as we shall see below. Before we assess the cultural significance of the narratives of power and noise in describing quality data, let us examine the ways the social and the ethnographic influence the dynamics of collaboration.

FRENCH DNA: ETHNOGRAPHIC NARRATIVES

The science of diabetes has inspired a series of critical philosophical interventions, the most famous of which is likely Canguilhem (1991 [1966]).[17] A more recent one warrants specific attention. In the early days of fieldwork, Gary initiated a discussion about Rabinow's book *French DNA*.[18] French DNA describes the moral and philosophical vexations of the use of biological material. It details the souring of a diabetes collaborative venture between Millennium Pharmaceuticals and the Centre d'Etude du Polymorphisme Humaine (CEPH). Rabinow proposes we look at science as a cultural construct that can be used to imagine something new or make sense of something old. Echoing decades of scholarly critiques of science, Rabinow argues that science must not be reduced to truth about nature. Blood in France, Rabinow explains, is a biosocial substance par excellence. The central story line is of the French reactions to their DNA being acquired by an American pharmaceuticals firm. Ownership and identity, in Rabinow's account, are revealed as constituent elements of blood samples in France.

For the first time, argues Rabinow, the materiality and sociality of blood ruptures the ethical imagination about the potential partnerships. The national scandal detailed in Rabinow's account illustrates how DNA acquired a French nationality. The tainted blood scandal of 1983-85, in which shortages of blood led to a system for prisoner donations and hence HIV contamination, was illustrative of how blood was imbued with nationalistic and altruistic value sets. French social scientists liked the idea of participation and belonging that donation enabled for prisoners. Prisoners liked the perks of donation (wine, food, time away from their cells, etc.), and the French government benefited by adding to its stock of blood supply. The issue, writes Rabinow, is that blood has a special status because it implies "the person who is the source and, in a more abstract manner, the representation that is made of humanity."[19]

As a key figure in the diabetes world, on par with Rabinow's informants, Gary was mostly interested in discussing the gossipy aspects of Rabinow's text. I had first heard of "Francois' book," as Gary liked to call it, when Gary promoted it from the podium at an ADA miniconference dedicated to the genetics of diabetes. Francois played a major part in Rabinow's multiactored account. Francois is a member of the consortium and was known by most of the conference attendees. Gary, Nora, and most of their collaborators attended. Researchers from Glaxo, Parke-Davis, and other pharmaceutical firms were present as well. There were scientists from land grant universities, the ADA, private research organizations, the NIH—including Francis Collins—and from several countries.[20] Gary's talk was on the story of the discovery of one of the diabetes genes, NIDDM1, and the most recent genetic findings that implicated a calcium protease, calpain-10. He joked with the audience and recommended they all get "Francois' book." It took me awhile to figure out that he meant *French DNA*, and I looked forward to eventually talking to him about it.

One day in the initial weeks of my visits to his lab, Gary beat me to the punch and asked what I thought of Rabinow's book. I was not ready to discuss it with him. In fact, I had not sorted out my own thoughts about it and was reluctant to have the conversation with Gary so early on in my fieldwork. I thought to myself, "Times have changed when informants have read and [as I was soon to find out] have criticisms of ethnographic work that at least provisionally claims to discuss the informants' lives."[21] I knew that Gary knew more about the topic than I did. What is more, Rabinow had not made the informant-collaborator-ethnographer cross-talk easy because of his robust engagement with French philosophy.

However, I was a visitor and an ethnographer. Thus, if Gary wanted to talk Rabinow, I was obligated to talk Rabinow. "He got the story fairly correct," Gary told me, "but all that philosophy shit really detracted from the book." Bracketing his pejoration, I acknowledged that for a reader like him the philosophical and historical arguments were not well articulated as part of the story of the power play between two central figures of the deal. I, of course, was more interested in Rabinow's cultural analysis as an explanatory device than whether or not it fit with the narrative. This fit issue, was, after all, what Gary was commenting on. He wanted to be entertained by the narrative. He was.

Some weeks later, I told Gary that I had e-mailed Prof. Rabinow to discuss my work. I was now ready to defend his use of philosophy and to use it as a way to further explicate my work in his lab. I wanted to make clear to Nora and Gary that I, too, would be doing more than writing an entertaining read. My work would have philosophical aspects as well.[22] Gary's custom was to launch into discussions with me at his whim. In one instance, he wanted to discuss Rabinow's *Making PCR*.[23] Gary did not really want to discuss the book but, rather, what Rabinow had not said about the personal life of one of the scientists. Gary is a friend of an ex-wife of one of Rabinow's informants, and hence I won't detail Gary's extremely partisan perspective. "'Smith' is a brilliant guy," he said. "He could anticipate the end, but couldn't do the day-to-day routine of seeing it through." Then, in his customary self-deprecating manner, Gary continued, "I must be the simple molecular biologist because my science is about routine, making sure it's perfect, each step, each experiment, over and over. I've got Nora, who's the smart one. I'm the dumb one. My job is to keep her happy."

This exchange illustrates Gary's simultaneous evocation of the rhetoric of objectivity and its perversion. On the one hand, Gary critiques Rabinow for attempting to situate the *French DNA* scientific story within a broader context of meaning (i.e., "philosophy shit"). On the other, when discussing *Making PCR*, Gary desires to fill out the ethnography with details of Rabinow's informants' personal lives. As a text,

Rabinow's *French DNA* is an actor in the diabetes enterprise that required me to account for its influence. I do not mean to overstate the case of this one book. Rather, I intend to situate it as an estranged familiar in my attempt to understand the collaboration within the diabetes enterprise. Gary's use of "Francois' book" brings to life the way science narratives, ethnographic or genetic, are multiply layered texts with personal, scientific, and philosophical registers.[24] Situating these registers into the knowledge produced by the enterprise is the task at hand.

THE BIG UNKNOWN: PHYSIOLOGY AT THE FUNCTIONALIST CROSSROADS

"Situated knowledges," argues Haraway, "require that the object of knowledge be pictured as an actor and agent, not as a screen or a ground or a resource, never finally as slave to the master that closes off the dialectic in his unique agency and his authorship of 'objective' knowledge."[25] We read above how an anthropological narrative sheds insight into the inner workings of the enterprise. There are, of course, dozens of narratives that influence knowledge production. Accounting for them all is not possible. However, for a condition such as type 2 diabetes, at this postgenomic moment, the objects of interest are the exact mechanisms that cause diabetes or, at minimum, the genetic contribution to a causal pathway.

On this score, Nora and Gary are appropriately modest. Their modesty expresses itself in several ways. Gary's self-deprecation serves to both bolster his alliance with Nora and to remind everyone that Gary does not need to posture. He is a powerful scientist who can afford to self-deprecate. Such are the "structured dispositions" of those endowed with immense social, cultural, and material capital. More than this, Nora and Gary are both uncomfortable with the human genome hype. As Nora noted after Collins's talk at the mini–genetics conference, "You know, I'm certain that we'll all look back at what we are doing today and see that it is sloppy, crude work. But it is the best we can do for now." Nora and Gary both reiterate the modesty of their contribution to understanding diabetes at every opportunity. "The really hard work has yet to be done," remarks Nora to me in our first meeting. This is a refrain that Gary also frequently deploys. Both she and Gary speak of the research that comes after the genetics work has been done, after the susceptibility genes have been identified. They refer to the work to characterize the triggers, pathways, and other physiological mechanisms of diabetes. They speak of physiology.

Nora's and Gary's genetic epidemiological research effectively redirects the research efforts from statistical susceptibilities derived from genetic analyses to the effects of calpain-10 at the cellular level. Diabetes physiology is most frequently described as a condition affecting processes of blood sugar regulation that involves insulin secretion and insulin reception by muscle and fat tissue. Within the accounts of the physiology of diabetes, which is an outgrowth of the genetic epidemiological guidance offered by Nora, Gary, and colleagues, we read of several shifts in scale.

The physiology of diabetes is a world inside of a world. It is imbued with a taxonomic polyglot and a complex interactive function for each actor. To explain this bioscape requires the narrator to mediate from community to the universal body, to specific body (phenotype in genomic parlance), to genetic signs of physiologic possibility expressed as statistically derived susceptibilities, to an enzyme (calpain-10) interacting with an uncertain series of endocrinological processes.[26] To represent this world requires the creation of models that mediate between extracellular and intracellular systems "conveniently characterized as *in vivo*, *in situ*, or *in vitro*."[27] I would add to this *in silico* to reflect the ways Sun County lifeworlds are powerfully reduced to data sets transmitted via e-mail and run through countless software programs. This form of symbolic abstraction of Sun County DNA donors extracts the meaning of diabetes from those most affected by it. As Emily Martin writes, "In the change of scale, something very minute, discovered by science, comes to play a deciding role in human questions or concerns that are very large."[28] Let us further examine the narratives of physiology for the consequences of such shifts in scale in diabetes science.

A most recent turn of research into diabetes has been the quantification of genetic codes for the purposes of locating susceptibility markers that might guide physiological research. But genetics is before physiology, or rather genetics informs physiology by pointing to an ever finer biological mechanism that may underlie the phenotype, the measurable manifestation of glucose metabolic impairment. Physiology is the study of basic biological processes and functions. The physiological research spawned by the work of Nora and Gary, as well as most other physiological characterizations, are functional. There are dozens of molecules, substrates, elements, tissues, genes, and hormones that interact. Research papers on diabetes slice these actors into different pieces, isolate, experiment, measure, and test. They use specific cell types, such as pancreatic islet cells, skeletal muscle, or adipose tissue, or tissues of various species, in this case various mouse and rat models.[29]

The polygene discovery pointed to a gene that codes for an enzyme, calpain-10. Calpains are a common cytosine protease (calcium-activated neutral proteases) expressed everywhere in the body. Researchers are unsure what calpains do. A year after the polygene paper, Gary handed me two unpublished manuscripts from his collaborators. He had tipped them off about calpain-10 when the polygene results were quite preliminary. His colleagues had busied themselves in preparing publications about calpains. In the manuscripts, the researchers hypothesized that calpain regulates insulin secretion by modulating the movement of insulin secretory granules through the plasma membrane in the beta cell. In other words, when calpain-10 was inhibited, beta cell membranes released less or more insulin depending upon the duration of exposure to the inhibitor. The modulated amount of insulin made available by the beta cell is further affected by the hypothesized caplain-10 function on glucose uptake in muscle and fat tissue. Researchers found that in the presence of the calpain-10 inhibitor, muscle and fat tissue had impaired glucose metabolic responses, narrated as glucose utilization and oxidation. They hypothesized that impairment in the signaling pathway, a message system to the cells to use or break down glucose, occurred as a result of the inhibitor-induced reduction of calpain-10 action. What interests us here is not the truth claims of these hypotheses. Rather it is the metaphor of impairment and error.

The physiological narratives of impairment or error have a long history within diabetes science. In *The Normal and the Pathological*, Canguilhem scrutinizes the philosophy of error inherent in biological life sciences. Deconstructing the physiological science of diabetes from the nineteenth century, he exposes the philosophical roots of the normal and pathological. What were once quantitative measures in excess of normal physiological functions have now found expression in finer and finer understanding of what those measures would examine. Canguilhem argues that the model of pathology has shifted from that which is different from the norm to that which is erroneous. Canguilhem traces the origins of the concept of pathology from early French physiology, in which pathology was but a quantitative deviation from a norm. However, the norm is in fact elusive. The final analysis is that "normal" is a context-bound condition that changes according to a dynamic between the environment and the organism. Disease, he concludes, is really just another way of living.

Canguilhem orients the present discussion toward a critique of the pathology narratives of diabetes. If we do not take for granted the narratives of "normal and pathological" metabolism and endocrinological function, we are permitted to disassemble the layers of cultural meanings that surround the condition referred to as diabetes. We are enabled, for example, to interrogate the narratives of diabetes physiology and the practices of knowledge production that generate them. Of Canguilhem's method, his student Michel Foucault expresses an epistemological modesty applicable to both subject and objects of inquiry. He writes:

> The history of science can consist in what it has that is specific only by taking into account the epistemological point of view between the pure historian and the scientist himself, this point of view is that which causes a "hidden, ordered progression" to appear through different episodes of scientific knowledge: this means that the process of elimination and selection of statements, theories, objects are made at each instant in terms of a certain norm; and this norm cannot be identified with a theoretical structure or an actual paradigm because today's scientific truth is itself only an episode of it—let us say provisional at most.[30]

In this light, the epistemological juxtapositions that follow are provisional representations of diabetes. They are meant to explicitly illustrate a moment, an episode of knowledge production, within a sociocultural context. To reiterate what has been stated elsewhere, the project of epistemological critique is not to achieve a superior understanding per se as much as to practice playing "other cultural realities off our own in order to gain a more adequate knowledge of them all."[31] This analytical strategy enables a kind of conceptual agility through which multiply assembled concepts can be used to explain diabetes knowledge production.

NARRATIVES AND REPRESENTATIONS: METAPHORS AND MEANINGS

The Mendelian gold rush of single-gene phenomena is over, and an infinitely more complex research proposition has emerged. In the parlance of the diabetes enterprise, diabetes is referred to as a complex disease because to understand it biologically will require sets of tools and analytical strategies that must also manage the environmental triggers while searching for genetic ones. The complexity cannot be overstated. The trajectory of structure-functionalism in biological sciences appears in the history of the milestones of diabetes science where hormonal mechanisms lead to cellular functions, which lead to genetic localizations, which lead back to proteins and cells. Table 2 shows how physiologists first isolated the hormonal mechanisms responsible for glucose regulation (insulin), then moved to the cells that produce insulin followed by

TABLE 2   MILESTONES IN DIABETES RESEARCH

1877—Claude Bernard's *Lectures on Diabetes and Animal Glycogenesis* details his
  physiological postulates that diabetes' symptoms are but variations on normal
  physiological states (in Canguilhem 1991: 68).
1920—Banting and Best isolate islands of Langerhans in the pancreas.
1921—Discovery that pancreatic extracts lower blood sugar. Insulin is discovered.
1962—Neel's "thrifty gene" hypothesis
1971—Insulin receptor defined
1972—Beginning of recombinant DNA era
1975—Links between HLA and diabetes susceptibility proposed
1977—Insulin gene cloned
1985—Method for amplifying DNA, polymerase chain reaction (PCR) developed
1991—Maturity onset diabetes of the young (MODY) 1 mapped
1996—MODY 2 and 3 genetically mapped
1999—Non-insulin-dependent diabetes mellitus (NIDDM) 1 and NIDDM 2 genetics
2000—Polygene discovery

SOURCES: Dr. Morris White, Lily Lecture, ADA meetings in 1999; Canguilhem 1991 [1966]; Feudtner
2003.

the current search for the genetic material responsible for a diabetic
phenotype.[32] Genetics researchers expend years of energy and capital
just to give molecular biologists a specific physiological target, the function of which, in turn, requires years of energy and capital to figure out.
Researchers remark that each element of this complicated set of factors
contributes a small portion of the risk for the disease. Postdocs often la-
ment the complexity of their task after Gary and Nora poke holes in
their research presentations at lab meetings and journal clubs. Citing
both Wes Craven's popular *Nightmare on Elm Street* and James Neel's
(1976) *Diabetes Mellitus—A Geneticist's Nightmare*, several postdocs
after a lab meeting exclaimed, "The nightmare continues."

The nightmare is made of metaphors that have yet to be made material. Leys Stepan and Jordinova argue separately that science is built
on metaphors and analogies that mediate between representations of
nature.[33] A metaphor evokes association, writes Leys Stepan, and "per-
mits us to see similarities that that metaphor itself helps constitute."[34]
But these are representations of the natural world, not direct and mir-
roring descriptions, argues Jordinova. Their power lies in the ability
to convey complex ideas to different constituencies in ways that rhe-
torically conflates representation with description. In situations where
the natural and the cultural are still being contested, as in Gary's

postdoctoral research projects, nightmares are appropriate representations of the uncertainties of diabetes knowledge.

In a similar way, Haraway argues that between 1920 and 1940,
functionalism and systems theories finally achieved a legitimacy that
supported the autonomy of the social sciences in universities.[35] It was
the period of the birth of social engineering, in which the science of society was used to speak of the rational management of populations. At
the same time, primatology and animal sociology deployed experimental techniques upon (against) populations of animals through which
conclusions about the human social order were produced. The conclusions drawn were that the "true social order must rest on a balance of
dominance, interpreted as the foundation for cooperation."[36] Emily
Martin likewise illustrates how metaphors of war and flexible late capitalist production influenced the field of immunology.[37] Researchers and
the public alike came to view immunity as a series of pitched battles
against enemy intruders such as microbes and viruses that were imminently flexible in their offensive and defensive maneuvers.

Haraway, Leys Stepan, Jordinova, and Martin illustrate the way
meanings reflect and emerge from the metaphors and analogies used to
describe the objects of scientific inquiry.[38] Far from sociologically neutral, the cultural work of scientific mediation[39] calls our attention to the
relationship between scientific ideas and approaches and the context of
their development. The case of diabetes science is no exception.

At its core, insulin and blood glucose are the central metaphors for explaining the pathological condition called type 2 diabetes. As one National Institutes of Health Web site reads, "Type 2 diabetes is a condition
characterized by high *blood glucose levels* caused by either a lack of *insulin* or the body's inability to use insulin efficiently."[40] What interests us
here is the persistent metaphor of biological functionalism used to explain
diabetes, a metaphor that remains unchallenged even amid uncertainty.

The history of biological sciences is often narrated as biologists' attempts to "peel back successive layers of organization to ultimately reveal the molecular interactions that take place within the living cell."[41]
Traditionally, physical structures were depicted in relation to their function within the system (e.g., heart to circulation). By the 1830s this
structure-functionalism had moved into the microscopic. Things too
small to be observed by the naked eye were proposed as the basic units
of physical structures. Organs were composed of cells, and cells were
composed of even smaller functional parts. In the 1930s, when Pauling's
atomic models for molecular chemistry were put forth, the structure-

functionalism moved precipitously into the molecular realm. For genetics, the functional terrain was that of heredity, which moved from Darwin's populations to Mendelian trait theories, to chromosomal action, to biochemical and DNA interactions, and then to molecular structure.[42] While certainly not a linear process, as the present case will illustrate, the developments moved from smaller to smaller apace with the technological capacity to "see" into the deepest and presumed most basic forces behind the physiological world.

Consortium members' scrutiny of the data sets, protocols, and markers still leave intact the presumption that failures of biological processes are responsible for diabetes. That is, the failure to produce or use insulin, currently narrated as genetic regulation and receptor function, respectively, are blamed.

The metaphors of resistance to a regulating force which results in an excess of energy is a trope of modern governance par excellence. As Jordinova illustrates, the social imaginary is tapped into by scientists as a kind of shorthand explanation.[43] In a process she terms "mediation," Jordinova demonstrates how, through the use of language and semiotically open representations of nature, the historical specificity of a scientific truth claim can be assessed.[44] That is, there is a dialectical relationship between the world and accounts of it that explains the ways science and culture are coproduced. For diabetes, it is worth noting that the key physiological processes responsible for diabetes are reduced to a biochemical interaction between two molecules: glucose and insulin. Glucose is a basic sugar and is most often narrated as the body's source of energy, while insulin is described as the trigger or regulator of the body's use of glucose. Additionally, diabetes and obesity are linked in as yet unknown mechanisms, but an excess of fat is thought to contribute to "insulin resistance" through an immune inflammatory response.[45] Thus, the key metaphors of diabetic pathology describe the failures in the body's use of energy.

Reminiscent of Martin's analysis of war and labor metaphors in immunology in the 1980s through 1990s, diabetes metaphors of resistance and energy use evoke the economic transformation from production to (over)consumption in particular, but not exclusively, related to the economies of sugar.[46] In the narratives of diabetes, the pathology occurs because the body resists the regulation of its source of energy. The metaphor of resistance mediates a condition similar to unruly workers or colonial subjects resisting the disciplining power of manual labor or external rule, respectively. While major labor and independence movements predate the metaphors of insulin resistance, it coincides precisely with the consumption-driven market logics of neoliberalism circa 1980 and forward. Too much glucose, after all, is predominantly delivered via the overconsumption of food relative to caloric need. Thus, the pathology occurs when the body resists the power (energy) derived from overconsumption in both the literal (ingestion) and the economic (buying power) senses. In this metaphoric narrative, consumption is the energy behind privatization, capital market liberalization, and social reforms—the key ingredients of neoliberalism.[47] Insulin resistance thus might better be understood as the embodied expression of the contradictions of these market logics. The former is the overconsumption of harmful and substandard foods that have resulted in premature death from obesity and related illness. Of course the two forms of consumption are related.[48]

Zooming in to the objects of scientific inquiry within the diabetes enterprise reveals a search for the functional mechanisms of glucose resistance: that is, functional activities at the level of molecular chemistry for which a "therapeutic agent" (read drug) may be developed. To the possibility of having a finding turn out to be useful in developing a drug, one genetics lab director said emphatically, "I wish! That would be great." Yet, what does the case of calpain-10 specifically tell us about our world? That it is complex and interactive. That the production, distribution, and consumption of insulin occurs through a concatenation of secretion, signaling, transport across boundaries, reception, and utilization of vital elements. Also, as in the dominant metaphor of controlling diabetes via constant glucose monitoring, the physiological mechanisms of control are also central to the functioning of the system of glucose regulation, cellular capacitance, and secretory potential.

Beyond the mechanistic functionalism of these key metaphors lies the making of data sets that are required for diabetes science.

For instance, within the diabetes enterprise, we read from the quantitative geneticist's presentation, that the power of research depends both upon the sheer volume of various research factors and with a reduction of noise in data sets. Noise is that which impairs the standardization of data. Power is data with the highest N (response rates, number of samples, individuals, likelihood scores). Noise is a term used to describe data sets that contain errors or are weaker than wished for variations within a sample of blood, a genotype, or results from a computer simulation. The more populations, the more DNA markers, the more SNPs, the more controls, the more randomization, and the least noise, the more powerful the data. Power, thus, in this light signifies a kind of mass efficient silence.

Taking a coproductionist tack on these biological and social narratives enables us to juxtapose the social context of the lives of DNA donors with the description of a good statistically "powerful" data set with "low noise."[49] I am also reminded of Thacker's insight that biomedia conditions embodied subjectivities through technology, as well as social, cultural, and political mediation.[50] Of the research subject whose data points appear in computer simulations, Thacker writes, "The body of the subject is therefore always scripted in part by scientific-medical modes of knowledge production."[51] In this light, a powerful and noise-free data set is at once large and quiet, silent and bulky, noiseless and numerous.

Haraway reminds us that the objects of scientific knowledge are intimately linked to their broader social worlds. She writes, "Accounts of such objects can seem to be either appropriations of a fixed and determined world reduced to resource for instrumentalist projects of destructive Western societies, or they can be seen as masks for interests, usually dominating interests."[52] Thus, if we travel back out of the microcellular, out into the world of "skin and bones," and apply the notions of expanding and silencing power, the critically social nature of diabetes research reiterates a familiar theme. In conversation after conversation, grant after grant, paper after paper, DNA donors are data points, objects of research, not actors. Participants are "schedules," "controls," or referred to by the title of the research grant, "a GR" for genetics of retinopathy and so on. As Carl relays the history of the research, "I looked for who carried the genes. Gary focused on the physical map of chromosome 15. We [geno]typed the larger population." A docile population that endures generations of social inequality, the ostensible effects of the excesses of capitalist expansion, is required for diabetes knowledge but only as a silent mass.[53] Like the shift between cyberspace and bricks and mortar,[54] the political implications of the assemblage of subcellular research complexity with the conditions of life for DNA donors cannot be sundered. In other words, biopolitics[55] and diabetes science are hand in glove.

CONCLUSION

In this postgenomic era, the collaborative practices of diabetes scientists represent scientific knowledge production writ large. Trans- and interdisciplinarity is now de rigueur for the sciences funded by the NIH.[56]

Collaborative practices hold the potential to transgress the dualism of mind-body, human-machine, and good-bad. Ethnographically unpacking technoscientifically infused social practices is both a method and theoretical orientation. It is also an expression of the consequences intended for this project. It orients the reader toward what is at stake in the research endeavor presented here. Haraway expresses what is at stake as follows:

> Taking responsibility for the social relations of science and technology means refusing an anti-science metaphysics, a demonology of technology, and also means embracing the skillful task of reconstructing the boundaries of daily life, in partial connections with others, in communication with all of our parts. It is not just that science and technology are possible means of great human satisfaction, as well as a matrix of complex dominations. Cyborg imagery can suggest a way out of the maze of dualisms in which we have explained our bodies and our tools to ourselves.[57]

I am less interested in the imagery of the cyborg than I am in Haraway's provocative suggestion that technoscientifically infused social relations can be both oppressive and liberatory. Hence, in spite of the critical intervention that as ethnographer-cum–cultural critic I hope to advance here, it would be a mistake to interpret this account as either a simplistic apology or as dismissive antidiabetes science. To be sure, the tensions between the legacies of racism and the humanistic impulses of implied or overt antiracism that appear in the diabetes scientific enterprise are not contrivances. They are constituents of the vexations of (1) diabetes science, (2) this ethnographic project, and (3) the society in which both were produced.

Finally, I have aimed to illustrate the ways that cross-disciplinary collaboration requires a kind of articulation work characterized by the regulation of data and which affirms a particular social order.[58] Articulation work is often an invisible facet of cooperative work and is concerned with managing contingency.[59] In Nora's illustrative case, articulation work manages the ontological frameworks that define diabetes as foremost gene based and thus an enterprise that requires rich and extensive data sets. Recall that the impaired metabolic interactions involved in diabetes are often narrated as insulin resistance. A person produces ample insulin but her body resists it. I am here interested in the proposition that insulin resistance may be a corporeal manifestation of a broader social or occasionally political resistance to the indignities of social inequality—a resistance that is metaphorically reflected as massive silent data sets. In this light, the metaphors of powerful data afford an explanation of diabetes science that cognitively and perhaps politically requires the silencing of the ever-expanding population of Mexicanas/os and other poor populations with elevated risk of diabetes in the United States and elsewhere.[60] To open the metaphorical frame more broadly, the mass silences required of good data and good border subjects fit the needs of market-driven solutions of consumer capitalism under neoliberalism. It is a situation in which markets (agribusiness, contraband, and fast food) are leading forces for consumption in a region where ownership (land, contraband) are freighted with human suffering. We ignore the links between the narratives of insulin resistance and the social context of lives affected by diabetes at the risk of trivializing both. To expound upon this proposition, let us turn now to the ways DNA data sets operate as a kind of currency within the networks of diabetes knowledge production.

CHAPTER 5

Recruiting Race

*The Commodification of Mexicana/o Bodies
from the U.S.-Mexico Border*

On the "Beldon Farms" in Northern California, the local chapter of the
American Diabetes Association staff and volunteers (one social scientist
included) conduct a free screening for diabetes among farmworkers.
Translating for the English-speaking monolingual public health nurse,
several of us would fill out a card for each employee that lists his or her
name, weight, age, sex, and time of last meal. The men and women
would line up to get their finger lanced and fill a tiny pipette with their
blood. The blood would then be transferred to a glucose meter that would
calculate sugar levels. While waiting for the results, workers were
screened by the Lion's Club volunteer ophthalmologist for retinal ab-
normalities. Of the hundred or so workers we screened that day, the
public health nurse referred two to a doctor.

Screening is an important element in diabetes surveillance. For type 2
diabetes, many of the effects of blood sugar abnormality are not de-
tected until retinopathy, angiopathy, or neuropathy has developed. Damage to the eyes, nerves, kidneys, and feet are the most common complications. Because diabetes can be stealthy, screening takes place around the
world as a preventative measure. Mr. Beldon had welcomed the volunteers, providing lunch and many expressions of gratitude. On this day he
donated $10,000 as a way to say thank you to the Lions and ADA.

The donation symbolizes that the health of his workers is important
to the landowner. Of course, anything that prevents laborers from missing work because of illness has the added benefit of making the harvest

go smoothly. Yet the exchange of screenings for money is emblematic of a larger set of technoscientific relations. Arguing that Mexicans have for more than a century endured the imposition of an identity as commodity, Vélez-Ibañez writes, "In a capitalistic economic system, things such as labor, materials, and processes can be bought and sold for a price, and conditions are created in which some populations may be regarded primarily as a type of price-associated group to be used and discarded not unlike disposable materials or any used manufactured goods."[1] To be sure, diabetes research practices conform to Vélez-Ibañez insight, but they are much more. Ethnographic evidence illustrates that as both subjects of state-corporate interpellation and as necessary actors in disease research, U.S. minority and immigrant DNA donors serve as a form of global human capital. However, they also are participants in their own biological commodification, and this requires closer analyses of both their participation and the processes of that commodification.

This chapter will deploy the theory-method intervention of following DNA samples and data sets through time and space to illustrate how the ethnicity of donor populations becomes a valuable commodity in the world of genetics research. Unlike Mr. Beldon's screening and donation in the fields of Northern California, no such benefactor exists in Sun County, and screenings are coupled with the taking of DNA samples. Further, as the samples are circulated to research partners in wet labs around the globe, their value to the careers of sample handlers grows.

It has already been shown that diabetes is framed as a racialized disease and that this reflects the unequal weight given to the incidence rates of diabetes at the expense of its prevalence. The consequences of this slippage must be understood as the first step in transforming the political and social conditions for Mexicanas/os in Sun County into attributes of the Mexicana/o body itself. Portrayals of epidemics such as AIDS, Black Death, or kuru, Lindenbaum notes, predictably create carriers who become scapegoats in the collective political and ritual actions that precede the eventual fading of the disease from our consciousness.[2] Diabetes, as a disease already framed by race and ethnicity, has additional implications in the era of genetic epidemiological research.

I argued in chapter 2 that the incidence of diabetes in the Mexicana/o populace must be viewed as strongly associated with the national political and economic transformations on the border over at least the last three decades—transformations that are a result of the mechanization of agricultural production, urban industrialism, corporate agribusiness, and the concomitant regimes of labor control.[3] Also noted earlier is the fact that Mexicanas/os are now used for a genetic research enterprise that is directed by Anglos funded by the state. This chapter explores the consequences of a scientific enterprise that fits the pattern of Anglo-Mexican relations in the U.S. Southwest over the past century and a half. The pattern is one of exploitation, in this case the unequal distribution of benefits accrued from the extraction and circulation of DNA from Sun County Mexicanos/as. To begin, let us turn to the various ways that racialized DNA samples operate as commodities within research transactions.

RACIALIZED PROPERTY

Samples are the raw material of the diabetes enterprise. Their possession, their collection, and their conversion to a data set for use in wet lab experiments and dry lab computational analyses operate within an economy of scientific knowledge production infused with Carl's humanistic ideals of finding a cure for future diabetics. Carl's sampling occurs as a result of a complicated relationship with his research participants. His care for the people is expressed in his protocols that require referral to a physician whenever necessary. He often hounds his staff to follow up with participant care issues. Yet the samples are not given freely. In exchange for their participation, people get a cotton tote bag, some pens, a monogrammed beverage cup, and a free ride to the field office and home again (which for about one-third of the participants means crossing the border). They receive food, some receive money, and those who need a referral to a doctor and diabetes education classes receive it. Participants get screened for diabetes and a host of other conditions determined by what research is funded at the time. For most, this screening is the only way they can keep track of their blood sugar. In Sun County, health insurance is a luxury few can afford.

For the consortium, Carl's field office is the initial moment in a long chain of research processes. The collection of Mexicana/o DNA samples forms the backbone of the collaborative exchanges for consortium scientists. However, DNA samples are not readily exchangeable. We saw in chapter 4 how blood samples are quickly converted into stable currency for laboratory research by field staff in the tiny lab with kitchen counters for bench space. At this stage in DNA processing, staff transform the samples into bits of purified protein placed in microcentrifuge tubes, which, if filled, hold 2.mL (about half a thimble) of material. In this form, the arrays of samples are placed in Styrofoam or plastic trays and arc labeled with various population identifiers, the name of the recipient and other data. Samples are divided up and shipped to collaborators around the country who then test and sequence the samples for a variety of diabetes-related experiments. The transformation from a wet lab material into a dry (computational) lab data set enables, with a few keystrokes, the global circulation of the genetic information derived from the DNA.

In their analyses of the ways scientific knowledge is standardized, Fujimura and Fortun observe that molecular biologists must convert their data into the language of genetic sequences "in order to cooperate and collaborate"[4] with scientists across disciplinary social worlds. Befitting this observation, the thousands of samples Carl has collected in the past three and a half decades have always traveled across social worlds. The present collaborative venture includes, among others, physicians in Mexico, epidemiologists in Texas, statisticians in Michigan, quantitative geneticists in Chicago, molecular biologists from Sweden, and postdocs and researchers in wet and dry labs from the NIH, academic, and corporate laboratories. It also includes Mexicana/os who participate through donations of blood and time.

I earlier described the ways Mexicanas/os are continually recruited for Carl's research. Most participants have done so for many years and thus do not need the reminder calls each staff member offers. However, at any given time, there are as many as four different research projects taking place. To accommodate work schedules, participants begin arriving at 7 A.M. and are seen into the evening and on weekends. Each research protocol requires its own set of measurements and attendant forms. For a diabetes and blood pressure study, there are 20 pages of forms that staff are required to fill out. Enrollment data, health history, medications, doctors, one form called Sun Female Form, a physical activity and lifestyle form, family history, blood pressure, and laboratory test forms are part of the packet. Judi and her staff spend hours on each participant. Their days are spent making appointments, arranging transportation, and in many cases driving to their homes or fields to collect follow-up blood samples or to bring the participant to the center for tests. The labor of collecting participants is a necessary part of the production of diabetes knowledge, as is the labor of participating in the research.

Contemporary research of late capitalist cultural transactions and power relations increasingly attend to the interaction of the material and semiotic, of the human and the nonhuman. Organs, networked devices, cell lines, data sets, prostheses, weapons, infectious agents, and drugs increasingly orient our analyses and research practices. Yet, mapping the ways the social and the material are co-configured begs reconceptualizations of the novel and persistently unequal distributive and consumptive networks through which material matters are produced. The present chapter assesses the ways that blood samples taken from racially marked populations operate within a regime of value production and are transformed into commodities.

The mix of voluntary donation, of humanistic disease prevention, and of material exchanges within the diabetes enterprise affords an opportunity to retheorize the manner in which value is produced. In this instance, value refers less to the ethicomoral questions of the donation encounter and more to the material, symbolic, and social capital that are bundled into the exchanges of donated DNA.[5] To examine this process requires that we follow the life history of a sample from its original donation into wet lab collaborative networks and out into the broader context of the corporate uses of knowledge derived from research partnerships. Following Clarke's and Fujimura's attention to the objects of scientific research directs my own thinking to what the materials (blood samples) within the diabetes enterprise reveal.[6]

In his analysis of the circulation of indigenous art forms in Mexico, Garcia Canclini points out that the meanings of an object as it moves between producer, consumer, and broker make tracing the social course of an object ideal for understanding "the manner in which capitalist development redefines identity as it combines various forms of production and representation."[7] This process is made all the more visible when the objects at hand are racialized population DNA samples, the biography of which this chapter will detail.

Discussion of the extraction of biological samples from vulnerable populations attained new visibility with the debates about the treatment of the Yanomami peoples. Thrust into the academic headlines by journalist Patrick Tierney's account of blood sampling by James Neel and his colleagues for genetics-based research, the discussions were inflammatory, heated, and politicized.[8] Among the issues that surfaced in the debates and formal investigations was that of the ethics of sampling for genetics research. Within the American Anthropological Association's formal report was the finding that Neel's team followed the new informed consent and ethical guidelines in place in 1968, the year the samples were acquired. However, members of the Yanomami people reported that "they (or their parents) had assumed that they would receive short-term health benefits from having their blood drawn in 1968."[9] In another case, the Havasupai people of Arizona prevailed in legal action against Arizona State University for using blood samples in ways not officially approved or without individual consent.[10] These debates and lawsuits highlight that the donation of biological samples is fraught with concerns about exploitation, most notably that informed consent and an equitable exchange occur between donor and recipient.[11]

Andrews and Nelkin survey the disturbing ways the body has been and continues to be configured as a commodity.[12] This oftentimes results in immense profitability for some and great distress or even harm for others. Whether it is the now famous case of *Moore v. Regents of University of California*,[13] genetic tests for rare diseases made unaffordable by patent royalties, forced forensic sampling, or organ snatching, the common theme is one of a profit made from the bodies of vulnerable or incognizant donors. Andrews and Nelkin highlight the political, ethical, and legal vexations of a science too closely wedded to commerce. They write, "The body has become commodified, reduced to an object not a person."[14]

In their analysis of a new materialism for an anthropology of the body, Lock and Farquhar remind that the discrete, structured, individual body mythologized by European modernity inaccurately portrays the social multiplicity of bodily life.[15] Further, drawing our attention to post-Cartesian materialism, they note that in scholarly and practical life, human experience must be imaginable as "at once subjective and objective, carnal and conscious, observable and legible."[16] Earlier analyses of the body include the social, experiential, and political body; the production of bioengineered tissues; the trade in organs for donation; and, what concerns us here, the interrelations between the body and political economy for which Paul Farmer's structural violence is a notable founding concept.[17] With special attention to the materiality of the body, we might ask; What can be learned when the objectification of racialized bodies evoked by Andrews and Nelkin, but not fully explained, is fleshed out ethnographically?

THE LIFE HISTORY OF A RACIALIZED BLOOD SAMPLE

One morning, Lena draws blood from Jaime, a farmworker, in the backseat of the minivan. The crews are weeding the peppers at dawn. We had stopped to get Jaime some tacos to break his fast, and the smell of chorizo filled the van on our drive along nameless dirt roads that abut the Rio Grande. Five vials are drawn; three are placed in the portable centrifuge, the rest on ice in a cooler. Before week's end, the vials of whole blood or buffy will be labeled, added to a shipping container, placed on dry ice, and shipped to awaiting lab techs. "Mex/Am" reads the label on the Styrofoam shipping cube containing Jaime's sample.

Like clockwork, samples are processed according to protocol. At Gary's lab, techs handle everything but genotyping and analyses. Postdocs take over once the samples are ready to run through the sequencer. Once sequenced, Nora's team takes over converting the genotypic data into data sets that she sends to collaborators or compares with genotypes developed by collaborators in England, Japan, Utah, or Massachusetts. Jaime is now a subject number on a data set with other "Mex/Ams," although now ethnicity might be coded by numbers like those that identify the researchers who collected the data, a specific study, or eventual storage catalogue number.

By examining the life history of a sample in the diabetes collaborative research enterprise, I am adapting Kopytoff's cultural biographical approach to the process of DNA commodification.[18] Kopytoff advances the notion that a thing's biography, the shifting meanings it carries through time and space, reflects the broader social structure and cultural values of its origins. He argues that the shift in a thing's status—as a commodity to one person at one time and not a commodity at another time—reveals a "moral economy that stands behind the visible economy of visible transactions."[19] By tracing the biography of DNA, the nonhuman actors[20] in the diabetes gene research enterprise, the symbolic and material value of a sample emerges. The production of value, as revealed in the exchange situations, troubles the bipolar rhetoric of persons versus property and offers ethnographic insight into the value generated within scientific practices. In this section, I will begin with a review of diabetes and DNA sampling. Then I will discuss the ways biological samples from racialized populations are transformed into materially and semiotically valuable objects within various corporate, academic, and state-funded collaborative research transactions.

The DNA collection process is so central to genetics research and pharmaceutical developments that the *Wall Street Journal* featured it on the front of its business section. The article describes the collection of DNA in rural Texas and was written by a staff reporter assigned to developments in the pharmaceutical industry. While no drugs are mentioned, the human-interest coverage speaks volumes as to entanglements of the industry's financial and social interests. Webster's definition of a commodity, "Something useful or capable of yielding commercial or other advantage," illustrates the wholesale fetishization of things exchanged for other things. For to say that a thing is "capable" is to impute agency to an inanimate object. Such a definition denies the human role in the process of commoditization. It thus ascribes, as Marx said, "a social relation between objects, a relation which exists apart from and outside the producers."[21] Unfortunately, such a fetishized definition also permeates discussions of biopiracy, bioprospecting, and critiques of patent case law and benefit sharing. The present analysis seeks to unpack the practices of DNA acquisition and exchange by suggesting a more anthropologically robust definition of a commodity: an object in which a social, cultural, and material investment is made with the expectation of a return on that investment.[22] This definition seeks to highlight rather than take for granted the social requirements for and of commodification and thus prevent the objectification of bodies and the fetishization of DNA.

Appadurai (1986) argues that "a commodity is not one kind of thing but one phase in the life of some things."[23] Further, he avers that politics, the social relationships that control the flow and desirability of a thing, "is what links value and exchange in the social life of commodities."[24] I have thus far briefly sketched the political and historical context of Carl's sampling along the U.S.-Mexico border, that is, the politics of the initiatory exchange of DNA. I now turn to the symbolic and material regimes of value generated in the next stages in the life history of blood samples.

MATERIAL, SYMBOLIC, AND CULTURAL CAPITAL

Carl's NIH biographical sketch reveals that his career has been enriched by his U.S.-Mexico border samples. Ninety-five percent of his publications and all of Carl's research grants are based upon his collection, exchange, and analyses of "Mexican American" samples. Additionally, Carl's research has been funded by grants from the state of Texas, the American Diabetes Association, and the NIH. His annual budget for the period I reviewed exceeds $1 million. Commenting on his current budgets Carl remarked, "I've got more money than I can use right now." I witnessed Carl practically begging his field office staff to spend money to replace equipment. "It costs you nothing to replace the global positioning system and blood pressure units," he would scold his all

Mexicana staff, for whom doing without was easier and more familiar than the luxury of buying something new.

Samples are part of a material and symbolic economy that profoundly shapes and is shaped by a researcher's relationship to the diabetes enterprise. Carl ships his samples to collaborators who are part of numerous research grants in Carl's portfolio. In fact, the geographic distribution of DNA samples maps perfectly onto the collaborative partnerships indicated on various research grants. These grants form a complicated web of state, corporate, and privately funded research enterprises that require the collection, storage, exchange, and sale of DNA samples. Carl is not alone. Many researchers profit by providing DNA samples to others in exchange for being credited as a coauthor of an article.

A postdoctoral fellow in Gary's lab recounted a story about the leveraging of samples for her career advancement, which will illustrate the point I am making. Pilar, a postdoc who is from Mexico, called Gary, by then a renowned diabetes geneticist, in search of a job in the United States. Gary called her the next day inviting her to his lab. Pilar said that she motivated Gary to accept her as a postdoc because of her rare Zapotec samples. Pilar recounted that she had heard rumors of a doctor who was doing work with Zapotec peoples. She tried unsuccessfully to contact him and decided to just go to Oaxaca, a region in south-central Mexico where she had heard he was working. She found him and, after some negotiating, was able to collect 23 samples of his (note the possessive pronoun) diabetic patients. Of the potential for collecting more samples in Mexico for genetics research, Pilar said emphatically, "Mexico es una riqueza" [Mexico is a treasure].[25] However, after some time conducting her postdoctoral research, Pilar needed some additional samples to use as controls. Pilar and the doctor were in conflict, she reported. A combination of Mexican medical establishment red tape and Pilar's assertiveness in accessing the population had caused a strain in their relationship. As a consequence, she could not access "her" samples, "mis muestras." The doctor was resistant to forwarding them to her, Pilar explained, but warmed up to the idea when she informed him that by providing the samples he would get published in *Nature Genetics*. While "Pilar's" 23 samples were used in a groundbreaking publication, no nondiabetic Zapotec samples were used, and the doctor was not listed as a coauthor. Pilar, however, was a coauthor.

Carl's and Pilar's sampling practices are emblematic of the ways DNA and the data generated from it are exchanged for other forms of professional wealth. The polyvalence of biological samples is exemplary of the confluence of economic and symbolic capital in the sense espoused by Bourdieu by virtue of their translatability from one into the other and back again in a perpetual life cycle of circulation and value accumulation.[26]

"Exchange," concludes Appadurai, is not "a by-product of the mutual valuation of objects, but its source."[27] Many significant exchanges occur with DNA samples after Carl or Pilar have acquired them. As Marx (and Appadurai) reminds us, value is the result of the amount of labor necessary to produce the commodity.[28] Thus acquiring samples and bringing them to market are part of the labor required for their exchangeability. However, as the case of racialized diabetes DNA samples illustrates, both the political conditions of acquisition and the labor required for their production, acquisition, and exchange are concealed in the value they are given during their circulatory life history. Hence, a sample's value is taken for granted. That is, the physical labor required to produce Mexicana/o DNA blood samples is concealed within the requisite transactions of scientific collaboration and career advancement. After all, Judi and her staff are not listed as coauthors on Carl's publications, yet their labor is certainly required.[29]

Additionally, the meanings assigned to DNA do not reflect the social relations that made the donation possible in the first place. For example, blood samples circulate with only the ethnic taxon as a semiotic reference, "Mexican American." Carl's staff collects and processes samples for shipping according to weekly quotas. A shipment of samples is a sign of productivity. The deadline and quota are mere motivators against Carl's ever-feared heightened scrutiny of the sampling operation.

Once at the wet lab, it takes ethnographic prodding to elicit the story of samples. Pilar's story would not have been revealed had I not queried her. Additionally, one German physician, Klaus, painstakingly took two years collecting samples from his patients before coming to Gary's lab as a postdoc. Only after some months, when I asked him about the data set, did he tell me the hours-long details of collecting samples. Both Pilar's and Klaus's stories demonstrate that in spite of the unseen labor required to collect them, the story of the samples is one that those responsible for collection are more than eager to tell.

The standardization of the biovalues of DNA samples as occurs in their exchanges for an array of professional wealth illustrates how *exchange* is the source of the value of a sample: It is not, as the dominant commodification theorem implies, the result of some inherent or potential downstream worth of the DNA. Understanding this biovalue requires attention to the processes of its generation but also of its consequences. "The bodies and vitality of individual and collective subjects have long had a value that is as much economic as political—or, rather, that is both economic and political," write Nikolas Rose and Carlos Novas.[30] In other words, to hold that DNA is inherently valuable is to default to a supply-side economic formula that fetishizes—read de-labors—the material exchanged (Mexicana DNA) and the social processes at work that imbue the codified information-rich genetic texts with meaning as it becomes a data set or scientific publication.

The labor required to bring DNA to its point of exchange has not by any means been fully delineated here. Still it is worth asking: Whose labor is involved in the production of a biological sample *before* it is extracted from a body? What are the material conditions that confer a value upon this sample? The answers preliminarily lie in the political and social context of the exchange relationship noted earlier. Further, I suggest that the circulation of blood samples within the diabetes research enterprise troubles the oft-used supply-and-demand formulas of value creation for scientific knowledge.[31] The default to supply-side economics plays into the fetishized definition of commodification. The reductionistic parsing out of biological or technological processes with immediate exchange or downstream use values in this biocapitalist era is not novel.[32] Enclosure and ownership have always gone together. What is new about the creation of biovalue is that this is done while articulating different forms of meaning—for example, individuals and groups are, as Sunder Rajan puts it, "bundles of genetic variations that can be targeted, tested, monitored and changed in new ways,"[33] while structurally concealing that the biocapitalist enterprise writ large is working upon the meanings of "the biological" and life itself.

The work of biovalue creation and its appropriation requires both the materiality of biological samples and the data-rich information generated from it, although it is often thought that only the information is the important part of value creation.[34] However, as Franklin and Lock so accurately observed, it is the reproductive potential of the biological samples—that the cell can be converted to a cell line that can be sequenced or synthesized for further study and that a finding might affect subsequent generations—which gives biological materials the allure of something special.[35] Helmreich's classification of the concept of biocapital is useful here.[36] My use of biocapital and biovalue is equal measure formalist and substantivist. That is, I am interested in the logics of value creation, their meaning systems, as well as the ways such substances as DNA or blood samples operate within, through, and because of those logics. [37]

We read in chapter 3 about the disturbing purity and admixture discourse that exists amongst diabetes geneticists. The case of sampling along the border shows the complex social and political conditions that allow Mexicanas/os to be targeted for disease research. In this light, the Mexicana/o population's "race"—or bioethnicity, as I will discuss in the conclusion of this book—is itself a necessary part of the exchangeability of their samples. Put another way, without a history of conquest and dispossession, without the border as a zone of race wars, and most recently without the impoverishing conditions that have resulted from the permanent economic stagnation along the border, the extraction of DNA from Mexicanas/os would not likely exist because Mexicanas/os as a social formation would not exist in its current form. This is to say, the relational aspects of Mexicana/o history that have subjected border inhabitants to 150 years of racialized conquest and which, as was discussed in earlier chapters, must be implicated in diabetogenesis, would not exist.

I do not mean to infer that the mere existence of Mexicanas/os along the border caused them to be sampled. Rather, the argument is that each set of samples is acquired through a complicated set of social and political conditions that, for the most part, are rendered invisible once the sampling has occurred. These conditions include those that created the ethnic identity to begin with, the scientific rationale for sampling, the humanitarian justifications for sampling, and the local circumstances that make donors willing to participate in research practices. While all human groups are potential DNA donors, not every group has an equal chance of being targeted for genetics research.

TO MARKET, TO MARKET

Mexicanas/os are by no means the only racially targeted population for genetics research. Coriell, for example, contains a catalogue of numerous ethnically labeled sample sets for sale.[38] Recall from the introduction to this book that the abstracts from 1998, 1999, and 2000 American Diabetes Association's annual meetings showed that the different kinds of populations used jumped 15 percent, from 153 to 179 distinct ethnically labeled groups. Further, there was a 36 percent increase in the use of population-based data, with a 60 percent and 30 percent increase in such uses by geneticists and epidemiologists, respectively. The increase in ethnic labeling reflects an emergent trend in genetic science of complex diseases, in pharmacogenomics, and in forensics. Why is it that at the moment "race" is pronounced scientifically dead by many in the scientific community, researchers need population-based specificity to advance their research agendas?

One reason is that the use of populations reflects the race to join the human genome project. As Pilar's "ownership" of her Zapotec samples illustrates, a rare data set can gain an investigator access to the rights and privileges of publication, collaboration, and research. A reportable finding derived from an ethnically labeled group can thus attract further opportunities and possibly serve to validate or confirm the findings of other researchers. As Carl's field office indicates, DNA sampling is a capital-intensive enterprise for which some return on one's investment is expected. For example, several of the authors on the polygene paper hold a patent on the discovery. The patent for the polygene notes, "Using this method, the inventors show that the interaction of genes . . . makes a major contribution to susceptibility to type 2 *diabetes* in Mexican Americans from Sun County, Texas." The patent document is an exhaustive detail of every facet of the polygene discovery, including a myriad of wet and dry lab techniques and their potential application in the detection, selection, or alteration of a number of proteins and in the development of drugs.[39]

In this section, I will explore the ways that the use of population DNA is driven by the search for professional and other forms of profit. But more specifically, I will argue that DNA sampling along the U.S.-Mexico border is deeply infused with the acquisitive interests of the pharmaceutical industry. To be sure, pharmaceutical company representatives were present at consortium meetings. They were not special participants, however. They were involved in collaborations with Nora, took the lead on projects, and sponsored special meetings on current scientific topics, for example, the genetics of diabetes. Industry-sponsored research projects and its participation in collaborations of all kinds ensures their access to the latest research, if they choose their partners wisely.

More broadly, drug companies are abundantly represented in the diabetes literature, in patient cookbooks, and in pamphlets of all kinds. But nowhere are drug companies more visible than at the American Diabetes Association's meetings, which are the quintessential marketplace of diabetes knowledges and products. The industry's role is most interestingly manifest in the exhibit hall for these meetings. The "product theater" as it is called, comprises six thousand square feet oozing with products, promotional gimmickry, 3-D simulations, and ritual enactments, all designed to capture the largely physician market share for an array of products and services. At the meetings in 2000, 114 corporate exhibitors compete for conferees' attention. The 20 or so nonprofit exhibitors also vie for attention, but they are no match for the six-figure budgets of the biggest and brightest pushers in this surreal corporate technological "drugscape." Two-thirds of the hall is dedicated to the product theater, the other third to the poster panels. Exhibits are packed into this carefully planned space. The largest exhibits occupy approximately three hundred square feet each and are spaced so as to capture maximum visual and interactive contact. Logos bombard the hall. Lilly, Bayer, Pfizer, Bristol-Myers Squibb, Merck, Becktin-Dickinson, Novartis, and Glaxo all beckon a consumptive gaze and ultimately a prescription, subscription, or clinical adoption in physicians' practices. Smaller names abound. As the morning meetings of the drug and medical technologist representatives conclude, music fills the hall and, like the start of trading at the New York Stock Exchange, a voice—this one a woman's—announces the opening of the exhibitions over an omnipresent PA system.

The biggest attraction was the five-hundred-square-foot exhibit for Bristol-Myers Squibb's heavily promoted Glucophage. Set up to mimic ABC's 1999 game show sensation, *Who Wants to Be a Millionaire*, the exhibit was a showstopper. Designed like a roundabout, the set was an open-air studio at which contestants "win" prescription pads for answers to clinical trivia. True to its original British version, Regis Philbin had been replaced by a British actress who seamlessly managed the choreographed music, trademark heartbeat bass soundtrack and all, to the game show format. What was it about that exhibit that enabled it to attract both physicians and health educators to Glucophage in a venue organized by an association devoted to curing diabetes?

If Regis Philbin's prime-time ritual enacted for television audiences is the hyperreal simulation of the dot.com American dream,[40] that which stock portfolios soon demonstrated was a bubble soon burst, Bristol-Myers Squibb's "Millionaire" product theater is, in Beaudrillard's words, "an idealized transposition of a contradictory reality" par excellence.[41] For, if—as is the case—the stated objective of the American Diabetes Association is to end diabetes, and diabetes is a disease created by overconsumption, overproduction, overdevelopment, and excess upon excess, then the spectacle of the Glucophage product theater operated as a good simulacra must. It enacted the contradiction of disease through excess by celebrating the excess in a venue designed to eliminate the disease.

The disease no longer is the point, but rather the excess, the fantasy of getting rich quick, as the ultimate foil for social dis-ease.

But more than the playful juxtaposition of materialist recuperations inspired by Marx or the messier explication of the "rules of the game in the fields of racialized knowledge production" that Bourdieu's analyses enable, or even my rhetorical enactment of a simulacrum too salient to ignore, I mean to elaborate the relationship between the material and cultural forces at work within, upon, and constituent of the diabetes enterprise. The product theater, in which the Millionaire showpiece is only one of hundreds of displays, instantiates the blurring of natures and cultures occurring with increasing frequency in biomedical research writ large. A scientific conference is funded in part by its sponsors and the registration fees of the (captive) audience that stroll through the exhibit halls between scientific and other sessions. The audience are scientists and practitioners who likely accept the economies of conference finance and are unaware of the influence of product placement. The blurring of knowledge and capital accumulation can scarcely be more apparent than the product theater at the American Diabetes Association meetings.

By tracing the life history of DNA samples as they come to be valorized within the regime of scientific accumulation embedded in the shopping and swapping of DNA, I have tried to characterize a process that reiterates not only familiar forms of material exploitation but also unfamiliar mechanisms of sociopolitical and cultural meaning making.

The product theater can also be understood as an apparatus of biocapitalization that resocializes—denatures, so to speak—the bios in an effort to convert DNA into currency. Paradoxically, this requires both an erasure of the process of capitalization and the contingency of any knowledge claim derived with and through the population samples. And it is interesting that this conversion process also erases any ethnic specificity of diabetes: the drug works on all bodies, for all diabetics. Surely the drumbeat of tailored medicines now thrumming the corridors of disease enterprises writ large complicates this rhetoric.

Recall my working definition of a commodity, an object in which a social, cultural, and material investment is made with the expectation of a return on that investment. My point here is that racially marked DNA samples function, like all products of diabetes knowledge, as a kind of currency. It is a currency derived from bodies and fashioned to meet biomedical and economic ends. The value of samples and of the process of their commodification is derived in the social relations through which they are produced, exchanged, and consumed. For example, we have seen that samples are exchanged for rights, privileges, goods, and services. If a researcher has a set of samples, even a very few, they can apply for grants to conduct experiments upon them. Samples can be parlayed into a careerlong research program or into the keys to membership in cutting-edge research consortia. Samples can get a researcher's name in print and they can be stored, banked, processed, and sold. For example, the Sun County DNA samples can be purchased at Coriel for $50, the cell culture is $250.

CONCLUSION

In thinking about the social, economic, and political consequences of DNA sampling, it would be easy to argue at this point that the samples and all knowledge derived therefrom belonged to the donors. The chair of the European Ethics Committee of the Human Genome Organization, Bartha Knoppers, argues that patent policy initiatives must focus on the equitable material transfer agreements between donors and scientists.[42] But this would be acquiescence to the logic of possessive individualism often invoked in patent case law by suggesting that cells, organs, or tissue (and anything derived from them) were owned and could be exchanged—as if by magic—by one party or another depending upon their relationship to the biomaterial or its cognitive byproduct.

Further, in their critique of the ways biological samples are becoming like minerals, crops, and land referred to in the language of science as extracted, harvested, or procured, Andrews and Nelkin write, "Such language reflects a set of cultural assumptions about the body: that it can be understood in terms of its units, and that these units can be pulled from their context, isolated, and abstracted from real people who live in a particular time, at an actual location, in a given society."[43] Though these criticisms are important, they do not elucidate the process of value production that occurs long before patentability and in spite of any consent issues.[44]

The focus on profit taking or benefit sharing so removes the DNA samples from the conditions of their extraction and processing that no claim can be made for a benefit having occurred as a result of the acquisition and development of population samples in the first place. Thus, Andrews and Nelkin's and Knoppers's supply-side notions of valuation and critiques of unfair or nonexistent benefit sharing practices, while fundamentally important, misrecognize the social relations that make possible the production and circulation of DNA samples.[45] Inattention to the social context of sampling and the *social* life of a sample overlooks the regimes of value generated by its exchange. This reification plays directly into the interpellative power of the academic-industry-state enterprise to enlist research subjects and their ethnicity as global human capital. Instead, I follow Strathern's insight that one modality of making property out of bits of biological organism (animal or plant) requires the delinking of the product from its origins.[46] This enables the reassignment of ownership at each stage in the development of knowledge. This is not magic. It is the emergent form of property relations manifest in intellectual property rights discourses.

Blood samples, like all things, did not appear out of nowhere. They must be understood in a context, which, as Johannes Fabian reminds us must be relative to "individually and therefore historically situated practices."[47] The context of DNA sampling does, I think, help explain the process of creating value. That DNA from certain populations enables the cultural process of valuation is the point. Why Mexicana DNA? Why now? Why from South Texas? The question is not what makes DNA valorization possible, rather, what does the valorization of DNA produce?

These questions are both broader and narrower than arguing that donors have rights. Corinne Hayden's analysis of benefit sharing has carefully unpacked the problematics of this simplistic ethical claim.[48] Rather, this book argues that DNA sampling produces a form of epistemological biopolitics that traverses the palpably local conditions of DNA donation and the regimes of genetic knowledge production. The biovalue generated in this life science biocapitalistic enterprise is an instance of Sunder Rajan's biocapital par excellence.[49] This case illustrates the means through which, like other manifestations of the making of wealth within capitalism, acceptable levels of ethnic differences in morbidity and mortality of disease are reinforced rather than addressed. That this occurs under the guise of universal incontrovertible good of the human genome projects, of the concern for public health along the border, or in an event organized around preventing disease, demonstrates both the perduring processes of social stratification *and* the quotidian means through which the processes of the accrual of return on investment are manifest within the research enterprise.

CHAPTER 6

Bioethnic Conscription

In the 1960s and 1970s, scientists immortalized a unique line of cancerous cells from Henrietta Lacks.[1] The cell line was celebrated for its unique contributions to research but later became the source of great controversy when it became the presumed source of laboratory contamination. Landecker's account of the HELA (a name formed from the first two letters of the donor's names) cell line details how metaphors of miscegenation overtook this once-venerated cell line when the source of contamination was thought to be the polymorphous expression of an enzyme believed to occur only in people of African ancestry.[2] Human biologists, reports Landecker, confused race for population, even though the evidence of contamination would have been more conclusive without reference to racial difference.[3] The case of the HELA cell line poignantly depicts the ways "race" promotes the uptake of social worlds into biological ones. This chapter explores this process further through an assessment of the representations of race in scientific publications, in collaborative discussions between scientists, and in the ways ethnicity appears in pharmaceutical marketing materials.

In the preceding chapters, I explored the acquisition of DNA and examined the cultural consequences of DNA sampling when viewed in sociopolitical context. I assessed the collaborative practices through which diabetes knowledges are produced, and I evaluated the criticisms of the use of population-specific labels for their potential to reinscribe biological division between human groups. Having examined the *production* of diabetes knowledge, I am now in a position to revisit some of the issues raised earlier from the perspective of the consumption of diabetes knowledge.

"Consumption," writes Bourdieu, is "a stage in a process of communication, that is, an act of deciphering, decoding, which presupposes practical or explicit mastery of a cipher or code."[4] Bourdieu argues that "reading" art, for example, is an act that requires a level of cultural competence born of specific social location. In the quote above, Bourdieu referenced works of art as the objects in need of deciphering. This chapter explores scientific representations of diabetes knowledge as artifacts that, like art, can be subject to cultural analyses. Keeping focused upon the key polygene "discovery" and then on to the corporate representations of diabetes will shed new light on the consequences of the use of racialized DNA.

As a complex disease, type 2 diabetes is, according to Nora, "the poster child for gene-environment interaction" because its putative risks lie in both environmental and biological domains. Further, a researcher at the American Diabetes Association remarked that, "environmental triggers could lead to the precise mechanisms [for diabetes] as genetic triggers could."[5] The dichotomy of genes and environment will serve as a narrative device throughout this chapter to make visible the geneticization of disease and the configurations of Mexicana/o ethnicity that appear in diabetes knowledge production. To decipher the biologisms in diabetes knowledge products, I will adapt Bourdieu's analysis of consumption, his "social critique of the judgment of taste," to explain the ways representations of race and ethnicity reflect broader social relations.

Specifically, in this chapter I will advance the concept of bioethnic conscription as the process whereby ethnicity comes to be constructed as meaningful for scientific research. By examining how concepts of race and ethnicity appear: (1) in genetics research (2) in the process of scientific publication and (3) in the marketing of pharmaceutical products, the ideological fault-lines between genes/environment, biology/society and race/ethnicity are revealed. The case of diabetes challenges the anthropological distinctions between race and ethnicity, complicates the characterizations of race/(R)ace in science, and shows how the social and political context of ethnic identity is variably expressed at each stage of biomedical research and development. From this vantage point, diabetes science becomes intelligible as an instance of a racially inflected project[6] that sustains social inequalities through the circulation of racialized genetic material and through the representations of ethnic populations as disease prone.

Recall that diabetes is a complex of diseases characterized by elevated blood glucose triggered by a combination of poor insulin production, insulin resistance in skeletal muscle and lipid tissue or both. Recall also that geneticists, epidemiologists, government analysts, and journalists also frame diabetes as an ethnoracial disease and cite a well-worn set of references that confirm the unequal burden of the disease on certain ethnic groups. We will begin by reviewing the origins of the notion of genetic susceptibility to diabetes in ethnic groups and compare them with the environmental causation narratives for health disparities between ethnic groups. The epistemological comparison between genes and environments will be useful in the interpretation of various representations of race and ethnicity in diabetes knowledge.

EPIDEMIOLOGY OF RACE: GENES AND ENVIRONMENTS

In chapter 2, it was shown that diabetes is represented as a public health epidemic in the popular press. Recall the *Newsweek* (2000) story that describes Sra. Benitez as a "representative victim" of diabetes. But what does Sra. Benitez represent really? Demographically, if we use population estimates to figure the total number of diabetics by ethnic group as defined by U.S. Census Bureau, 6–8 percent of the U.S. white population is 18 million people. Suspending for a moment the plus 4 million variance this figure has with the CDC estimates of all diabetics, 18 million white diabetics is four times greater than all African American diabetics, three times greater than all Hispanic diabetics of any ethnicity, and 37 times greater than the estimates of American Indians and Alaskan Native diabetics.[7] Or, put another way, by reconciling the epidemiological and census ledgers, there are 1.6 times as many white diabetics as African American, Hispanic, and Native American diabetics combined. The representation of diabetes as a racialized disease reflects the unequal weight given to the prevalence rates of diabetes at the expense of its incidence. This representational slippage is emblematic of a series of practices, examined below, that configure people of color as diabetes prone. The CDC and the World Health Organization report that diabetes affects different populations at varying rates. Yet the numbers merely describe the patterns of disease in various populations but do not explain them.

We have seen throughout this book that the presumption of genetic susceptibility is the backbone of the diabetes enterprise demonstrating that many have joined the sweepstakes characterized by Neel.[8] This explains why, in reporting on the polygene, one science reporter for the *LA Times* hailed the discovery as "strikingly consistent" with Neel's thrifty gene hypothesis.[9] Genetic explanations vie with environmental ones, however. In a critique of the thrifty gene hypothesis, McDermott shows how the conflation of genes and race within this paradigm elides the consideration of the social determinants of the disease.[10] McDermott's conclusions warrant extended citation: "Diabetes in Aborigines has been defined, by non-Aboriginal scientists, simply as a problem of 'race' and 'genes' in a changing environment. Race becomes a biological entity and an independent risk factor, reified over and over again in repeated studies of disease which take no account of socioeconomic status, history or culture."[11]

Interrogating the thrifty gene hypothesis as a biological determinism, McDermott counters with evidence that intrauterine environments and nutritional factors in early infancy and childhood evince a U-shaped relationship between birth weight and diabetes. That is, both low and high birth weight are associated with the disease.[12] Hales and Barker propose a "thrifty phenotype" hypothesis of diabetes arguing that "poor nutrition in fetal and early infant life are detrimental to the development and function of the Beta cells,"[13] especially when coupled with childhood food deprivation and later caloric excesses. Though the specific causal mechanisms are still being investigated, the principles behind the fetal origins hypothesis, later life conditions, and health outcomes have proved to be robust.[14] Further, in an interdisciplinary review of the thrifty genotype hypothesis, Paradies, Montoya, and Fullerton demonstrate unequivocally that there is no evidence that the differential rates of diabetes across global populations are a result of a thrifty genotype.[15]

Such studies offer support to an extensive body of research that demonstrates the predictive effects of poverty, unequal access to health care, stress, discriminatory experiences, and social inequality for low birth weight, poor fetal and postnatal nutrition, and complex diseases such as heart disease, diabetes, and hypertension.[16] However, the differences between genetic and social epidemiology research epistemologies do not explain the process of racialization that occurs in genetics research into complex diseases.

The purpose of this chapter is not to offer an alternative causation hypothesis or to critique the epistemological shortcomings of genetics or epidemiology.[17] Rather, what concerns us here are the conditions that make possible the racialization of diabetes. The remainder of this discussion will thus describe instances of the use of race and ethnicity, will assess its social consequences, and will explain the ways scientific configurations of racialized groups reconstitute U.S. race relations.

FISSURES IN THE VEIL: SCIENTISTS ATTEMPT TO SITUATE DIABETES KNOWLEDGE

It is tempting to dismiss the use of folk taxonomies within the diabetes genetic enterprise as illogical, unethical, harmful, or insensitive. However, to do so would miss the extraordinary insight into the processes of racialization within the scientific practices under study. A close examination of these practices reveals that the use of ethnically labeled groups in diabetes research is fraught with instances of contestation and justification, as well as misrecognitions of the social determinants of the disease and the social constructedness of the research variables. These practices, which are examined below, are not part of the official representation of diabetes knowledge, but serve as both background information and moments of ideological disjuncture. Ethnographically, attending to these disjunctures reveals that at issue are the social conditions and implications of knowledge that skirt the dichotomies of gene-environment, social-biological, and race-ethnicity.

The search for genetic contributions for diabetes begins, as has been shown in previous chapters, with the collection of DNA samples, which are converted into data sets. The consortium data sets are organized and labeled by geography, by institution, by population, and by sampling and diagnostic criterion used to select research subjects. One handout at a consortium meeting lists data by contributor as follows: "Chicago–Mexican, Fusion, Glaxo–African American, Pima, St. Louis, Wake Forest Caucasian." In instances in which populations or one specific data set are discussed, labels include "Native Americans, whites, African Americans, Japanese Americans, Mexican Americans," with Amish and Pima as subset populations for whites and Native Americans, respectively (see also the introduction to this book for the list of labels from the American Diabetes Association abstracts, shown in figure 1). And yet, contrary to the critique that these labeling practices are simple reifications of biological taxonomies or that the use of such population labels reinforce a long line of racial stereotypes, labels and the usefulness of the populations they reference were at times questioned by scientists.[18] For example, while discussing a data set for inclusion in one experiment, one researcher corrected a colleague who was considering Puerto Rico as a source of DNA comparably admixed as the Mexican American samples. The researcher interrupted her by saying that the comparison wouldn't work because "the native populations on Puerto Rico were wiped out."[19]

This was not the only time I witnessed a researcher referencing an aspect of social history to inform the selection of populations for research. Another occurred when a scientist came to give a lecture in the genetics department. As is the custom, researchers interested in a visitor's work sign up for informal meetings. At one such meeting, the people of Haiti were extolled as the ideal ancestral proxy for U.S. African Americans because Haiti, the researcher argued, was a hub of the slave trade where many Africans remained. The researcher's implicit assertions that Haitians are genetically purer than African Americans were followed by some inconclusive talk about who was sampling in Haiti and how those samples might be secured for genetic analyses. However, unlike the case of native Puerto Ricans, the construct of Haitian genetic purity, the geopolitical role of Haiti for the slave trade, and the utilitarian manner in which researchers discussed the acquisition of Haitian blood samples was never questioned. Most glaringly absent was a sense of the profoundly social factors that Farmer has connected to the mortality and morbidity of Haitian people: poverty, gender inequality, political upheaval, urbanization, and intense structural challenges of the Haitian economy.[20]

Over the course of my conducting participant observation with scientists, there were moments when my questions would rupture the black box of population labeling. Often after a meeting between scientists, I would pull one aside for a debriefing. Among the questions I would ask were queries about data sets and methods. Once when I gently questioned the use of skin tone as a measure of Amerindian ethnicity, one epidemiologist remarked, "Well, yes, skin tone is just one measurement among many that we use. We know the classification is not ideal, but we had to have some kind of replicable measurement."

Researchers, when directly queried, do not argue that the labels represent biological differences. Theirs is a pragmatic claim.[21] Though imperfect, the classificatory labels have coherence. Why are population data sets so important? As explained in chapter 1, the more homogeneous a population is, the easier it is to detect genetic variation that is statistically more likely to be related to a trait of interest. In trying to find diabetes genes, researchers must compare people with diabetes with those without diabetes. However, they need family data to increase the homogeneity of the study population in order to decrease the likelihood that the candidate genetic material that researchers are searching for is not simply a family specific SNP.

The search for candidate genes for type 2 diabetes began with the "discovery" of a single gene NIDDM1 on chromosome 2 that increased susceptibility in Mexican Americans. The polygene reported in October 2001 is the effect of NIDDM1 in combination with a gene on chromosome 15, CAPN10. It is actually a combination that requires haplotype heterozygosity at both sites to confer the increased susceptibility, the article reports. Homozygotes for either of the specific NIDDM1 or CAPN10 haplotypes confer no increased risk. Increased risk was determined through computer simulation in which researchers compare the genes at a particular region, or genomewide scans, to detect differences between diabetic and nondiabetic people. But this would not control for population variation. If comparing so-called whites with African Americans, the differences could be ascribable to evolutionary population structures. According to geneticists (and some biological anthropologists), each population has its own evolutionary history that is different enough, one from the other, to inform genetic analyses. Thus, scientists explain, by using population data sets, the likelihood that the observed genotypic differences arise from different ancestral genes is minimized.

The rationale for the use of these population categories is occasionally problematized by consortium members—on their own or through ethnographic interlocution. However, the ideology that true biological differences exist between populations labeled with folk taxonomies endures. No scientist I spoke with would openly argue that his or her use of population-specific data reiterated biological distinctions between humans, however. Yet neither did any question the fundamentally social nature of the labels used to identify the populations. One need only look at the labels "African American" and "Mexican American" to understand that these taxa are social: there is nothing biological about the slave trade, the Spanish Conquest, Mexican statehood, or the conditions that made possible "gene flow" from white males into enslaved females' offspring or Mexico-to-U.S. migration, without which neither label would exist.

The finding of the polygene disrupts the putatively benign nature of the diabetes genetics enterprise as the geneticists describe it, however. Recall that a polygene is a statistically observed genetic effect that is the result of an interaction between two genes working together. Chapter 1 detailed the process of this research. However, one aspect does warrant further explanation. A complex disorder such as diabetes requires more than one component to confer risk on a given individual. Finding genes by comparing those affected with those who are not is relatively easy when the culprit is a single gene and immensely easier than when environmental factors are added to the analyses. This "discovery" is newsworthy because now the doorway is conceptually and methodologically open for polygenetic traits to be added to the genetics bandwagon of disease causation.[22] That is, until this discovery, gene-gene interactions were thought to be too complicated to find. Beyond pointing toward a possible physiological pathway, the *Nature Genetics* piece offers conceptual and methodological avenues for subsequent investigators to pursue.

The representation of type 2 diabetes appearing in *Nature Genetics*, the popular press, and the CDC literature obviates the social context of the disease. Following Farmer's call to view disease sociologically,[23] we should recall that the DNA used by diabetes researchers came from Mexican Americans who live in a very troubled place. Sun County's unemployment rate, which hovers around 20 percent, has been precipitated, as noted in chapter 2, by historical shifts in agricultural labor practices, shifts that are deeply imbricated in the formation of the U.S. frontier, nation building, and race relations between Anglos and Mexicans in the American Southwest.

Aspects of Sun County political economy are arguably connected to diabetogenesis. In particular, over the past 60 years, shifts to the pesticide-laden and mechanized production practices of corporate agribusiness have led to an influx of farmworker families into the urban areas.[24] Recall, if you will, the sedentary lifestyle hypothesis. And of diet, as one Sun County land development agent in the 1930s is quoted as saying, "The white people won't do the work and live as the Mexicans do on beans and tortillas and in one room shacks."[25] This same sentiment is used to justify present-day efforts, most notably by Mexico's former president and Coca-Cola executive Vicente Fox, for a new worker amnesty or *bracero* program and to explain why Mexican immigrants are permeating rural U.S. communities. Mexicanos/as are needed to do the work.

Thus, under the conditions of poverty, dispossession, and capital dislocation, Sun County diabetes etiology takes on a starkly sociological register. In this light, diabetes is a profoundly social condition for Sun County residents. It is endured by certain groups brought about by forced migration from rural to urban settings, by an overdetermined reliance upon certain foods or foods with limited nutritional value, by the restrictions of physical movement required of wage labor, by poverty, and by unequal access to health care. It should come as no surprise that these sociopolitical conditions correlate to diabetogenesis.[26]

By the mid-1970s Sun County had caught the attention of epidemiologists who documented that of Texas's 254 counties, Sun County had the highest rates of diabetes. By 1983, the *American Journal of Epidemiology* reported that Sun County "Hispanics" were three to five times as likely to have diabetes as the general U.S. population. In a statement that appears to contradict his own work, the researcher who gathered the early epidemiological data and continues to collect DNA and provide free screening to Sun County residents told me that poor access to health care is the primary cause of diabetes in Sun County.

By noting Sun County's political history, by reintroducing a robust social element as a countervailing aspect of diabetes genetic research, a more balanced understanding of Sun County and of diabetes is possible. Of the disconnect between social inequality, AIDS, and tuberculosis, Farmer writes, "That [these] are not widely viewed as indissociably linked is in part a result of the limitations of epidemiology and international health—disciplines that increasingly take shelter behind 'validated' methodologies while ignoring larger forces and processes that determine why some people are sick and others are shielded from risk."[27] That the evidence for the genetics of diabetes risk is mounting in spite of (or at the expense of) the social context of the disease merely demonstrates the ability of the biogenetic view to trump the sociological one. After all, genes lead to proteins, proteins to drug targets, drug targets to new drugs and immense payoffs.

More precisely, though, are the boundary infrastructures that support the enduring dominance of diabetes science as a racial project writ large.[28] The concept of a genetic contribution to type 2 diabetes simply meets the needs of too many communities of practice and their politically salient apparatuses to be discarded for something else. That type 2 diabetes, or any socially determined disease for that matter, is considered an etiologically genetic condition is a classificatory act that entails the sorting of the genetic from the social, the behavioral, the moral, psychological, or political.[29] It is precisely because, as Lock and Farquhar observe, "the human body is a fulcrum around which an economy of everyday life is enacted and communities, polities, and civilizations are formed,"[30] that genes, not life conditions, will endure as the dominant etiological framework. Genetics, plain and simple, holds more nodes in the architecture of capitalist social organization and thus captures a dominant share of analytical imagination.

This is not to suggest that researchers who make up the diabetes consortium are ignorant of the effects of proper diet and adequate exercise. "Take away the television and the automobile, and diabetes would all but disappear," quipped the head of one lab. Nor are researchers unsympathetic to social inequality in the United States. Their career interests lie elsewhere. In fact, this case illustrates how, in spite of the sympathies of diabetes scientists, arrangements of U.S. racial inequality find their way into diabetes research publications and drug company promotional campaigns. I present two tales from the field, one dealing with the production of diabetes knowledge and the other with the marketing of a leading diabetes drug.

MEXICAN AMERICAN GENES

In this ethnographic project, I do not intend to argue that human biological variation is unimportant or nonexistent. Rather, what concerns us here is whether the labels used by researchers in their conversations and publications articulate population differences as biological or social. What these examples from scientists' discussions about labels demonstrate is that the process of biological reductionism of ethnicity into race is not a simplistic black box that scientists never question. Not only are labels contested differently for different populations, scientists are aware of the multiple readings of their science by its consumers. As we explore further the careful ways Mexicana ethnicity is used by scientists within the diabetes genetics enterprise, the problem of the use of ethnic labels will become even more complicated.

Lee and colleagues argue that population variation and genetic medicine is often the result of a "naïve genetic determinism"[31] on the part of its practitioners. That is, the genetic differences now discernable with SNP and other mutation analysis technologies are used to explain the patterns of disease between populations as the differences between the populations themselves and not as the varying social and historical environments in which they live. However, is the absence of an explicit definition of race evidence of such naïveté? The previous exemplar of the ruptures and reported rationale for "racialized" labels suggests that diabetes researchers deploy ethnic labels advisedly. And yet their caution does not necessarily indicate an understanding of the fundamentally social nature of population taxonomies to which we now turn.

Nora, the quantitative geneticist who welcomed me for the most extensive observations during my fieldwork, was ignorant neither of the social history of donor populations nor of the realities of U.S. race relations. For instance, she asked me to lunch one day because, I learned, she was concerned with the way Mexican Americans were being represented in her work. That week her computer simulations suggested that a particular *combination* of white and Asian/Native American genetic material increased the carriers' susceptibility to diabetes.[32] Recall from chapter 1 that the search for candidate genes began with the discovery of a single gene labeled NIDDM1 on chromosome 2, which increases the susceptibility for diabetes in Mexican Americans. The polygene discovery is the effect of NIDDM1 in combination with a gene on chromosome 15, CAPN10. It is actually a combination that requires haplotype heterozygosity at both sites to confer the pattern of increased susceptibility. The admixture of Mexican Americans, it is hypothesized, make the heterozygosity more prevalent in Mexicanas/os than in people of European descent. Homozygotes for either NIDDM1 or CAPN10 haplotypes confer no increased risk as determined through simulation.

Sitting in the hospital cafeteria one day, Nora wondered aloud to me if someone might use her findings in a way that could harm Mexican Americans. I asked her if she was worried about objections she imagined *I* had or those of some unspecified reader bent on feeding ideas that support racial prejudice. "I wouldn't want to do anything that could be used by someone to negatively portray the Mexican Americans who donated their time and DNA for our analyses," she clarified. Similarly, Gary addressed the issue at his lab meeting. Commenting to me afterward, Gary remarked, "You know we should be careful. These things are sensitive. . . . It could be construed as an argument for antimiscegenation and such."

A couple of months later, my jotting of field notes was interrupted by stereophonic groans from Nora and Gary. Nora had just read an e-mail from the editor at *Nature Genetics* who had been assigned to their submission. "We've had trouble getting published even though we've replicated our sample in Mexican American populations," Nora explained. "And now," she said with sarcastic emphasis on the "now," "we are told that because our work has been confirmed in two white populations, that we can take the 'Mexican American' out of the title of our paper." This was accompanied by a further meaning, which was that one of the impediments to publication had been overcome and publication was closer. With disgust, Nora and Gary talked over each other to explain to me how their original paper had been population neutral; it had not labeled the population from whom the DNA had come. *Nature* had told them that since the DNA came from Mexican Americans, the title needed to reflect this fact. Nora and Gary were incensed that their work was being ghettoized in this way. "We do [universal] human genetics, for Christ sake," Gary grumbled. "They are treating millions of Mexican Americans and the millions more Mexicans like the Amish, some small population isolate!" Two collaborators, a Swedish and a German researcher, had confirmed the findings in their population samples. Gary and Nora inferred that because *Nature Genetics* had allowed them to take Mexican American out of their title based on the "confirmation" that in the journal's editorial eyes what had been a Mexican American genetic condition had been transformed into a universal human condition. Nora and Gary were clear that *Nature's* editorial coercion was wrong, that their work needed no such confirmation. But further, their last and most biting objection to the titular dispute was that if it affects only Mexican Americans, then it is not fit to publish in *Nature Genetics*. But if it is a genetic condition found in "whites," well, that makes it a human gene and thus worth publishing. "It's not replication they wanted, its confirmation," Gary said cynically.

In this last complaint, Nora and Gary were clearly unloading some of their frustrations at the delays in publication. Many scientists report that their experience with article and grant reviewers is not always pleasant, and diabetes lore has it that it becomes downright nasty at times. However, the fact that Nora and Gary marked the irony of the editor's concerns noting the implicit denigration of Mexican Americans therein speaks to their recognition of the political implications of scientific knowledge production. Not only was the debacle an insult to them as professionals (Gary felt the editors should have "taken the chance two years ago") it referenced the wider context of race relations in the United States. It marks a science in which certain bodies count more than others, in which knowledge about "white" bodies holds more weight and sells more journals, and in which subtly pernicious notions of Mexicans as a racial human subspecies persist. Nora's and Gary's protests actively disrupt the privileged Eurocentricity of *Nature Genetics* and demonstrate their politicized engagement with the contested boundaries of what counts as human. Far from cut-and-dry racialization, Nora and Gary are here demonstrating that their use of a population at "high risk" for diabetes cannot be reduced to the group's ethnic identity.

The same month that Gary and Nora informed me of their exchange with *Nature,* the journal published an editorial explaining a new policy on the use of race in the publication. Citing the American Anthropological Association's statement on race, *Nature* noted that "race" is not a scientific term and that it is commonly used with poorly defined lay terminology. As a consequence, the editorial states that *Nature Genetics* will "require that authors explain why they make use of particular ethnic groups or populations, and how classification was achieved."[33] In the paper by Gary and Nora and colleagues, admixture was specified, and Sun County was mentioned as having a relatively homogeneous population, which meant homogenously admixed.[34] Other populations used in their paper (Pima [Native American peoples], German, Zapotec, Botnia) were "specified" to a similarly vague degree. However, the justification for the use of population DNA was implied, and the reasons for using these specific populations were not adequately detailed.

In this case the quibbling over the words "replication" versus "confirmation" is not trivial. It is about the struggle over what counts as rational knowledge. The ethical and political struggle over the title of Gary's and Nora's article is an instance of knowledge production that is cognizant of subjugated positions and the responsibility of science. Nora seemed to be operating—*pace* Haraway—with a sense of a "power sensitive conversation"[35] and an organic sense of the responsibilities of positioning. It is a form of knowledge making that does not blindly rely upon the "god trick," the force of objectivity, but rather upon the strategic positioning of the scientist, of his or her work product, and of the lives of the people whose donated DNA made the knowledge work possible. In other words, Nora and Gary were deliberate in their representation of Mexican Americans and paid special attention to the consequences of the knowledge they produced. Reflecting the potential miscegenation messages that could be read into his and Nora's piece, Gary remarked, "We only included what was absolutely necessary." The paper excluded any reference to genetic admixture even though it is the alleged mixing of Native American/Asian and Caucasian genes that makes the polygene possible in the first place.[36]

FROM SCIENCE TO MEDICINE

In another instance, race and ethnicity are deployed very differently. While attending the meetings of the American Diabetes Association, I immediately noticed the marketing and promotional tactics of dozens of companies. Like most science conferences with medical ties, ADA meetings abound with corporate logos, products, and drug representatives. Amid the visual bombardment of product placement that nearly envelops the conference venue, the ad campaign for Amaryl caught my attention. Amaryl is an oral sulfonylurea that lowers blood sugar by stimulating the pancreas to release additional insulin.[37] The campaign's signature artwork pleases the eye. It depicts a man wielding a sickle mid-stock on a sugar cane. Behind him, purple mountains accentuated by white cumulus clouds starkly contrast with the orange sunset and thick cane field in the foreground. The block relief artwork, more cartoonlike than realistic, shows this lone cane worker filling the clapboard bed of a trailer with downed canes headed for production. The worker has been busy. The midground, between the stacks of prostrate cane in the trailer filled by the worker and the distant mountains, shows hillsides of cleaved cane stubs that mark the landscape.

The maker of Amaryl is Aventis Pharmaceuticals. The pharmaceutical division's principal area is in prescription drugs. It contributes about three-fourths, 13.9 billion Euros, of Aventis's sales. The remainder comes from Aventis's agricultural, animal, nutrition and other life sciences products.[38] (Aventis received publicity in October 2000 when its bioengineered corn was found to have been illegally incorporated in taco shells, allegedly causing severe rashes.) It is difficult to say what Aventis Pharmaceuticals spends on this one ad campaign. "That's proprietary information," one marketing professional said when queried. However, the Amaryl brand permeates the American Diabetes Association's conference materials. The cane-worker image appears on the back of the Program and Abstract book for the conferences and is one of only 16 color ads in the 550-page volume. It also appears in glossy brochures, on T-shirts, and in numerous medical and scientific journals. The Amaryl name and its chemical name, glimepiride, are branded to the backs of the conference nametags, exhibition hall I.D. cards and numerous other items. This ubiquity could explain the overwhelming success of this ad, as measured by product recognition studies with physicians.

The construction of meaning in an advertisement relies upon "mutual knowledge" between its creators and the intended audience. As Chavez notes in his analyses of magazine covers, "The communication carried out by cultural objects relies on the same mutual knowledge as talk, or the casual conversations carried out in everyday settings of

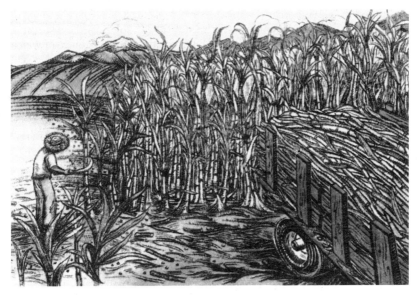

FIGURE 5. Amaryl® advertisement image: Silkscreen T-shirt of sugar cane worker. Photo by the author.

social life. When people talk to each other, they are connected cultur- ally by the setting and mutual interaction."[39] A Caribbean cane worker, beautifully depicted, struck me as more than coincidence. The Amaryl ad campaign's image of the cane worker makes visible the contradic- tions that inhere within Nora's work and the genetic epidemiology of diabetes more broadly. The ad shifts the meaning between the biologi- cal need addressed by the drug and the bodies it targets while capital- izing on the social semiotic cache that the image carries. For example, I was immediately struck by the social meanings conveyed in the ad. Stylistically the ad evokes the popular Mexican protest art of the Taller de Grafica Popular: its relief print motif could just as easily have been employed to protest monocrop agriculture or indentured labor.[40] What is more, the ad's vibrant orange, yellow, brown, and green evoke the palette made popular by artist Diego Rivera.

Recalling the coca colonization hypothesis, the setting was clearly a plantation, somewhere in Latin America or the Caribbean, with a lone brown-skinned laborer who works to feed our appetite for sugar. An image of a place, a relationship, where, in anthropologist Sidney Mintz's words,

Europeans. . . . imported vast numbers of people in chains from elsewhere to work. These would be, if not slaves, then men who sold their labor because they had nothing else to sell; who would probably produce things of which they were not the principal consumers; who would consume things they had not produced, and in the process earn profit for others elsewhere.[41]

"It's cutting sugars" the Aventis's product manager for Amaryl defensively assured me after I queried him about the ad campaign, its history, and the meaning of the image. Standing in the middle of the Amaryl exhibit at the ADA science meeting's "product theater," we examined the five-foot-tall depiction of the cane-worker scene like two art critics at the Getty. The presumably British employee had gotten protective because I suggested that one reading of the ad could be a racialized one. I was curious, I told him, if the ad was intended to link people of color to the product. In my mind, I saw a powerful installation of the emerging majority (Latinos, African Americans, Indians, Asians) in the role of the market for Amaryl.

Marcus, as I will call Amaryl's product manager, denied the connection. In fact he interrupted my query with an anxious defense of the ad's potential messages. "I've only heard of three negative comments since we started this ad," he said. One was mine, that it could be read as a linkage to an emerging market of ethnoracial patients; another he himself suggested: that the cane worker could be seen as subservient. He listed a third "negative" interpretation, "that the image is inaccurate because you've got to burn sugar cane before harvest." Marcus's own interpretation—that an image of a cane worker could be seen negatively as subservient—is surely the most critical of these alternative readings. In my query, I had not implied that an emerging market reading was "negative."

As I looked further into Aventis and Amaryl, I found Marcus's denial that there was any ethnoracial intent behind Amaryl's ad campaign at variance with other evidence. On November 10, 2000, some months after my meeting with Marcus, an Aventis press release read, "Amaryl tablets provide significant reductions of HbA1c and fasting plasma glucose in Mexican Americans with type 2 diabetes." The release noted that "10.6 percent of Mexican Americans are diabetic, that Mexican Americans are twice as likely to develop diabetes than whites and that since 1990 there has been an alarming 38 percent increase in the prevalence of diabetes among this population." It goes on to document a randomized trial that shows that Amaryl outperforms diet and exercise in lowering blood glucose—a finding that contradicts alternative research on white populations and a report released by the U.S. Department of Health and Human Services in 2001. Additionally, Aventis is a featured company in a March 2002 conference on marketing to multicultural audiences. Because each product line is tied to stock valuations, bonuses, departmental expansion, and advancement up the corporate ladder, Marcus's denials seem all the more puzzling. Could he have overreacted to my query in response to the impending press release?

Amaryl presents Aventis with a problem. In the wake of a new generation of products, how can the market for Amaryl be sustained? As the press release implies, one apparent strategy is to link the drug to Mexican American diabetics. Yet Amaryl cannot be directly marketed to Mexican Americans; the text of those ads would not be socially or politically tolerated or scientifically defensible.[42] Instead, Amaryl is aggressively marketed to physicians deploying what could be called cross-cultural signposts to repeatedly reinforce the connection between Amaryl and its intended consumers. For example, Aventis, like many drug companies, sponsored a party during the 2000 ADA meetings.[43] The slick ad-quality invitation depicted a chameleon on a yucca blossom with the words, "Come show your true colors at the coolest party in town. Arriba, baby!" On the inside of the foldout invite were the Aventis logo and party particulars, and the sign-off that read, "Don't Miss It—It's Muy Caliente!!"

The six-year-old ad came out before the recent press release. And the ADA meetings at which the party invitation was used was held in San Antonio, Texas. Yet, whatever site-specific marketing gimmicks Aventis used during the ADA meetings do not diminish the long-standing association of diabetes with ethnoracially defined populations. After all, the connection of diabetes with various "ethnic peoples" is at least as old as Neel's thrifty genotype hypothesis. What is more, marketers and the artists they employ are well trained in the arts of persuasion. Social, clinical, visual, and scientific information and symbols must all work together to be effective.[44] While Amaryl may be effective in lowering the blood sugars of Mexican American diabetics, the implication that it is more effective than when used by other ethnic groups is a specious one.

Such cross-cultural marketing has cultural side effects, however. While the images in the Amaryl ad work to link the (formerly) colonized and enslaved to Amaryl, the Anglicization in the party invitation reconstitutes a Spanish-speaking subsegment of that group into social subordinates. Linguist Jane Hill, in her 1993 *Hasta La Vista, Baby: Anglo Spanish in the American Southwest*, points out that the jocular, ironic, and parodic register of this kind of Anglicization forms an important part of the subordination of Spanish-speaking people. Linguistic evidence has shown that Anglo's predominant borrowing of Spanish in boldly parodic registers "distances utterers from the voice which issues from their mouths (and texts) and serves to denigrate the source of that voice, constructing this source as ridiculous and contemptible."[45] Hill's argument is aptly put. If the public use of Spanish language is mostly Anglicized in a vulgar way, as in the bold parodic nature of "Hasta La Vista" or "Arriba, Baby," then the ethnic insult behind this linguistic practice is all too apparent. Imagine an English reversal in which the word "y'all" was consistently overemphasized to stress the social position of those who use this colloquialism. Or, closer to home, if in articles in the *Chronicle of Higher Education* about the social sciences, anthropology was always written "anthro-apology" to reference our ceaseless disciplinary public controversies and reflexive analyses. Further, because mistakes and variants in the use of English are markers of social stratification, if not ridicule and discrimination, the overt flaunting of this bold parodic Anglicization reinforces the notion that Anglos can get away with linguistic mistakes in ways not open to Spanish-speaking groups.[46]

BIOSOCIALITY AS A RACIAL PROJECT

If we evaluate Nora's and Gary's work alongside the Amaryl ad campaign and public relations materials, what are we to make of the simultaneous sensitivity to, yet deployment of, racial inequality within the diabetes research and development apparatus? Nora's organic sense of the possible negative effects of her work on her Mexican American donors and her own and Gary's objections to the implications of the *Nature Genetics* titular dispute presents a unique form of what Rabinow calls "biosociality." Biosociality, a concept with many productive and evocative meanings, speaks to a phenomenon whereby individuals appropriate biogenetic discourse as part of their identity.[47] The case of diabetes illustrates that the phenomenon also works in reverse. Instead of biology informing notions of self, it is the case that the social narratives of colonialism, eugenics, slavery, and conquest—as embedded in population constructs, code switching, and imagery—inform the portrayal and selection of the biological units of analyses for diabetes research. The inversion of biosociality, from the biological informing the social to the social informing the biological, is an effect of the multiple levels of analyses inherent in complex disease gene research. In this case, Mexican racialized DNA "actants" operate as material semiotic actors.[48] That is, the biogenetic material is so loaded with social meaning that those who handle it are required to reattach, in the form of an ethnic label, the sociohistorical context of its production as it extends outward from the lab.

In other words, it matters where the DNA came from. In the lab, there was never a mention of the labels used for the units of analyses. It only came up when (1) the populations were being evaluated as potential donors; (2) Nora and Gary were struggling to get this particular knowledge published; and (3) physicians and their patients were being enlisted as allies in the diabetes enterprise. In fact, we see in the case of Amaryl and the publicity that Nora's and Gary's "discovery" received that the farther away the ethnoracial knowledge circulated from the labs, the more it reflected ethnic donors and thus the more encumbered it became with meanings forged out of racialized social inequalities.

The differential pattern of diseases between and among human populations is an important topic for research. To dismiss variations in disease incidence and prevalence among ethnic groups because it threatens to biologize race and thus offends our long-standing political battle against biological determinism is a mistake. I locate myself as an ally to my ethnographic interlocutors, but as one with epistemological premises and political commitments different from theirs. The different morbidity patterns for diabetes might well be researched as consequences of the different environmental (life) conditions of groups whose ability to live among and mate with other groups has been socially, geographically, legally, and often violently constrained. More succinctly, epidemiological differences between racially classified groups "might be a proxy for discriminatory experiences, diet or other environmental factors": social factors that should be closely investigated along with genetics.[49]

Presented here are the nuanced practices of scientists who are not only sensitive to the social context of their knowledge, but who work against the ways their science could reinforce long-standing notions of European biological superiority. However, in spite of their efforts, diabetes is already a racialized disease that informs the targeting of socially defined groups for pharmacological interventions. In so doing, pharmaceutical marketeers reinscribe race and ethnicity as biological, a process I call "bioethnic conscription." Bioethnic conscription, as here detailed, instantiates the complex dynamic between race as a key symbol of identity, race as biological myth, and race as a geoterritorial concept. Bioethnic conscription thus also explains why the ethnoracial differences are part of the requisite narrative of diabetes in venues as diverse as government publications, scientific journals, grant applications, and the popular press, to wit, social inequalities are needed to make the knowledge.[50] Likewise, when Carl, Nora, and Gary package the Mexicana/o DNA within their research findings, they too conscript the social and political history of Sun County and the broader U.S. race relations between Anglos and Mexicanas/os into their scientific practices. Thus, in conscripting the ethnic identities and social contexts of disease patterns into the production and consumption of scientific research, researchers and marketers naturalize racial social inequalities.

As a racially inflected project, the diabetes research-and-development enterprise serves as a proof of principle for Omi and Winant's racial formation.[51] Race is a "fundamental dimension of social organization and cultural meanings in the US"[52] occurring through the linkages between social institutions and representation. Scientific institutions and related representations are not exceptions to this process. However, Omi and Winant's insistence that race is an overtly political phenomenon overlooks the mundane processes of the production of cultural meanings of race in biomedical milieus. I have attempted to ethnographically assess and retheorize these "fundamental dimensions" of race in diabetes research by simultaneously attending to its historical, political, and bioscientific aspects. What is more, the uptake of ethnicity within genetics discourse, its conscription into the biological, come into clearer view when the process of "discovery" is examined at the moment DNA samples are acquired, when they are made into novel biogenetic insight, and when they are disseminated through publication and product promotion.

CONCLUSION

The case of the diabetes enterprise adds real-time ethnographic evidence to the pathbreaking work that has shown—after the fact—that social categories get mapped onto emergent scientific knowledge. The contribution of this chapter to analyses of the narratives, metaphors, and politics of knowledge production as discernable through the texts scientists produce is less temporal than methodological, however.[53] For example, one cannot with certainty know through analyses of the end product of research what shaped the scientists' choice of words, selection of research subjects, or choice of publication venue. However, the practices analyzed here do detail concrete instances of what goes into the black boxes of DNA samples labeled with folk taxonomies.

Additionally, the emphasis I place on the relationship between the *production* of diabetes knowledges and the *consumption* of the findings produced extend the analyses of the human and nonhuman networks configured in scientific milieus, of the organizing force of theoretical and methodological assemblages scientists enlist to advance their work, and of social metaphors used in immunity and conception narratives.[54] By focusing on the practices of racialization as part of racial formation within the context of U.S. race relations, I have worked to offer a conceptual and empirical foothold that scholars, public health workers, and activists can use to contest the use of racialized representations in chronic disease research.

Further, the diabetes genetics enterprise lends empirical support to studies that argue against the uncritical use of race as a variable in epidemiology, medicine, and social scientific quantitative analyses.[55] While vital in the efforts to call attention to the social relations beneath racial statistics and taxonomies, these studies do not interrogate *why* and *how*; in spite of repeated reminders, scholars and the scholarly journals in which they publish consistently deploy race as a static attribute or as a biological category. For such an interrogation, a broader epistemological frame is required, one in which the context of the production of scientific knowledge is analyzed along with the content.

As an instance of a racial project *in vivo*, the deployment of racial labels and symbols within the diabetes research-and-development apparatus shape, as much as they are shaped by, the political context of their production. Thus, as racial formation theory correctly posits, diabetes scientists and marketeers simultaneously structure and signify. Researchers, editors, and drug marketeers circulate representations of human variation and create their own rationale for the use of bioethnically conscripted groups of people. This in turn structures further research practices. The consequence of a racial project that traffics in biologically, socially, and historically crafted data is that the meanings of social inequality take the form of individual pathology, which invites new forms of genetic surveillance and predetermines the hegemony of biological solutions for a chronic sociological dis-ease.

Finally, SNP-based research, as deployed by Nora and her Chicago colleagues, do not create biological race. To reinterpret a familiar aphorism, "SNPs don't make races, people make races." The trick is buried in the tautology that Duster so ably exposed. Researchers find biological differences between groups of people based on social differences they have found between groups of people. Therefore, the racialization occurs in the grouping of populations sampled for research, not only in the scientific knowledge made from that grouping or the predicted consequences of that knowledge. That said, a population with a high incidence and prevalence of an important disease is sampled "as if" they constitute a homogenous population in order to investigate the contributions of small genetic differences to large health consequences. If social conditions were always given such attentive investigation, their differentiated effects might also speak to population vulnerability. However, in this case it would be the burdens of racial discrimination, of poverty, of inequity that would surely be revealed.

Beyond Reductionism

Bioethnicity and the Genetics of Inequality

Explaining how race comes to be a site of commonsense truth claims, popular truth claims, and scientific truth claims about diabetes and human difference writ large is one of the aims of this book. Race and nature, or at times race as nature, comprise an assemblage of productive associative relationships, as Donald Moore and colleagues rightly aver, that are at once material and semiotic. That is, there are real social relationships that affect us all, that are shaped by and that shape the way we work, play, live, and learn while also molding our experiences and our understandings of our world. Scientists, Mexicana/o DNA donors, fieldworkers, and health professionals of all types are participants in the composition of this social milieu. These sometimes novel and at other times socially reproductive composites require an explanation of their articulated formations when and where they appear. Here I have aimed to build upon the insights of Moore and his colleagues with an analysis that details the ways "race and nature are constitutive features of modern power."[1] What captures my attention in this book is the uneasy terrain of a scientific milieu in which racial politics of difference, and dare I say cultural politics of meaning, are impossibly entangled in liberal humanism, community development, identity politics, disease prevention, careful scientific practices, and sincere concerns about the health of the chronically underserved and disenfranchised.

In this realm, a critical politics of race that is discernable in the diabetes enterprise requires an attention to more than critical analytics of modernity and power. Offering such a critique of the diabetes enterprise might be satisfying, but it ends where it must begin. It is precisely the ways old and new meanings of racial difference emerge in the production of biogenetic knowledge making forged from new and not so new technoscientific practices and processes that is the challenge before us. In other words, understanding power, the productive and reproductive structures, objects and meanings that emanate out of technoscience, cannot occur if we already predefine the cultural politics we expect to find. A serious analysis of all things racial, especially in the United States, amply demonstrates that Moore and colleagues are correct to place social injustice and political technologies of violence at the center of their analytic of race and nature.

My project seeks a slightly different path without diminishing the power analysis of race in the twenty-first century. It seeks to produce an account of a specific articulation of race that demonstrates why and how our critical analytics, no matter how convinced we are of their validity, have failed to interrupt the nonrandom patterns of injustices and inequities that are always already embedded in all things racial and racialized at this historical moment. In other words, what requires explanation are not the processes and practices that technoscientists reiterate in the making of the three or five "races of man." Although necessary, this is an unsatisfactory level of resolution if we are to understand and transform those material and semiotic assemblages that perpetuate inequity. Rather, what demands explanations are why this occurs in spite of the scientific, ethical, social, and political consequences so carefully detailed by scholars and analysts from a spectrum of fields across the social and biological sciences and humanities.

Diseases that involve complex gene-gene-environment interactions (e.g., asthma, diabetes, heart disease, cancers, etc.) are the next frontier for genetic medicine. However, the Mendelian gold rush of the previous single-gene model has given way to an infinitely more complex scientific venture. Researchers must now transform "the environment" and at-risk "populations" into variables that fit biological analyses while keeping in mind the speculative futures of potential drug markets, public health concerns, and individual scientific career imperatives. Whether carried out in the name of genetics, public health, molecular epidemiology, epigenetics, or some other epistemological assemblage, there is no built-in protection from the deployment of knowledge claims or artifacts that amplify rather than redress inequity. The antipolitical effects of reductionism, determinism, scientism, biologization, or other crude links between genotype and phenotype, individuals and groups, or biology and human illness remain even under the most careful of human intentions. The specific effects of this constellation of social and biophysical forces have been discussed in the preceding chapters. This concluding chapter reexamines the use of racialized population DNA in diabetes research and evaluates the broader social consequences of complex disease research in the postgenomic era.

In their erudite treatment of classifications, Bowker and Star detail the hermeneutic circle that helps bundle the various slices of race, genes, and diabetes detailed in the preceding chapters.[2] Drawing upon Cicourel's[3] observation that researchers begin with broad classification schemata that are expected to fit the data and then elaborate those categories as if they were derived from the data in the first place, they write,

> There is no simple unraveling of the built information landscape, or, *pace* Zen practice, of unsettling our habits at every waking moment. The moral questions arise when the categories of the powerful become the taken for granted; when policy decisions are layered into inaccessible technological structures; when one group's visibility comes at the expense of another's suffering.[4]

To be sure, the conundrum of race, of disease, of "the Mexicano/a" within the social milieu that I have called the diabetes enterprise naturalizes unequal power relations. However, the moral questions, the "gotcha politick" of epistemological critique, are by now tired exemplars of interventions into the problems of race in science. I have attempted here to detail the ethical and scientific conundrums of race within the social milieu of the diabetes enterprise. And I have attempted to do so in a manner that makes it difficult to simply dismiss diabetes genetics and complex disease genetics in general, opting instead at explaining how race comes to be thought and made material. As the barrage of race-based medical findings with genes de jour indicate, pointing out the consequences (ethical, moral, scientific, logical) in themselves have been pathetically unsuccessful in raising the discussion of biological variation beyond shouting matches and finger pointing. What, then, has this project attempted to contribute to the problematic bundling of race, science, medicine, and "Mexicanness" within the diabetes enterprise?

The preceding chapters examined various aspects of the academic-, corporate-, and state-funded alliance of molecular, biological, computer, and clinical scientists who are conducting research into the genetic epidemiology of type 2 diabetes. We saw that because type 2 diabetes affects populations differently, researchers use racial taxonomies to parse populations and social history to rationalize their categorical choices. However, in spite of the use of racial labels for the populations used for research, it was clear that a simplistic reproduction of biological subspecies arguments does not occur in diabetes epidemiology. Still, Durkheim and Mauss observed, "Every classification implies a hierarchical order."[5] Unearthing that order is the easy part. Explaining how that order produces classification systems and, more systemically, produces types of people to fit certain politically configured classification systems is the greater challenge of this book.

THE PRODUCTION OF DIABETES KNOWLEDGE

By following DNA from Chicago back to its point of acquisition along the border, we were able to reassemble the cultural meanings that are produced and then concealed in diabetes knowledge productive practices. Pertinent to the critiques of reductionism, determinism, and essentialism, it was shown that the use of population-based data sets by researchers results in critically nuanced reiterations of human variation that blend past and present arrangements of social inequality into future-oriented scientific knowledge. Such reiterations do not biologize race per se. Rather, they prepackage diabetes data sets in a manner that is easily translated into representations that construct de facto biological differences between human groups labeled with social categories.

The analytical tack taken here has been to examine the process of diabetes knowledge production through various stages of research. Beginning with the identification of populations to be sampled, the prepackaging of ethnicity fits long-standing patterns of so called "race" relations along the U.S.-Mexico border. The relationships between Mexicanas/os and Anglos have been structured by dispossession, exploitation, war, and white supremacy. Anglo institutions such as settlement, agribusiness, and now science demonstrate a consistent pattern of extracting value from the bodies of Mexicanas/os. The diabetes enterprise differs only in the level and ontological framework of its exploitation. Instead of an external enemy whose land was needed or an unwanted Other from whom cheap labor could be extracted, diabetes science requires Mexicana/o bodies as a source of cheap embodied biocapital to accomplish its objectives.[6]

Yet, because this new entrepreneurial force imposed upon Mexicanas/os is biomedical, it has different requirements but with similar results. First, Mexicanas/os are reduced to a form of ethnic purity through the collection of genetic pedigrees and the homogeneity presumed of the Sun County population. This is the initiatory moment of the reductionism critiqued by the authors cited above. However, it is not the science per se, isolated from the culture in which it is produced, that imposes the reductionistic consequences. It is the constellation of social and historical relationships between Anglos and Mexicanas/os in the border region that prefigures the Mexicana/o population. That is, what is crucial here are the linkages between the racialized justifications for discrimination and dispossession[7] and the emergence of a people who are cast as biologically informative for diabetes research. To reiterate, the scientists are not reducing Mexicanas/os to a pure ethnic stock; the reductionism existed even before the public health workers identified the higher diabetes risks in the population.

BIOETHNICITY

Perhaps the most dynamic aspect to the use of racialized DNA samples within this biogenetic enterprise is that the racial and ethnic identity ascribed to the donor populations is made to do symbolic labor. The conditions of a donor's life, those events that shaped his or her physiological condition and the social and political history that attached itself to the donor's life in the form of an ethnic identity, are deployed to serve the biogenetic disease enterprise. In the preceding chapters, we have seen the multifold ways through which the symbolic enrollment of "Mexicanness" transpires within the products of diabetes research. It must be noted that it is not "race," the fictive biological concept, that is being conscripted. Rather, it is the social and political formation that configures donors' bodies as different, in this case "98 percent Mexican American," that is conscripted into the diabetes genetic enterprise. The social configuration of Mexicans, as distinct from other social groups (most notably Anglos in the Southwest) is drafted into the material and symbolic service of the biogenetic enterprise as a necessary part of producing diabetes knowledge and its hoped-for downstream pharmaceutical products.

Instead of academic arguments on whether racialized groups create de facto biological subspecies or biologically distinct human groups labeled with folk taxonomies, it should be recognized that the uptake of ethnicity into biological science creates something new, what I call "bioethnicity."

Operating at the confluence of biology and society, bioethnicity simply recognizes that biological races do not exist and that all knowledge derived from racialized populations is in fact the social histories and life conditions of those populations pressed into service of biomedical discourse. For diabetics on the U.S.-Mexico border, it is thus the history of migration, of reproduction, of transformation in labor and agribusiness production, and the nutritional, emotional, and physiological burdens of war, poverty, racialized violence, and prejudice that are being refracted within these particular biomedical knowledge claims. Of course, also embedded in this knowledge are the myriad ways that Sun County Mexicanas/os have created successful thriving lives in spite of all these challenges.

Thus "bioethnicity" is a term that does not presume a difference between biology and society. It more accurately expresses the class of racialized thing produced within biomedical discourse that is, like all such things, a sociocultural conception. Bioethnicity is what González Burchard and colleagues[8] explicitly attempt to "discover" by finding the biological basis for parsing ethnic groups, and it is what "Mexicana/o" means within the diabetes research milieu. Technically, each use of bioethnicity should be examined for its particular biologistical configuration. If, for example, a researcher is simply using a label to describe a specific group, and that use is not meant as proxy for anything other than that specific group, and the biological variation of that group is merely an estimate based upon the continuous clinal distribution of biogenetic variance that has resulted from drift, flow, founder effects, bottlenecks, selective or other evolutionary pressures, then the search for biological human variation and the use of a descriptive label for the population under examination should not warrant concern. However, the problem with this set of qualifications is that they are rarely part of a scientific claim about biogenetic human variation.[9]

Thus, having sampled Mexicanas/os for the diabetes genetic epidemiological enterprise, Mexicana/o ethnicity is conscripted into the capital-intensive research apparatus. What I have termed "bioethnic conscription" is a process whereby the descriptor of a population is conflated with an attribute of that population. Another way to explain this slippage is that in preparing a data set for use in biomedical enterprise, Carl and his colleagues must translate the descriptive statistical profile of Mexicanas/os in Sun County into the raw material suitable for experimental analyses. The process of preparing the DNA samples for various experiments is the site of such translation. While it travels through the mail to Nora or any other collaborator, the DNA sample loses its descriptive nature and is received as if it represented an attribute of the donors' bodies.

Sociologist Tukufu Zuberi surveyed leading social scientific journals and came to the same conclusions. He writes: "Using racialized census, survey, or other social data is not in and of itself problematic. The racialization of data is an artifact of both the struggle to preserve and to destroy racial stratification. Before the data can be deracialized, we must deracialize the social circumstances that have created racial stratification."[10] This is why Carl's, Gary's, and Nora's good intentions and astute situated interventions fail. There is no doubt that diabetes scientists are genuinely concerned about the welfare of Mexicanas/os. Hence, in spite of Carl's stated objectives in grant applications and in meeting presentations that his work will benefit those born today by helping to find the causes of diabetes, the unequal impact of diabetes upon Mexicanas/os in his sample will persist. Similarly, Nora's and Gary's arguments with *Nature Genetics* and any other attempts to situate their representations of Mexicana/o bodies provides, at best, ambiguous messages about the causes of diabetes. As long as their research deploys bioethnically conscripted populations, it will support the notion that the differential incidence and prevalence of diabetes among Mexicanas/os is a function of an attribute of their bodies.[11]

The consequences for this technoscientific process are that disparities of health are converted to biological differences.[12] This enclosure of the biological constitutes a sociocultural black-box effect and ensures that social worlds of those who disproportionately experience chronic disease remain irrelevant and extraneous. However, scientists who use bioethnicity in their research cannot be cast as simplistically reductionistic or essentializing. The example I present of the *Nature Genetics* editor insisting that Nora and Gary title a publication as "Diabetes loci in Mexican Americans" because they didn't have any Caucasian samples that confirmed their findings shows the complicated ways "race" is taken up in scientific literature. In this case, even though my collaborator-informants knew this to make no genetic sense in view of their findings, they were coerced as a condition of publication—against their vociferous objections—to present their findings as de facto proof of genetic variation between "Caucasians" and "Mexican Americans" as essentialized populations. During revisions, they received confirmation from Finnish and German populations and immediately took the words "Mexican American" out of the title.

However, because Gary and Nora's primary data set came from a known population labeled as "Mexican Americans," their polygene discovery is inextricably bound to the array of conditions that made the acquisition of their DNA data set possible. As was discussed in the preceding chapters, the sociological conditions for this include dispossession, war, and labor inequality keyed to the historical and ongoing political and economic exigencies of the Mexico-U.S. frontier. The local conditions include the disposition that engenders sufficient *confianza* to acquire DNA samples from affected bodies. And the scientific conditions include a well-funded genetics-based science interested in homogeneous populations. Together, these conditions form the constellation of material conditions that are coproduced by the racialized logics of genes, disease, and human variation.

I am not arguing that genetic frequency distributions across populations do not exist. Surely such variation exists. In the case of transplantation, for example, it is precisely these attributes of the person's body that are sought after. Unlike chronic disease, in which there are acknowledged environmental influences, finding a match for organ or tissue donors is seldom about the context of a donor's life. For transplantation, there are reasons to genetically screen people or screen people by blood group or by other physiological/biochemical attributes to mitigate an immunological response to the transplantation or transfusion. However, when "race" is used as a selection factor, the need for a physiological attribute (a genetic marker, a blood type, a protein, etc.) is conflated with a descriptor (Asian, African, Caucasian, Mexican) that bears relatively little physiological relationship to the attributes in question. This is especially true of chronic diseases in which social conditions, life experiences, and family history manifest in a local biology.

This study has revealed instances of a slippage in the use of ethnoracial labels from "descriptors" of human groups to "attributes" of human groups. And as we have seen in the preceding chapters, the sociocultural consequences of this slippage are tremendous. It leads the biomedical enterprise to pathologize ethnicity. This then creates the conditions whereby the consumers of such knowledge (physicians, pharma, patients themselves, insurance carriers, "the public") can easily confuse the descriptor with the attribute. What is more, it obscures the social and the cultural aspects of human variation (identity, language, cultural forms, class, gender, historical experiences, etc.), aspects that are deeply and historically implicated in who gets sick and who does not.

Bioethnicity is a cultural phenomenon bearing no essential connection to physiological attributes of human variation and no origins in the scientific production of knowledge. Racial reductionism was there all along.[13] It is not that there is no empirical connection between disease and group membership. There is. But the implicit causal models used to explain why are counterfactual. Genes do not cause chronic disease. Genes in certain bodies under certain conditions contribute to disease susceptibility.

We can observe different prevalence rates between populations. But, affirming Duster's critique, to then study the disease by examining the differences between populations rather than the different environments is to merely affirm what you already know.[14] That researchers continue to do so is the result of the implicit causal model in the biomedical research enterprise: human biological variation drives disease. As the *Newsweek* article and the Amaryl ad campaigns examined in this book illustrate, whatever is found in the group's body is associated with the disease, and then group membership itself is associated with the disease.

PROBLEMS OF KNOWLEDGE AND THE KNOWLEDGE OF PROBLEMS

This book assembles different analytical and epistemological perspectives on the configuration of race, borders, and medical science. The conversations I am entering into include critical race theory; health disparities (epidemiology, public health); critical medical anthropology/sociology; Chicana/o–Latina/o studies, especially assessments of borders and the nation state; and, of course, long-standing anthropological interests in human variation, intergroup relations, and social inequality. It is a project that issues an anthropological challenge. In a complicated field of capital-intensive cultural formation, how are we to conduct research and retheorize our findings in ways that exemplify our disciplinary expertise without foreclosing the linkages to analyses less committed to—and less experienced at—empirically documenting and connecting the quotidian, the particular to the larger social and material forces that coproduce the behaviors, objects, and meanings that occupy our ethnographic attention?

I have tried to refine our understanding of social reproduction in scientific practices without being overly deterministic. To do this requires finding the cracks within and between these analytical perspectives as a way to integrate what I find to be disparate yet isolated conversations.

For example, in chapter 5, the dominant ethical discourse of profit sharing was shown to adhere to the logics of possessive individualism and presumes the inherent integrity of the scientific products.[15] Value is already generated in the diabetes enterprise, and new commodity forms are produced even though pharmaceuticals are years away from developing drugs based upon physiological and clinical research of the diabetes enterprise. However, I have pointed out that an ethics discourse that misrecognizes the inherently exploitative nature of population use in biomedical research is a function of its epistemological blinders. They are not intentional acts.

Equally important to this account are the ways I have attempted to redress the effects of privilege within the social and cultural studies of science, technology, and medicine and the social and cultural anthropology from which this book is derived. Privilege, like ignorance, is invisible to itself. I have tried to prevent this invisibility in several ways.

First, I have included, as part and parcel of this research, a description of my political and analytical commitments. Reflected in the autobiographical sections in the introduction and in the anti-anti-science conclusions throughout, I have tried to avoid summary dismissals of scientific work simply because I assess it to support racial prejudice or biological reductionism. Like the present project, diabetes knowledges must be understood in context. A scientific claim may inflect ideas of racial prejudice, but not because the scientists are racists. Rather, the assemblages I have examined here invite negative racialized interpretations because of their antipolitical decontextualization. That is, the claims conceal the social conditions of their production and make possible the characterization of Mexicanas/os as a public health threat by virtue of their bioethnicity. Therefore, I have taken great pains to report—affirm, even—the good intentions of diabetes researchers because failure to do so would conflate a description of their practices with an attribute of science and scientists themselves. Doing so would miss the point of this book entirely.

Moreover, this book is constructed as an interdisciplinary project that opens, rather than forecloses, possible applications and readership of its findings. Bridging ethnic studies, history, public health, genetic sciences, anthropology, critical epidemiology, and other fields is an attempt to make possible a cross-grain reading from which common alliances or even sharper areas of disagreement might emerge more clearly. My refusal to cast only in negative terms my collaborators, my commitment to implicate myself as collaborateur,[16] and my work to contextualize the diabetes enterprise and this project are meant to open up those spaces of possible intersections between those with overtly different disciplinary, political, and scientific commitments. That is, to understand the problems of knowledge while simultaneously grappling with the knowledge of problems.

THE GENETICS OF INEQUALITY

My hope for this project is that it illustrates the linkages between disease, capitalism, U.S. race relations, and the organization and production of science. As a study of diabetes, the larger project links the politics of sugar, both blood glucose and cane/beet varieties, to the colonial and thus racial histories that produce it. It examines the U.S.-Mexico border less as a geographic place than as a space of contested boundaries of identity and nation-statehood. This border story, like so many before it, illustrates, albeit in contemporary forms, the ways frontiers are created through racializations, the movement of people and the material and semiotic embodiments that sometimes counter and at other reinforce interethnic conflict.[17]

This book has also argued that DNA sampling for chronic disease within ethnoracial groups is a highly developed system of appropriation, classification, and technocratic governmentality. As such, the diabetes genetic enterprise may very well be a blueprint for bioprospecting worldwide. Characterized by enclosure of the material and symbolic aspects of the body, supported by the state, funded by multinational corporations, and carried out by a select group of experts in the name of some universal incontrovertible human good, the acquisition and commodification of DNA alienates donors from the social and political context of their lives and reproduces long-standing structural inequities. Symbolically, Judi's matter of fact "It's in our blood" reply demonstrates that the social and political determinants of disease are kept from the realm of our descriptions of diabetes etiology, even from those who convince us they know better. Instead, diabetes is seen and thus acted upon not only as biologically determined, but also as wedded to the purported biology of our ethnicity.

Sampling, it is argued, is the grossest form of surplus value accumulation yet invented by capital. In exchange for a few pens, a cotton bag, a monogrammed cup, and some life-saving glucose monitoring, people give their DNA. Meanwhile, mounting evidence exists that if all Mexicanas/os on the Texas-Mexico border had decent health care, access to a full complement of food, and time and space to exercise, they would not likely have diabetes in the first place.[18] Yet, we search for the genes because it is, as critics of genetic determinism have observed, one of the few options imaginable.[19] As a result, research in critical public health and critical epidemiology must perpetually compete with the emerging genetics stranglehold on explaining disease causality. Further, once Glaxo, Pfizer, Aventis, Squibb, or another launch its diabetes-fighting bioengineered drug with the bioethnically conscripted genetic samples funded by the ADA and the numerous branches of the NIH, the hegemony of genetic notions of curing and disease treatment will be further reinforced.

Finally, this "modest intervention"[20] illustrates that such genetic narrations of complex disease biology are profoundly social. Thus, the genetics of diabetes susceptibility among Mexicanas/os and other disadvantaged groups must be understood, at least for now, as genetic differences made meaningful by social, historical, and political processes that affect unevenly distributed rates of disease. In short, what the postgenomic disease gene enterprises "discover" are nothing less than the genetic manifestations of local biology. What they find are the genetics of inequality.

Epilogue

As this book goes to press, the polygene discovery featured herein has failed to be replicated by other scientists. The preponderance of evidence points toward some evolutionary significance, but the association with type 2 diabetes susceptibility remains elusive. Nora is a sought-after speaker on methodological matters, and her message is always the same: "Proceed with care and with caution." Diabetes genes have been reported in Icelandic populations that do not rely upon racializations or "admixture."[1] Whether these findings stand the test of confirmation, replication, or the weaknesses that result from sociocultural black box effects, remains to be seen.[2]

The race debates continue, and the attempts to find genetic contributions to chronic health inequities of minority groups runs relatively unhampered.[3] Further, the theoretical rationale for ethnic-specific genes for diabetes, particularly the thrifty genotype hypothesis, has been challenged, and the fields of epigenetics, systems biology, and fetal origins have steadily been uncovering evidence in favor of their approaches to chronic disease disparities.[4] In spite of this, the moment, methods, and myopia of chronic disease genetics remain in full force.

Glossary

ACTANT (ACTOR): A term that reflects a central tenet in actor network theory, which states that humans are not the only relevant actors in the social world. In this way, "actant" expands the term "actor" in order to include the role of objects and non-humans in the production of social phenomena.

ACTOR NETWORK THEORY: A method of inquiry that does not limit in advance the types of beings populating the social world or the shape, size, heterogeneity, and combination of associations related to a particular topic under investigation. It allows the researcher to follow actants (actors) as they continually create new associations.

ADMIXTURE: The conglomeration of genetic material purportedly present in specific human groups due to the interbreeding of two or more groups often ethnoracially labeled. It is based on the assumption that distinct racial groups exist because they were geographically isolated from one another.

ADMIXTURE-SUSCEPTIBILITY HYPOTHESIS: The notion that members of admixed groups possess genetic material that makes them more susceptible to particular diseases than (pure) members of major racial groups.

ALLELE: The alternative form of a gene or DNA sequence that occurs at a given location on a chromosome. Some loci have only one allele, some have two, and some have many alternative forms. Alleles occur in pairs, one on each chromosome.*

BIOBANKS: Places where biological material and health-related information of individuals of a given population are stored for the purposes of medical and genetic research.

Note: Definitions marked with an asterisk are taken from the American Anthropological Association, Race: Are We So Different? resource glossary, http://www.understandingrace.org/resources/glossary.html.

BIOCAPITAL: A form of capital that involves turning biomaterial into a commodity with both material and symbolic value.

BIOETHNIC CONSCRIPTION: The process whereby the social origins of human difference are folded in to a biogenetic or clinical claim.

BIOETHNICITY: Refers to the resultant product of the ways ethnicity comes to be constructed as meaningful for scientific research. Bioethnicity emphasizes that biological races do not exist and that ethnicity is conscripted into biological science stripped of its social meaning and origin.

BIOGENETIC (BIOGENESIS): The claim that biology is the origin of what is in fact a complex phenomenon.

BIOLOGICAL DETERMINISM: The philosophy or belief that human behavior and social organization are fundamentally determined by innate biological characteristics, so that differences in behavior within and between groups are attributed to genetic variation rather than influences of environment, learning, or social arrangements.*

BIOLOGICAL FUNCTIONALISM: The tendency in the biological sciences to describe physiological structures and processes in utilitarian terms.

BIOPOLITICS (GOVERNMENTALITY): Biopolitics posits that modern governance operates through biopower, which is the organization of power over life centered on two sites: the individual body and the population. The individual body is disciplined to fit the norm through various methods (i.e., routine) at institutions like schools, hospitals, and prisons. Populations are regulated through the use of statistical information (i.e., life expectancy and mortality rates).

BIOREDUCTIONISM: Process whereby a complex phenomenon (e.g., disease) is presented strictly in biological terms.

BIOSOCIALITY: Describes a type of sociality and individual identities that have resulted from information made possible by genetic technologies.

BIOVALUE: Value generated through the exchange of biological material and information, which results in various forms of professional wealth in the field of genetics.

BLACK BOX: A term used in social and cultural studies of science to refer to taken-for-granted assumptions which are left (oftentimes deliberately) unquestioned and unexamined.

CELL: The smallest unit of life. Our human bodies are composed of more than 100 trillion cells. Inside the cell membrane is the nucleus. The cell nucleus is surrounded by cytoplasm.*

CHROMOSOME: Long strands of DNA found inside the cell nucleus. Human cells each contain 23 pairs of chromosomes, inherited from our parents.*

CLASSIFICATION: The ordering of items into groups on the basis of shared attributes. Classifications are cultural inventions and different cultures develop different ways of classifying the same phenomena (e.g., colors, plants, relatives, and other people).*

CLINE: A gradual, continuous change in a particular trait or trait frequency over space.*

COMPLEX TRAIT: A physical trait affected by more than one loci, which interact with environmental conditions. Most studied human traits are complex (e.g., height, body size, and skin color).*

CULTURAL CONSTRUCT: An idea or system of thought that is rooted in culture. It can include an invented system for classifying things or for classifying people, such as a racial system of classification.* .

CULTURE: The full range of shared, learned, patterned behaviors, values, meanings, beliefs, ways of perceiving, systems of classification, and other knowledge acquired by people as members of a society; the processes or power dynamics that influence whether meanings and practices can be shared within a group or society.*

DIABETOGENESIS: The factors that contribute to the onset of diabetes.

DNA (DEOXYRIBONUCLEIC ACID): The molecule that encodes heredity information composed of four base pairs of proteins. Base pairs constitute the rungs of the DNA ladder, which are composed of four bases in pairs that specify genetic instructions: adenine (A), thymine (T), guanine (G), and cytosine (C). "A" always pairs with "T", and "G" always pairs with "C".*

DOMINANT ALLELE: An allele that masks the effect of the other allele (which is recessive) in a heterozygous genotype.*

EPISTEMIC (OR KNOWLEDGE-CENTERED) APPROACH: An approach designed to examine the making and effects of policies within and beyond the state. It focuses on uncovering how the "truths" that underlie particular policies came into existence.

EPISTEMOLOGICAL CRITIQUE: A type of critique that challenges settled ways of thinking and conceptualization. It is an analytical strategy that allows other cultural realities to lie alongside our own in order to gain a more adequate understanding of the process through which concepts become taken-for-granted truths.

ESSENTIALISM: The idea that all things have an underlying or true essence. Racial essentialists argue that all members of a specific racial group share certain basic characteristics or qualities that mark them as inherently different from members of other racial groups.*

ETHNICITY: An idea similar to race that groups people according to common origin or background. The term usually refers to social, cultural, religious, linguistic, and other affiliations although, like race, it is sometimes linked to perceived biological markers. Ethnicity is often characterized by cultural features, such as dress, language, religion, and social organization.*

ETHNORACE/ETHNORACIAL: A term used to describe practices that draw from both ethnic and racial categories.

EUGENICS: From Greek *eugenes* meaning wellborn. The eugenics movement of the late nineteenth and early twentieth centuries sought to "improve" the human species and preserve racial "purity" through planned human breeding. Eugenicists supported antimiscegenation laws and more extreme measures such as sterilization.*

FOUNDER EFFECT: A type of genetic drift that occurs when all individuals in a population trace back to a small number of founding individuals. The small size of the founding population may result in allele frequencies very different from those of its original population. Examples of populations exhibiting founder effect include the French Acadians, the Amish, and the Hutterites.*

GENE: A unique combination of bases (see DNA) that creates a specific part of our body.*

GENE FLOW: A mechanism for evolutionary change involving genetic exchange across local populations. Gene flow introduces new alleles into a population and makes populations more similar genetically to one another.*

GENETIC DISTANCE: An average measure of relatedness between populations based on various traits. Genetic distances are used for understanding effects of genetic drift and gene flow, which should affect all loci to the same extent.*

GENETIC DRIFT: A mechanism for evolutionary change resulting from the random fluctuations of gene frequencies (e.g., from one generation to the next). In the absence of other evolutionary forces, genetic drift results in the eventual loss of all variation. See founder effect.*

genetic EPIDEMIOLOGY: The use of genetics to understand disease in populations.

GENETIC epidemiology: The use of populations to understand the genetics of disease.

GENETIC MARKERS: An identifiable physical location on a chromosome used to (a) look for genes known or suspected to be implicated in disease, and (b) to identify individuals or sort humans into groups.

GENETICS: The study of human heredity, its mechanisms and related biological variation. Heredity may be studied at the molecular, individual (organism), or population level.*

GENOME: One complete copy of all the genes and DNA for a species.*

GENOTYPE: The genetic endowment of an individual from the two alleles present at a given locus. See phenotype. The precise sequence of nucleotide base pairs.*

HAPLOTYPE: A series or combination of closely linked bits of genetic material usually inherited together.

HAPMAP: An international research effort to find genes associated with human diseases and those associated with response to pharmaceutical agents.*

HARDY-WEINBERG PRINCIPLE: The stable proportion of genotype frequencies that are the consequence of random mating in the absence of the genetic mutation, flow and drift.

HETEROZYGOUS: The two alleles at a given locus are different.*

HOMOZYGOUS: Both alleles at a given locus are identical.*

HUMAN GENOME DIVERSITY PROJECT: An international project that sought to understand the diversity and unity of the entire human species.

HUMAN GENOME PROJECT: An international research effort to sequence and map the human genome, all of the genes on every chromosome. The project was completed in 2003.*

IN SILICO: Anything reduced to data sets, transmitted electronically, and run through software programs.

INSTITUTIONAL RACISM: The embeddedness of racially discriminatory practices in the institutions, laws, and agreed upon values and practices of a society.*

INTERPELLATION (HAILING): A concept used to describe how individuals become subjected to the rules of the established order by behaving in accordance with the directives of a figurative authority or dominant norms.

LOCUS: The location of a particular gene or DNA sequence on a chromosome.*

MENDELIAN INHERITANCE PATTERN: The inheritance pattern based upon a single dominant or recessive allele at one location on a chromosome.

MUTATION: A mechanism for evolutionary change resulting from a spontaneous change in the base sequence of a DNA molecule.*

NUCLEOTIDES: DNA contains one of four nucleotide bases: adenine, cytosine, guanine, or thymine. Genotyping reveals the precise sequence of nucleotides.

ONTOLOGICAL: Inquiry about or concerning what exists, what is, the nature of being, and relationships between fundamental categories of things. E.g., What is "race"?

PHENOTYPE: The observable or detectable characteristics of an individual organism. A person's phenotype includes easily visible traits such as hair or eye color as well as abilities such as tongue rolling or curling.*

POLYGENE: Any two or more bits of genetic material whose inheritance pattern and action work together. As distinct from a single-gene Mendelian inheritance pattern.   .

POLYMORPHISM: A discrete genetic trait in which there are at least two alleles at a locus having frequencies greater than 0.01.*

RACE/RACIAL: A recent idea created by western Europeans following exploration across the world to account for differences among people and justify colonization, conquest, enslavement, and social hierarchy among humans. The term is used to refer to groupings of people according to common origin or background and is associated with perceived biological traits. Among humans there are no races except the human race. In biology, the term has limited use, usually associated with organisms or populations that are able to interbreed. Ideas about race are culturally and socially transmitted and form the basis of racism, racial classification, and often complex racial identities.*

RACIAL CLASSIFICATION: The practice of classifying people into distinct racial groups based on certain characteristics such as skin color or geographic region, often for the purpose of ranking them based on believed innate differences between the groups.*

RACIAL IDENTITY/ETHNORACIAL IDENTITY: This concept operates at two levels: (1) self-identity or conceptualization based upon perceptions of one's race and (2) society's perception and definition of a person's race. Ethnoracial is a term used to describe classificatory practices that draw from both ethnic and racial categories.*

RACIALIZATION: The process by which individuals and groups of people are viewed through a racial lens using a socially invented racial framework. Racialization is often referred to as racialism.*

RACIAL PROFILING: The use of race (and often nationality or religion) to identify a person as a criminal suspect or potential suspect. Racial profiling is one of the ways that racism is manifested and perpetuated.*

SICKLE-CELL ANEMIA: A genetic disease that occurs in a person homozygous for the sickle-cell allele, which alters the structure of red blood cells, giving it a "sickled" shape. These abnormally shaped red blood cells are less efficient in transporting oxygen throughout the body, which can cause pain and organ damage.*

SINGLE-NUCLEOTIDE POLYMORPHISMS (SNP; PRONOUNCED "SNIP"): A single base pair within a DNA sequence that can vary among individuals. An example of a SNP is the change from A to T in the sequences AATGCT and ATTGCT.*

SITUATED KNOWLEDGE: An account or narrative that makes explicit the multiple factors that contribute to knowledge claims made by the author in order to allow the reader to adequately evaluate them. It is based on the notion that true objectivity in all forms of knowledge production is an impossibility.

SUBJECTIFICATION (SUBJECTIVITY): Foucault's theory of the process through which various institutions (i.e., prisons) create subject positions (i.e., the prisoner) which are constituted by particular notions of normality. These institutions, through various methods (i.e., routine), discipline individuals to fit the norm. Through experience with these disciplinary practices, these norms become internalized to such an extent that individuals continue to behave and expect others to behave within the norm even when no authority figure is present. Each individual occupies a myriad of subject positions, and his or her subjectivity is the sum total of these subject positions.

TAXONOMY: The science of describing and classifying organisms. Taxa/taxon are units or a unit of classification.*

THRIFTY GENOTYPE HYPOTHESIS: This unproven hypothesis was proposed by James Neel in 1962 as an explanation for the increased prevalence of obesity, and by extension diabetes, in contemporary society. Neel argued that during 99.9 percent of human existence we existed as hunter-gatherers who experienced frequent cycles of alternating feast and famine. As a result we developed a genotype exceptionally efficient in the absorption, storage, or utilization of nutrients, which has now become maladaptive in a context of sustained energy (calorie) surplus. The initial form of the hypothesis was not racialized but was, instead, an attempt to explain the sudden rise in diabetes in the modified social environments of the modern world.

TOTIONTOLOGICAL: The concept that an object is not ontologically fixed. At different moments and under various circumstances a single object has the potential to be very different things.

TRAIT: A characteristic or aspect of a phenotype or genotype.*

WET LAB: In the biological sciences, a wet lab identifies the place where standard experiments using biological material take place, as opposed to dry labs where computer analysis occurs.

Notes

PREFACE

1. Karen Taussig, Rapp, and Heath 2003; and Rapp, Heath, and Taussig 2001.

2. Permission to conduct research is but one of the many institutional hurdles that ethnography in organizations entails.

3. Montoya and Kent 2011.

4. Rabinow 2005.

5. Haraway 1988.

6. Ibid.

7. Nader 1972. For other exemplar of ethnographic projects that involve the study of the powerful see Yanagisako 2002, Marcus 1988, Ong 1992, Emily Martin 1994, and Traweek 1988.

8. Ginsburg 2006.

9. Ibid., 491.

10. Zavella 1991.

11. Benjamin 1969, cited in Kim Fortun 2006.

12. Wagner 2001, Strathern 1991.

13. Gupta and Ferguson 1997: 35.

14. Haraway 1988.

15. See Maurer 2005, Strathern 1991, Wagner 2001, and Keane 2003.

16. Kim Fortun 2006.

17. Wiegman 2000.

18. Cf. Morgan 2001: 229.

INTRODUCTION

1. Nelson 2008 and Tallbear 2008.

2. In this book, I will keep race and ethnicity bundled because they are used together in the medico-scientific practices under discussion. "Ethnoracial" will be used as an unmarked term for both race and ethnicity until its more complete analysis in the last chapters of this book.

3. See Bonilla et al. 2005; Evans et al. 2006; Guo, Roettger, and Shih 2006; Beaver et al. 2009; and McHughen et al. 2009. The list of physical, behavioral, and clinical phenomena claimed to have genetic associations is extensive. See Montoya and Kent 2010 and Montoya and Howard 2008 for critical responses to associations between conditions that problematically implicate "race."

4. Greenhalgh 2008: 15.

5. Collins et al. 2003.

6. Palsson 2007.

7. Ibid., 5.

8. The terms "discover" and "cause" reference the usage by the scientists under investigation. This project will critically engage and show the consequences of the genetic determinism this usage implies. See Hubbard 1990; Hubbard and Wald 1993; and Lewontin, Rose, and Kamin 1984.

9. Centers for Disease Control and Prevention 2000.

10. Chaufan 2008. The title of the edited volume "Diabetes as a Disease of Civilization: The Impact of Culture Change on Indigenous Peoples" unfortunately privileges as "civilized" the social dislocations that underlie diabetes among indigenous peoples in North America. An alternative framing could be what Weiss and colleagues term "New World syndrome," which more clearly indicts the "New World" even if his use of the word "new" privileges the temporality of European conquest.

11. Centers for Disease Control and Prevention 2000.

12. Ibid., 2.

13. Complete list: University of Lund-Sweden, University of Texas, University of Pittsburg, National Institutes of Health, University of Michigan, Wake Forest University, Glaxo Smith Kline, Southwest Foundation for Biomedical Research, Virginia Mason University, University of Chicago, Institut National de la Santé et de la Recherche Médicale–France, Institut de Biologie de Lille–France, Joslin Diabetes Center, John L McClellan Veteran's Administration, Peninsula Medical School–UK, Institute Pasteur de Lille–France, Medical College of Wisconsin, Steno Diabetes Center–Sweden, University of Utah, Exeter University–UK, Royal London Hospital–UK, American Diabetes Association, Karolinska Institute–Sweden, University of Maryland, Oxford University–UK, University of Colorado, University of Cambridge–UK, Washington University, University of Michigan, Malmo University–Sweden, Newcastle University–UK, University of California–Los Angeles.

14. Ong and Collier 2005: 4.

15. Rabinow 2005.

16. Foucault 1991.

17. See Flyvbjerg 2001 (139) and Montoya and Kent 2011 for a description of a dialogical approach in research.

18. Riles 2006: 63.

19. Jasanoff 2004.

20. Ibid., 38.

21. Ibid., 14.

22. Hall 2002.

23. Jasanoff 2004: 275.

24. Stocking 1968.

25. Rabinow and Dan-Cohen 2005.

26. See Rabinow's description of "contending logoi" (2005: 51), which I take to mean contending cosmologies or sociocultural logics and their institutional apparatuses.

27. Subramanian et al. 2001.

28. Latour 1988.

29. Those interviewed were the director of research, director of genetics, biostatistician—Glaxo; geneticist, biostatistician, molecular biologist, physician, post doctoral fellows—University of Chicago; statistician—University of Michigan; epidemiologist, population geneticist, geneticist, public health workers—University of Texas; geneticists, public health workers, statisticians, physicians, post doctoral fellows—Exeter; population geneticist—Instituto Nacional de Nutrición, Salvador Zubiran; geneticist—Universidad Nacional Autonomia de Mexico; and physician—Hospital de Los Niños, Mexico.

30. ADA 1998, 1999, 2000; ADA—Genetics of Type Two Diabetes 1999; American Society of Human Genetics 1999.

31. See Haraway 1989; see also Goodman, Heath, and Lindee 2003. Operating at the confluence of biology and society, bioethnicity recognizes that distinct biological races do not exist in humans and that all knowledge derived from racialized populations is in fact the social histories and life conditions of those populations pressed into service of biomedical discourse. See the conclusion of this book for a full explication.

32. E.g., Hanson ct al. 1998; Gilroy 1991; Gregory and Sanjek 1994; and Omi and Winant 1996.

33. Gould 1981; Lewontin 1972; Lewontin, Rose, and Kamin 1984; Marks 1996b, 1998; and Montagu 1997.

34. Marks 1998: 4.

35. Duster 2002.

36. Ibid., 69.

37. See Osborne and Feit 1992 for an early iteration of these debates.

38. Duster 1990.

39. R. Hahn, Mulinare, and Teutsch 1992.

40. R. Hahn, Wetterhall, and Burnett 2002.

41. Goodman 1997.

42. Schulman et al. 1999.

43. Ibid., 622.

44. Institute of Medicine 2002.

45. Schwartz 2001, Nature Genetics 2000, Goodman 2001, Duster 2001a, and Chaturvedi 2001.

46. Tang et al. 2005.

47. See the Social Science Research Council Race and Genomics Forum, http://raceandgenomics.ssrc.org/, for a thorough response to these and other populist positions in support of racialized science.

48. Reardon 2001.

49. See, for instance, the Genographic project, https://genographic.national-geographic.com/genographic/index.html, and the International HapMap project, http://www.hapmap.org/ (last accessed March 26, 2009). There are also numerous biobank projects around the globe.

50. Reardon argues that to resolve the controversies within the Human Genome Diversity Project would require that all involved "do the work of sorting through the scientific and social/ethical issues raised by any organized effort to study human genetic differences" (2001: 381).

51. Reardon 2001: 363.

52. See also Hans Jörg Rheinberger 2000 for an insightful analysis of the connection between genotype and phenotype.

53. Cavalli-Sforza, Menozzi, and Piazza 1994; Mitchell 1993; and Molnar 1998.

54. Molnar 1998: 33.

55. González Burchard, Ziv et al. 2003 and Risch et al. 2002.

56. Graves 2001.

57. Harrison 1995: 65.

58. Templeton 1998.

59. Lewontin et al. 1984 and Serre and Paabo 2004. In an erudite and timely attempt at an interdisciplinary statement, Lee et al. 2008 outline the guiding principles on using geographically defined racial categories in the scientific characterization of human difference.

60. The full statement is available as an electronic document, http://www.aaanet.org/stmts/raceapp.htm, accessed May 22, 2003.

61. Weiss and Terwilliger 2000.

62. See, for example, Institute of Medicine 2003. In 2003, a proposition in California by a University of California regent, Ward Connerly, sought to eliminate racial and ethnic recordkeeping from most government agencies. This kind of "color-blind" policy capitalizes upon the rhetoric of fairness at the expense of the consequences of persistent unequal treatment.

63. Nature, Genetics 2000: 98.

64. Boas 1940.

65. Montagu 1997; Lewontin 1972; Lewontin, Rose, and Kamin 1984; and Marks 1995.

66. Lewontin, Rose, and Kamin 1984.

67. Haraway 1988, 1989; Schneider and Ingram 1993; and Harding 1986, 1993.

68. Duster 1990 and Krieger 2003, 1999.

69. Cavalli-Sforza 1994 and Cartmill 1998.

70. Omi and Winant 1994 and Arendt 1958.

71. Omi and Winant 1994.

72. E.g., Haraway 1991, Gilroy 1991, Haraway 1989, Harrison 1995, Wilson 1980.

73. See also De Genova and Ramos-Zayas 2003 and De Genova 2005, 2006.

74. Callon and Latour 1981, Callon 1986, and Latour 1987.

75. Fujimura 1996.

76. See Law 1999, Strathern 1999, and Latour 1999 for critiques of the various unexamined assumptions within actor network theory.

77. Latour 1987 and Fujimura 1996.

78. Haraway 1997: 35.

79. Epstein 2007.

80. Scheper-Hughes and Lock 1987: 8.

81. Ibid., 23.

82. Wilkinson 1992 and Williams and Collins 1995.

83. Cooper and David 1986 and Krieger and Fee 1994b.

84. Cooper and David 1986: 111.

85. Krieger and Fee 1994a: 272.

86. R. Hahn 1992, Ahdieh and R. Hahn 1996, and Osborne and Feit 1992.

87. R. Hahn 1992.

88. Just a few of which include Anzaldúa 1987, Batalla Bonfil 1996, R. Rosaldo 1997, Vélez-Ibáñez 1996, Flores and Benmayor 1997, and Canclini 1993.

89. According to the U.S. Census projections, by 2010 there will be more than 47 million "Hispanics" in the country, representing 15.5 percent of the population. In 2007, according to the census, there were 39 million blacks in the United States. These are conservative figures, since a statistically significant proportion of immigrant and low-income people in the United States are undercounted, and "Hispanics" and "blacks" are disproportionately represented in these categories. See http://www.census.gov/population/www/socdemo/hispanic/hispanic.html, and http://www.census.gov/population/www/socdemo/race/black.html (accessed October 17, 2010).

90. See for example, Fisher 2009.

91. Greenhalgh 2008: 16.

92. Hubbard 1990 and Hubbard and Wald 1993.

93. Hubbard 1990.

94. Hubbard and Wald 1993.

95. Lippman 1993.

96. Lewontin, Rose, and Kamin 1984.

97. Boas 1940: 34.

98. Cartmill 1998.

99. Ibid., 656.

100. See Blaffer Hrdy 1986 and Fausto-Sterling 1989, 1985. Blaffer Hrdy argues that theories of sexual selection in primatology constructed males as aggressive and females as coy because the male researchers saw what they were predisposed to see. In examining the work of female researchers, Blaffer Hrdy shows how the women researchers interpreted the behaviors very differently. For example, female primates were not coy (as the male researchers hypothesized),

but rather selective. They were not monogamous and controlled by the alpha males but instead were promiscuous, sneaking off to mate with males outside of the band. Fausto-Sterling (1985) showed how an artificial research environment was created for the science of embryology to advance. She argues that in embryology, the removal of the developing organism from its environmental context and the placement of the nucleus at the head of developmental control hierarchy have enabled the creation of chimeric organisms, genetic engineering, and clones. Such practice of solitary command and control fits, she asserts, within the development of weapons, the scientific management of labor, and the developmental prescriptions about the psychosocial norms for diverse North American populations in the early part of this century.

101. Haraway 2003 and Kleinman 1988.

102. Gravlee 2009.

103. Lock 1993: 39.

104. Goodman and Leatherman 1998 and Krieger 2005.

105. Taussig 2009: 16.

106. Ibid., 199.

107. Mol 2002: 146.

108. Serres 1980, 1994.

109. Hacking 1999: 53.

110. Haraway 1988 and Strathern 1991.

111. Strathern 1991: 9.

112. Mol 2002.

113. In their fructuous work on the increasing strategic reliance upon bioscientific ideas of difference, Comaroff and Comaroff (2009) similarly note the ontological polyvalence of ethnicity. Cultural identity, they write, is "neither a synthesis of primordial essence nor instrumental self fashioning, rather it is both ascriptive and instrumental. Both innate and constructed. Both blood and choice" (72).

114. Haraway 1991.

115. My thanks to Erin Koch and Peter Donovan for helping me clarify the conceptual allegory between stem cell totipotency and totiontological properties of race as here configured.

116. Palsson's (2008: 217) parallel between the presumption of insular genomes and the cultural islands presumed in some cultural anthropology evokes some of the tensions through which I imagine this discussion must traverse.

117. I borrow this usage of the term "lively" from Sunder Rajan (2006) to refer to the ways cultural forms within the life sciences are deeply adept at taking on a life of their own. That is, the authorizing epistemological maneuver is to conceal the conditions that enabled the production of technoscientific cultural forms.

118. Arendt 1958 and Omi and Winant 1996.

119. Duster 2001a, Lewontin et al. 1984, and Hubbard 1990.

120. Cartmill 1998.

121. WHO 2008.

122. Sankar 2006.

123. Duster 1990.

124. Lock 1993.
125. See, for example, Lock's erudite analysis of the nondeterministic promise of developmental systems theory (Lock 2005).
126. Scheper-Hughes and Lock 1987, Molina 2006, and Chavez 2008.
127. Haraway 1991.
128. Fujimura 1987.
129. Haraway 1991.
130. Appadurai 1986 and Kopytoff 1986.
131. Haraway 1988.

CHAPTER 1

1. Foucault 1972: 49.
2. Collaborators in Utah provided the data set.
3. Hutterites, Amish, and Mennonites are three Anabaptist groups formed during the Protestant Reformation in the sixteenth century. Between 1874 and 1877, Hutterites migrated to North America from Russia and founded three colonies in South Dakota (see Hostetler and Enders Huntington 1967).
4. Many of Nora's collaborators had genotyping errors discernable through a Hardy-Wienberg test that measures the genotyping results with the expected frequency of homo- and heterozygosity given the mating pattern and general allele frequencies known for the population.
5. A cline is the gradual geographically distributed continuum of human genetic variation (cf. Serre and Pääbo 2004).
6. Griffiths et al. 1993.
7. See Duggirala et al. 2000, Hanson et al. 1998, Hegele et al. 2003, Imperatore et al. 2001, Mitchell et al. 2000, and A. Stern 1996.
8. See Cox et al. 1999, Duggirala et al 1999, Ehm et al. 2000, Elbein et al. 1999, Frayling et al. 2000, Ghosh et al. 1998, Hanis et al. 1996, Horikawa et al. 2000, Kong and Cox 1997, Permutt 2001, and Stern et al. 1996.
9. The rationale that scientists use is part of a long-standing but increasingly pointed debate about the use of race in genetics research. What is important to emphasize here is that the debate about race in science, some of which will be taken up in later chapters, requires an analysis that describes multiple literatures from within population sciences, human biology, genetics, and epidemiology while at the same drawing upon analyses from the social sciences and humanities. Not only does this require cross-disciplinary conceptual agility. It requires that each analysis and description be assessed for its particular use of the word "race." The concept is not self-evident, and analysts approach it in myriad ways drawing upon biosciences, social sciences, and history, often in differing ways. For three especially useful outlines of these debates see Abu El-Haj 2007; Fujimura, Duster, and Rajagopalan 2008; and Gravlee 2009.
10. Neel 1962.
11. See Zimmet 1997. See also Neel 1962, 1982.
12. For a complete discussion of the medical racialization of sickle-cell anemia, see Duster 1990; Tapper 1995, 1999; and Wailoo 2003.
13. Neel 1962; Neel 1982: 284.

14. Neel 1982: 290.

15. Paradies, Montoya, and Fullerton 2007.

16. Ibid.

17. Neel 1999: S3.

18. A. Stern 1999: S67.

19. The chromosomal location of a piece of genetic material provided through linkage analyses points the way for subsequent associational studies that scientists use to look for the presence of the gene material in other data sets from the same or alternate populations. Physiological research is required to see the biological mechanism of a particular protein once identified through linkage or other analytical means (see fig. 1).

20. "Nature Genetics" 2000.

21. DNA contains one of four nucleotide bases—adenine, cytosine, guanine, and thymine. It is the precise sequence of these nucleotides that genotyping reveals.

22. Linkage analysis is used to determine the chances of inheritance of two or more nucleotides together when there are no known, let alone dominant, alleles to track between generations—that is, when Mendelian inheritance patterns do not exist.

23. See chapter 5 for a discussion of how this admixture narrative was consciously suppressed by socially conscientious researchers aware of the antimiscegenation discourse skittering around their findings.

24. Duster 2001b: 8.

25. Fujimura 1996: 5.

26. Duster 2001b: 14.

27. Duster 1990.

28. Duster 2001b: 15.

29. Templeton 1998.

30. While this discussion refers to allele frequency estimates, there are numerous other technologies that are used to quantify the three or five races of man (see Fullwiley 2007a, 2007b; Tallbear 2008). I reference Templeton's candelabra model as a technical challenge to them all.

31. The out-of-Africa replacement hypothesis posits that anatomically modern humans dispersed out of Africa one hundred thousand years ago replaced the distinct "racial" lineages of *Homo erectus*.

32. Allelic variation, genetic distance, and population and haplotype trees are different techniques of grouping individuals of the same species by measuring "patterns and amount of genetic diversity found within and among human populations" (Templeton 1998: 633). For allelic variation, individuals are typed according to which genes they carry for certain known phenotypic traits such as blood type. Genetic distance converts allelic differences within and among populations into measurements of evolutionary divergence, that is, it measures genetic relatedness according to the time (distance) each population diverged from the other. Haplotype trees are measurements of specific patterns of genetic inheritance that plot ancestral mutational differences within and among populations.

33. Drift is the random changes in a population's genetic structure. Flow is the change in population structure attributable to breeding patterns.

34. Fullwiley 2007a, 2007b; Montoya 2007.
35. Fullwiley 2007a.
36. Fullwiley 2007b: 234.
37. Fullwiley 2007a.
38. Fullwiley 2008: 699.
39. Fujimura 1996.
40. Templeton 1998a; Fullwiley 2008.
41. Duster 2001b: 10; Marks 1995.
42. Duster 2001b: 15.
43. See Reverby's *Examining Tuskegee: The Infamous Syphilis Study and Its Legacy* (Chapel Hill: University of North Carolina Press, 2009) and James Jones's *Bad Blood* (New York: Free Press, 1981).
44. See M. Annette Jaimes, "American Racism: The Impact on American-Indian Identity and Survival," in Gregory and Sanjek, *Race*.
45. E.g., Risch et al. 2002, González Burchard et al. 2003, González Burchard et al. 2004, and González Burchard et al. 2005.
46. E.g., Horikawa et al. 2000, Shriver et al. 1997, Cooper et al. 2000, and Drysdale et al. 2000.
47. Fullwiley 2008: 298.
48. Bolnick 2008; Duster 2001b.
49. Fullwiley 2008: 706. Deborah Bolnick, for example, analyzed leading papers (Bamshad et al. 2003; Rosenberg et al. 2002, both of which rely upon a computer program called STRUCTURE (Pritchard et al. 2000). Bolnick compellingly demonstrates the ways researchers can predetermine the results of their genetic analyses by setting the program to find the number of groups researchers define. The results do not find the most likely number of groups, nor do the results reflect new groups in to which the markers and loci most closely sort. The structure program finds the number of groups researchers predetermine.
50. See Smay and Armelagos 2000.
51. Ibid., 20.
52. Rhine 1990.
53. Brues 1993, Hinkes 1993.
54. Norman Sauer 1992, Kenedy 1995.
55. Smay and Armelagos 2000: 22.
56. To name a few, Armelagos 1995; Goodman 1997; and Marks 1995, 1996, 1998.
57. Armelagos and Goodman 1998.
58. Smay and Armelagos 2000: 23.
59. See Cole (2007, 2001) for analyses of the use and abuse of fingerprinting as a way to positively identify someone.
60. See chapter 6 for a full discussion of Gary's and Nora's attempts to produce universally applicable genetic susceptibility models for diabetes.
61. American Anthropological Association 1998 in Duster 2001b.
62. Duster 2001b: 13.
63. Ibid., 17.
64. Gravlee 2009; Duster 2001b, 2002; Paradies, Montoya, and Fullerton 2007; Krieger 2005.

65. Marks 1996: 131.

66. In Condit 2007 we read of the ways journalists often overstate the role genes play in human variation and disease. Examining race and genetics as they appear in the press and surveys of lay people about the meanings of race and human variation as they pertain to disease risk, Condit compellingly demonstrates that genetic determinism is a dominant way of thought.

67. Bakhtin 1996 [1981], quoted in Fairclough 1995.

68. Kress 1988, quoted in Fairclough 1995: 7.

69. Goodman, Heath, and Lindee 2003.

70. Canguilhem 1966 [1991]

71. Haraway 2003: 111.

72. See Clifford 1988, Boas 1963 [1911], Benedict 1942, and Montagu 1997 [1942].

73. Templeton 1998, Fullwiley 2007b.

74. Fullwiley 2007a, 2007b; Kahn 2003, 2004, 2005.

75. Harrison 1995.

76. Omi and Winant 1994: 55.

77. Duster 2001a; Omi and Winant 1994.

78. Foucault 1972: 216.

79. Visweswaran 1998: 77.

80. Ibid., 79.

81. Gilroy 1994.

82. Visweswaran 1998: 78.

CHAPTER 2

1. The protection of the research subjects mandates that the exact location and identities of those involved in the diabetes enterprise remain anonymous in this book.

2. The Rio Grande runs in a southeasterly direction into the Gulf of Mexico. My use of "north" and "south" is relative rather than a true directional reference. Still, the "south" side receives the brunt of the afternoon sunshine, which in planning the office determined the locations of the two freezers.

3. Research protocols that test oral glucose tolerance require that five tubes of blood be taken every 30 minutes. Participants must remain catheterized for two hours. In between blood draws, with the catheter still in their arm, participants will be checked for levels of blood pressure, glucose, and triglycerides; will undergo an electrocardiogram; and will give a full family history.

4. See Acuña 1981, Almaguer 1994, De Genova 1998, and Montejano 1997. Prior to September 11, 2001, residents of Sun County sometimes crossed back and forth several times daily. Immediately following September 11, border security was tightened. Field staff did not report that this posed a problem for the sampling efforts.

5. Lower Rio Grande Valley Community Health Survey 2001 (Perkins et al. 2001).

6. Limón 1994: 16.

7. See Arreola 2002, Arreola and Curtis 1993, Maril 1989, and Truett and Young 2004.

8. Johannsen 1985: 24.

9. Cf. Acuña 1981, Almaguer 1994.

10. Montejano 1997.

11. Limón 1994: 24.

12. Marcus and Fischer 1986.

13. See Whitmarsh 2008 for the ways race and genetics are configured in asthma research in the Caribbean.

14. The *Wall Street Journal* sent its science writer to Sun County to write a special interest feature story about the economics of diabetes. The piece appeared in the spring of 2002 and was written by the reporter assigned to the biotechnology beat, demonstrating that the world of investment capital is always interested in frontiers of nations and of science.

15. In Fisher's (2009) critical assessment of clinical trial participation, Latinos are noted for their compliance with trial protocols, showing up for appointments and follow-up visits. So compliant, Fisher finds, that clinical trial managers argue that the increased participation rates of Latinos far outweighs the added cost of bilingual staff.

16. Corburn 2005 and Tesh 2001.

17. See chapter 5 for a discussion of sampling and commodification processes.

18. More ethnographic analyses of Mexicana professionals, paraprofessionals, and executives would enrich our understanding of a whole host of sociocultural phenomena and contexts.

19. See Checker 2005; Corburn 2005; Hale 2006, 2008; Sanford and Angel-Ajani 2006; Farmer 2005; Rylko-Bauer, Singer, and Willigen 2006; Montoya and Kent 2010; Morgan 2001; Minkler and Wallerstein 2003; and Cole and Foster 2001.

20. Jasanoff and Wynne 1998.

21. Corburn 2005: 64.

22. In addition to center staff, I spoke with practicing or retired doctors, lawyers, nurses, teachers, veterans, business owners, city planners, numerous service workers (retail, hospitality, agriculture), and public servants.

23. DuBois 1990.

24. M. E. Cotera 2005 and M. P. Cotera 1976.

25. Ruiz 1998: 145.

26. M. P. Cotera 1976, M. E. Cotera 2005, Limón 1994, Vargas 2007, Montejano 1997, Ruiz and Sanchez Korrol 2005, and Ruiz 1998.

27. El propósito de esta investigación es comprender porque se desalloran las complicaciónes de diabetes. Entiendo que este estudio es una extensión de los estudios del genético de diabetes en que participaba. Me doy cuenta que mi participación no significa que yo obtendré (o mi familia obtendrán) un beneficio inmediato. Sin embargo, puede permitir una comprensión mejor de como los genes contribuyen a diabetes y las complicaciones del ojo y así poder ayudar a quienes lo necesitan (translation in original).

28. Freire 1968, 1970; and Minkler and Wallerstein 2003.

29. See Freire 1968 and Montoya and Kent 2011. To be sure, ethnographically acquired material is every bit as fraught with ethical and political entanglements; however, these considerations have been amply taken up elsewhere. See Abu-Lughod 1991, Rosaldo 1974, and Behar and Gordon 1995.

30. Tutton 2007.

31. Lewontin 1991.

32. Additionally, Jezewski and Poss (2002) found that Mexicana/o participants in focus groups listed heredity as the primary cause of type 2 diabetes.

33. Althusser 1971: 149.

34. Ibid., 155.

35. Pierce 1996.

36. Epstein 2007.

37. Ibid., 15.

38. Ibid., 201.

39. Althusser 1971: 163.

40. Althusser 1971.

41. Farmer 1992, 1997.

42. Epstein 2007: 18.

43. Schneider and Ingram 1993.

44. Cole and Foster 2001; Pellow and Brulle 2005; Singer 2005, 2006; Bourgois and Bruneau 2000; Duster 1990.

45. Trostle and Sommerfeld (1996) and especially Trostle (2005) detail the concept of cultural epidemiology as the study of the ways locally structured meanings of illness are manifestly potent explanations of patterns of disease.

46. Pierce 1996.

47. Ibid., 679. See also Navarro 2004 for an analysis of how class relations are specifically avoided in research agendas in the United States.

48. Harvey 1990 and Marx 1976.

49. Krieger and Fee 1994a.

50. Ibid., 276.

51. Cooper and David 1986, Osborne and Feit 1992, Krieger and Fee 1994a, Williams and Collins 1995, and Wilkinson 1992.

52. Cain 2003: 192.

53. Ibid.

54. Nazroo 2003, van Ryn and Fu 2003, Harrell et al. 2003, and Williams et al. 2003. See also www.unnaturalcauses.org.

55. Hanh 1992, 1995; Hahn, Mulinare, and Teutsch 1992; and Inhorn and Whittle 2001.

56. Krieger and Fee 1994a and Krieger 2005.

57. Paradies, Montoya, and Fullerton 2007.

58. Ferguson 1994: 254–256.

CHAPTER 3

1. Gardner et al. 1984.

2. Montoya 2007.

3. Chakraborty and Weiss 1988.

4. As Nora's explanation reveals, homogeneity and population structure generally are a central feature of human genetic sciences writ large. For example, Mike Fortun's (2008) work on deCODE genetics in Iceland evinces similar scientific and popular concerns with population homogeneity. Although in the case of the Icelandic people, it is the science of homogeneity, or the lack of diversity, which is called upon to validate the homogeneity of the people. See especially Fortun's chapter 18.

5. Molina 2006, Briggs 2002, Simmons 2008, and Tapper 1995, 1999.

6. Gould 1993, Graves 2001, Boas 1940, Montagu 1997.

7. Basu et al. 2008, Tang et al. 2006.

8. Basu et al. 2008.

9. Templeton 2003, Bolnick 2008, Graves 2001.

10. Fullwiley 2008. Admixture estimation is by no means the exclusive provenance of researchers working with and on Latino populations. Estimates of personal or groupwide genetic admixture, whatever one's ethnoracial identification, is increasingly ground zero in debates within recreational genomics, personalized medicine, legal claims, and forensics. See Fullwiley 2008, Nelson 2008, and TallBear 2007, 2008.

11. Menchaca 1993.

12. De León 1983.

13. Horsman 1998.

14. Ibid., 150.

15. Jacobson 1998: 157–158. See Haney López 1996 for a complete discussion of the legal construction of whiteness.

16. Brackette Williams 1995: 201.

17. See Allen 1994, Almaguer 1994, Dominguez 1986, Ignatiev 1995, Roediger 1991, and Sacks 1994.

18. See Rapp 1995 for a discussion of similar hereditary constructs in and through amniocentesis.

19. Lock 1993.

20. Lock 1993, 2005; Goodman 2001; and Krieger 2005.

21. Rapp 1999 and K. Taussig et al. 2003 offer additional examples of the ways biosociality is not an overdetermined process.

22. Foucault 1983.

23. Ibid., 208.

24. Ibid.

25. Escobar 1995.

26. Ibid., 10.

27. Yanagisako and Delaney 1995: ix–x.

28. B. Williams 1995: 232.

29. Scheper-Hughes and Lock 1987: 7.

30. Sunder Rajan 2006.

31. Rabinow 1992.

32. Foucault 1991.

33. See Mol 2002 for an in-depth examination of the ways medical practices ontologically configure the body and disease.

34. Rabinow 1996a: 99.

35. Miles and Brown 2003: 102.

36. Duster 1990.

37. For example, the Sun County data sets are central components of the ancestry informative markers for Mexicanos. See Tang et al. 2006, Basu et al. 2008, and González Burchard et al. 2005.

38. Knorr-Cetina 1999.

39. Hall 2002.

40. Cf. Fullwiley 2008.

41. Hall 2002.

42. Macpherson 1962 and Weber 2002.

43. Vélez-Ibáñez 1996.

44. Molina 2006.

45. Chavez 2001, 2008. For more information on hate groups and nativism in the United States, see the Southern Poverty Law Center http://www.splcenter.org/index.jsp, accessed March 26, 2009.

46. I thank Rayna Rapp for this important insight.

47. See Yanagisako and Delaney 1995 for their influential analyses on naturalization of social relations.

48. See, e.g., Frankenberg 1993, Lupton 1999, and Beck 1992.

49. Lupton 1999.

50. Frankenberg 1993, Williams and Collins 1995, Cooper and David 1986, and Krieger and Fee 1994a, 1994b.

51. See Trostle 2005, Goodman and Leatherman 2005, Krieger 2005, Gravlee 2009, Kuzawa 2007, Francis et al. 2002, Fausto-Sterling 2008, Wallace 2005, Jackson 2004.

52. Omi and Winant 1996.

53. Tapper 1999.

54. Burchell 1993.

55. Cf. Haraway 1997.

56. Chapter 5 examines the complex ways the polygene discovery was, and then later was not, framed as Mexican American. The *Nature Genetics* piece states that admixture is not the cause of the increased risk. And yet the increased frequency of the susceptibility haplotype in Mexican Americans over Europeans, 14 percent versus 4 percent, is a result of the increased frequency of the haplotype found in Native American—read genetically Asian—ancestry.

57. Gould 1981; Lewontin 1972; Lewontin, Rose, and Kamin 1984; Marks 1996, 1998; Templeton 1998a

58. A most recent manifestation of this is the U.S. Homeland Security's commitment to high-tech smart border enforcement. This policy and the U.S. Border Patrol's Operation Gatekeeper has made crossing the border more dangerous by pushing crossers to remote areas. This has resulted in hundreds of migrant deaths as a result of starvation, murder, dehydration, and crossing plans gone awry, including the suffocation in 2003 of migrants within a tractor-trailer in Texas.

59. Foucault 1991.

60. Yanagisako and Delaney 1995: 5.

61. Gupta and Ferguson 1997: 5.

62. Cf. Appadurai 1996.

63. Fausto-Sterling 1985, Haraway 1989, E. Martin 1987, and Schiebinger 1993.

64. M. Taussig 1992: 87.

65. See Bowker and Star (1999: 308–310) on the creation of bioscientific monsters.

66. Scheper-Hughes and Lock 1987: 30; and Taylor 2003.

67. Lock 1993.

68. Duster 1990.

69. Rabinow 1999: 25.

70. A person familiar with the operation cynically complained that Carl's research intentionally never includes treatment or prevention because it would ruin his natural experiment. Further research of social service professionals, health care workers, and nonparticipants might elicit additional criticisms but is beyond the scope of this book.

71. Helmreich 2003: 437.

72. See González Burchard et al. 2005, Risch et al 2002, Kittles and Weiss 2003.

73. Jasanoff 2004, Reardon 2005, Fujimura 1996.

CHAPTER 4

1. Haraway 1988: 18.

2. Haraway's (1988) notion of partiality applies here: to wit, incomplete and from a particular point of view.

3. Haraway 1988: 19.

4. Ibid.

5. Nora had recently secured lab space in a different department and building. The move was to have given her more autonomy from Gary, to be part of a promotion to associate professor, and would have given her a very large computational lab for postdoctoral fellows. However, before the space had been completed, other "collaborators" had chiseled away at her lab space.

6. Maurer 2005: 92.

7. Mauss 1990: 73.

8. I attended three American Diabetes Association meetings, a special ADA-sponsored genetics meeting, and the meetings for the American Society for Human Genetics, all in the United States. Collaborators attended meetings in Europe, Japan, and Mexico, but I did not follow them there.

9. As discussed in the introduction, I consider this book a collaborative project in its own right.

10. Diabetes education often is population specific. Its topic includes culturally appropriate blood glucose regulation techniques, screening and outreach strategies, and research on practitioner-patient interaction.

11. Meetings are also expensive. Registration fees for nonmembers at the time of this research were more than $400. These costs, plus the capital expenditures that enable the logistics of face-to-face meetings, definitely prohibit participation by researchers from Africa, Latin America, and India or others with less time and money.

12. Securing permission for a field site from scientists represents distinct challenges. Though increasingly common as ethnographers "study up" (Nader 1972), the particular kinds of veto power that scientists hold over their would-be ethnographic interlocutors is formidable.

13. This was 2002, before the completion of the human genome. The maps the consortium needed were finer grained and of higher quality, I was told, than those being used for the Human Genome Project.

14. McAfee 2003.

15. Beurton, Falk, and Rheinberger 2000; Haraway 1997; Lewontin 2000; Keller 2000; Goodman and Leatherman 1998; DeWitt and Scheiner 2004.

16. Star and Griesemer 1989; Bowker and Star 1999: 296.

17. Canguilhem 1991.

18. Rabinow 1999.

19. Marie-Angéle Hermitte, *Le sang et le driot: Essai sur la transfusion sanguine* (Paris: Editions du Seuil, 1996), 186, quoted in Rabinow 1999: 86.

20. Mexico, Sweden, the United Kingdom to name a few.

21. The consumption of ethnographic material by former research subjects or "native" subjects is not without precedent. Maurer 2005 discusses the implications of this in detail. Additionally, my own reading in 1986 of Paul Willis's (1977) *Learning to Labor* could be considered a moment of this. Similarly, the African Nuer people living in the United States are rumored to currently use the anthropological classic *The Nuer* by E. E. Evans-Pritchard (1940) as a way to represent their "culture" to younger generations.

22. I never had that discussion with Gary, at least not directly and not that day.

23. Rabinow 1996b.

24. Nora also recognizes that her work occurs within personal, scientific, and other social worlds. She agreed to my ethnographic fieldwork because I was a fellow scientist interested in seriously understanding her work. This will become clearer in chapter 6.

25. Haraway 1988: 19.

26. See Thacker 2004 for an excellent analysis of the ways biotechnology mediates lifeworlds.

27. Rheinberger 1994: 6. See also Jordinova 1989.

28. E. Martin 1994: 171.

29. See Haraway 1997.

30. Foucault's introduction to Canguilhem 1991: 16.

31. Marcus and Fischer 1986: x.

32. This thumbnail sketch of "discovery" is not complete. It is meant here to illustrate the shift from hormones to genes, and, more specifically, to illustrate the endurance of metaphors of structure and function within research.

33. Leys Stepan 1991 and Jordinova 1989.

34. Leys Stepan 1991: 368.

35. Haraway 1991.

36. Ibid., 18.

37. E. Martin 1994.

38. Haraway 1991, Leys Stepan 1991, Jordinova 1989, and E. Martin 1994.

39. Jordinova 1989.

40. The National Institute of Diabetes and Digestive and Kidney Disease, Diabetes Dictionary, http://diabetes.niddk.nih.gov/dm/pubs/dictionary/P-T.htm, accessed October 28, 2010.

41. Micklos and Freyer 1990: 4.

42. Ibid., 6.

43. Jordinova 1989.

44. See also Thacker 2004.

45. Shoelson, Lee, and Goldfine 2006.

46. E. Martin 1994.

47. Ong and Collier 2005.

48. Readers are directed to K. Weber 2009, Pollan 2006, Nestle 2002, Schlosser 2001, and Spero 2006 for analyses that detail the linkage between food production, overconsumption, and poor health.

49. Jasanoff 2004 and Reardon 2001.

50. Thacker 2004.

51. Ibid., 11.

52. Haraway 1988: 18.

53. Langford's (2002) trenchant analysis of Ayurveda demonstrates that physiological processes must always be anchored in social contexts and that docility is not an overdetermined semiotic implication.

54. See Heath et al. 1999.

55. Foucault 1991.

56. See NIH Roadmap: Accelerating Medical Discovery to Improve Health, http://nihroadmap.nih.gov/index.asp, accessed August 21, 2004, and Collins et al. 2003 for a vision of trans- and interdisciplinarity.

57. Haraway 1991: 181.

58. Bowker and Star 1999.

59. Ibid., 310.

60. See Chaufan 2008; Paradies, Montoya, and Fullerton 2007; and Schoenberg et al. 2005.

CHAPTER 5

1. Vélez-Ibáñez 1996: 7.

2. Lindenbaum 2001.

3. See Montejano 1997.

4. Fujimura and Fortun 1996: 168.

5. See Sunder Rajan 2006 for a discussion of the regimes of value in global biotechnology milieu.

6. Clarke and Fujimura 1992.

7. Garcia Canclini 1993: 69.

8. Tierney 2000.

9. Glenn 2002: 1.

10. See LaDuke 2005. See also Nature Genetics 2000.

11. In 2003, the membership of the AAA passed a referendum officially resolving and repudiating the claim that Neel and Chagnon started or abetted the lethal measles epidemic among the Yanomami.

12. Andrews and Nelkin 2001.

13. *Moore v. Regents of the University of California* was a landmark 1990 Supreme Court of California case wherein a commercial cell line was developed from a cancerous spleen removed from John Moore while Moore underwent surgery at UCLA Medical Center. Moore was not informed of the cell line and later sued the regents, his doctor, and the pharmaceutical firm that bought the patent. Moore lost the case. The court ruled that Moore had no right to any profits accrued from his discarded body parts.

14. Andrews and Nelkin 2001: 6.

15. Lock and Farquhar 2007.

16. Ibid., 13.

17. See Scheper-Hughes and Lock 1987; Hogle 1995, 1999; Cohen 1999; Sharp 2001; and Farmer 1997.

18. Kopytoff 1986.

19. Ibid., 64.

20. Latour and Woolgar 1986.

21. Marx 1976: 165.

22. This is, of course, an extension of Marx's definition of a commodity as an item "in which a specific amount of labor time is objectified and which therefore has an exchange value for a definite amount" (1976: 953).

23. Appadurai 1986: 17.

24. Ibid., 57.

25. In 2005, Mexico launched an ambitious race-based genome project. See Guerrero Mothelet and Herrera 2005.

26. Bourdieu 1977.

27. Appadurai 1986: 4.

28. Marx 1976 and Appadurai 1986.

29. Judi and her staff at the center are routinely thanked in the acknowledgments of many publications.

30. Rose and Novas 2005: 454.

31. E.g., Knoppers 1999.

32. See Strathern 1996.

33. Sunder Rajan 2003: 111.

34. Sunder Rajan 2003.

35. Franklin and Lock 2003, and Landecker 2000.

36. Helmreich 2008.

37. Ibid.

38. The Repository Web site reads: "The Coriell Cell Repositories provide essential research reagents to the scientific community by establishing, verifying, maintaining, and distributing cells cultures and DNA derived from cell cultures. These collections, supported by funds from the National Institutes of Health (NIH) and several foundations, are extensively utilized by research scientists around the world."

39. The patent section on Rational Drug Design reads: "The goal of rational drug design is to produce structural analogs of biologically active polypeptides or compounds with which they interact (agonists, antagonists, inhibitors, bind-

ing partners, etc.). By creating such analogs, it is possible to fashion drugs which are more active or stable than the natural molecules, which have different susceptibility to alteration or which may affect the function of various other molecules."

40. See also the book *Q and A* by Vikas Swarup (2005), and its Oscar-winning film version, *Slumdog Millionaire* (2008), written by Simon Beaufoy, directed by Danny Boyle and Loveleen Tandan, for a recent reenactment of the simulacra albeit in the Indian context.

41. Baudrillard 1988: 72.

42. Knoppers 1999.

43. Andrews and Nelkin 2001: 6.

44. See Andrews and Nelkin 2001 and Knoppers 1999. Also see Hayden 2003, 2007, and Parry 2004 for additional examples of failures of benefit sharing in other contexts.

45. Andrews and Nelkin 2001 and Knoppers 1999.

46. Strathern 1996: 27.

47. Fabian 2001: 51.

48. Hayden 2007.

49. Sunder Rajan 2006.

CHAPTER 6

1. Landecker 1999, 2000.

2. Ibid.

3. Landecker 2000: 62.

4. Bourdieu 1984: 2.

5. This remark was gathered for the research project "From Transplant Medicine to Tissue Engineering: Uses of Human and Animal Tissue," sponsored by the Greenwall Foundation, Linda F. Hogle, PI. My thanks to Linda Hogle for permission to use this quote.

6. Omi and Winant 1994.

7. Population estimates came from the U.S. Census Bureau. U.S. diabetic estimates were derived by multiplying the total population of whites by the prevalence estimates in my informant-collaborator's PHS grant application. Native Americans and Hispanics were estimated as 20 percent, equal to the highest in the 15–20 percent range of Mexican Americans, African Americans as 12 percent. Asians and Pacific Islanders were not calculated for this example.

8. Neel 1999.

9. Maugh 2000: A-1.

10. McDermott 1998.

11. Ibid., 1193.

12. Pettit 1993 and Hales and Barker 1992.

13. Hales and Barker 1992: 600.

14. Rasmussen 2001, Leon 2004, Benyshek 2005, Lock 2005, Francis et al. 2003, Francis et al. 2002.

15. Paradies, Montoya, and Fullerton 2007.

16. Auerbach and Krimgold 2001, Krieger 1999, Wilkinson 1992, Williams and Collins 1995, Cooper and David 1986, Schoenberg, Drew, Stoller et al. 2005.

17. See DiGiacomo 1999, Frankenberg 1993, Garro 1995, B. Hahn 1995, Gravlee 2009, Inhorn 1995, Rock 2003, Smith-Morris 2004, Hunt, Valenzuela, and Pugh 1998, Schoenberg, Drew, Stoller et al. 2005.

18. McDermott 1998, Lewontin 1991, Marks 1998, and Duster 2001a.

19. Relative to the original peoples of Mexico, the Taino of what is now called Puerto Rico were almost entirely eliminated. Since this statement, several studies claiming to quantify the percentage of European, African, and Native ancestry in Puerto Ricans have been published.

20. Farmer 1997, 1999.

21. For a discussion of the pragmatic uses of race by forensic anthropologists, see Smay and Armelagos 2000.

22. Fujimura 1996.

23. Farmer 1999.

24. Montejano 1997.

25. Taylor 1930, cited in Montejano 1997: 199.

26. Black, Markides, and Ray 2003; Kaufman and Cooper 2001; Kaufman, Cooper, and McGee 1997; Maty, Everson-Rose et al. 2005; Maty, Lynch, Raghunathan et al. 2008; Maty, Lynch, Balfour et al. 2002; Nader 1972; Oakes and Rossi 2003; Phelan et al. 2004; Raphael 2006; Rosmond 2004; Chaufan 2008.

27. Farmer 1999: 281.

28. Bowker and Star 1999.

29. Ibid.

30. Lock and Farquhar 2007: 489.

31. Lee, Mountain, and Koenig 2001: 37.

32. About a month earlier, Nora had preliminary data that suggested that it was the Anglo ancestry that triggered the susceptibility. However, as her analysis expanded, the polygene discovery transformed into the haplotype heterozygosity explanation. This underscores that scientific research is processual and provisional as early evidence and explanations are tested, discarded, and become the basis of new hypotheses.

33. Nature 2000: 98.

34. Gary and Nora et al. 2000 is the pseudonym for the polygene discovery paper discussed in chapter 2.

35. Haraway 1988: 591.

36. It is also possible that Gary knows the unstable foundation of a claim that relies upon biogenetic differentiation between human groups as they are currently labeled.

37. Amaryl: glimepiride has since been replaced by a new generation of drugs.

38. For a history and analysis of the mutual benefits inherent in the cooperation between academic and drug researchers, see John P. Swann, *Academic Scientists and the Pharmaceutical Industry* (Baltimore: Johns Hopkins University Press, 1988).

39. Chavez 2001: 41.

40. My thanks to Melanie Herzog, Edgewood College, for connecting the Amaryl advertisement's visual style to the broader context of art in Latin America.

41. Mintz 1985: xxiv.

42. See, for example, Duster's (2001) editorial in *The Chronicle of Higher Education* with regard to Bidil, a drug marketed as especially efficacious in African Americans. Alan Goodman (2001) has also examined the marketing of antacids as especially efficacious in Asians and Caucasians.

43. Subramanian, Adams, and Venter 2001.

44. Two colleagues in an art department confirmed my suspicion that Aventis's marketing firm, Tori Inc., knows exactly what it is doing. As one remarked, "Artists are trained to know what messages images convey." A drug marketing director further explained, "Our job is to translate clinical information into product promotional materials."

45. Hill 1993: 149–150.

46. See Bourdieu 1984 (255) on the ways intentionally breaking linguistic rules serves to reinforce the social position of dominant groups while perpetually fettering those who try to use language correctly.

47. Rabinow 1992.

48. Latour 1987 and Haraway 1997.

49. Nature 2000: 98.

50. See Epstein 2007 for an excellent analysis of the ways ethnic and racial peoples are conscripted into research apparatuses for the sake of the political values of inclusion.

51. Omi and Winant 1994.

52. Ibid., vi.

53. Haraway 1989, Harding 1993, Leys Stepan 1991, Nader 1996, and Schiebinger 1993.

54. Latour 1987, Fujimura 1996, and E. Martin 1992, 1994.

55. Hahn 1992; Hahn, Mulinare, and Teutsch 1992; Zuberi 2001.

CONCLUSION

1. Moore et al 2003: 15.

2. Bowker and Star 1999.

3. Cicourel 1964.

4. Bowker and Star 1999: 320.

5. Durkheim and Mauss 1963: 8.

6. See Helmreich 2008 for an illustrative examination of the use of the concept of biocapital. My use here clusters with those that address the alienation of bodily substances. See especially Franklin and Lock 2003, and Lock 2001.

7. Horsman 1998 and Menchaca 1993.

8. González Burchard et al. 2003.

9. I am indebted to the participants of the Genetics, Admixture, and Identity Workshop sponsored by the Wenner Gren Foundation and the British Academy, for making this clear to me over a few days of discussion. The February 2009

workshop was organized by Sarha Gibbon, Monica Sans, and Carlos Ventura Santos. See also Montoya 2007.

10. Zuberi 2001: 102.

11. Similarly, Gravelle (1998) concludes that the ecological fallacy exists whenever associations found at the population level are inferred at the level of the individual. This is known as the "aggregation problem" in econometrics. Gravelle argues that the primary weaknesses in social epidemiology are just such statistical artifacts created through the ecological fallacy.

12. Kahn 2006.

13. Fullwiley (2008: 729 n. 9) makes a similar point about ancestry informative markers, noting that the theoretical assumptions of race long preceded the invention of genetic technologies.

14. Duster 2001b.

15. Macpherson 1962.

16. As collaboraeur, I also benefit from the broader concern with race in science in the genomic era because of the past abuses of people of color. I am as indebted to the sociopolitical conditions of Mexicanas/os along the border as Carl is. This should not be read as apologia or reflexive preoccupation. The degree to which it does apologize for a science that reaffirms racial prejudice is the degree to which the double standard of accountability in science exists. On the one hand, a social analyst can critique scientific practices labeling the practitioners as racist with impunity. On the other hand, a social analyst who points out the good intentions of scientists is labeled apologetic or, worse, uncritical. As one early reviewer of this manuscript remarked, "[Gary and Nora] strike me as mushy American liberals whose ostensibly non or anti-racist stance perpetuates the machinery of racism." While I partially accept the conclusions of this reviewer, the labeling presumes a privileged corner on the truth of the matter. Such presumption sunders the situated claims this book makes.

17. Molina 2003, 2006; A. Stern 1999; Kraut 1994; Romero 1997.

18. See Garro 1995, Health and Human Services 2001, McDermott 1998, J. Martin et al. 2000, Mi et al. 2000, Schulz et al. 2005, Marmot 2005.

19. Hubbard 1990; Hubbard and Wald 1993; Lewontin, Rose, and Kamin 1984.

20. See Heath 1998 for a discussion of modesty in ethnographic interventionism with our scientific interlocutors.

EPILOGUE

1. Grant et al. 2006.

2. Mike Fortun's 2008 work on deCODE Genetics Inc., from whence this finding originates, and Icelandic biotech more broadly, could be read as an acute contextualization of this finding similar to the ways the polygene finding has been situated in this book. Although inflected with the speculative promises of high-tech industry in Iceland and thus different from the present case, Fortun 2008 demonstrates that local conditions matter a great deal in understanding genomics. See also Taussig 2009 and Palsson 2007.

3. See Braun et al. 2007; Bolnick et al. 2007; Payne, Royal, and Kardia 2007; and Fujimura, Duster, and Rajagopalan 2008.

4. See Paradies, Montoya, and Fullerton 2007; Lock 2005; Francis et al. 2006; Gluckman et al. 2008; Sauer, Heinemann, and Zamboni 2007; Kitano 2002; Hood et al. 2004; Kuzawa 2007; and Benyshek 2005.

Bibliography

AAA. 1998. American Anthropological Association Statement on Race. *American Anthropologist* 100: 712–713.

Abu El-Haj, Nadia. 2007. The Genetic Reinscription of Race. *Annual Review of Anthropology* 36(1): 283–300.

Abu-Lughod, Lila. 1991. Writing against Culture. In *Recapturing Anthropology: Working in the Present*, ed. Renee Fox. Santa Fe: School of American Research.

Acuña, Rodolfo. 1981. *Occupied America: A History of Chicanos*. New York: Harper and Row.

Ahdieh, L., and Robert A. Hahn. 1996. Use of the Terms "Race," "Ethnicity," and "National Origins": A Review of Articles in the *American Journal of Public Health*, 1980–1989. *Ethnicity and Health* 1 (1):95–98.

Allen, Theodore W. 1994. *The Invention of the White Race*. Vol. 1: *Racial Oppression and Social Control*. New York: Verso.

Almaguer, Tomás. 1994. *Racial Fault Lines: The Historical Origins of White Supremacy in California*. Berkeley: University of California Press.

Althusser, Louis. 1971. *Lenin and Philosophy and Other Essays*. London: New Left Books.

Andrews, Lori, and Dorothy Nelkin. 2001. *Body Bazaar: The Market for Human Tissue in the Biotechnology Age*. New York: Crown.

Anzaldua, Gloria. 1987. *Borderlands/La Frontera: The New Mestiza*. San Francisco: Spinsters–Aunt Lute Books.

Appadurai, Arjun, ed. 1986. *The Social Life of Things: Commodities in Cultural Perspective*. Cambridge: Cambridge University Press.

———. 1996. *Modernity at Large: Cultural Dimensions of Globalization*. Minneapolis: University of Minnesota Press.

Arendt, Hannah. 1958 [1951]. *The Origins of Totalitarianism*. Chicago: University of Chicago Press.

Armelagos, George. 1995. Race, Reason, and Rationale. *Evolutionary Anthropology* 4 (3):103–109.

Armelagos, George, and Alan Goodman. 1998. Race, Racism, and Anthropology. In *Building a New Biocultural System: Political Economic Perspective on Human Biology*, ed. Alan Goodman and Thomas Leatherman. Ann Arbor: University of Michigan Press.

Arreola, Daniel D. 2002. *Tejano South Texas: A Mexican American Cultural Province*. Austin: University of Texas Press.

Arreola, Daniel D, and James R. Curtis. 1993. *The Mexican Border Cities: Landscape Anatomy and Place Personality*. Phoenix: University of Arizona Press.

Auerbach, James, and Barbara Kivimae Krimgold, eds. 2001. *Income, Socioeconomic Status, and Health: Exploring the Relationships*. Washington, DC: National Policy Association Publications.

Bakhtin, Mikhail M. 1996 [1981]. *The Dialogical Imagination: Four Essays*. Austin: University of Texas Press.

Bamshad, M. J., S. Wooding, W. S. Watkins, C. T. Ostler, M. A. Batzer, and L. B. Jorde. 2003. Human Population Genetic Structure and Inference of Group Membership. *American Journal of Human Genetics* 72 (3):578–589.

Basu, Analabha , Hua Tang, Xiaofeng Zhu, et al. 2008. Genome-Wide Distribution of Ancestry in Mexican Americans. *Human Genetics* 124 (3):207–214.

Batalla Bonfil, Guillermo. 1996. *México Profundo: Reclaiming a Civilization*. Translated by P. A. Dennis. Austin: University of Texas Press.

Baudrillard, Jean. 1988. *Selected Writings*. Translated by M. Poster. Stanford, CA: Stanford University Press.

Beaver, Kevin, Matt DeLisi, Michael Vaughn, et al. 2009. Monoamine Oxidase a Genotype Is Associated with Gang Membership and Weapon Use. *Comprehensive Psychiatry* 51 (2):130–134.

Beck, Ulrich. 1992. *Risk Society: Towards a New Modernity*. London: Sage.

Behar, Ruth, and Deborah Gordon, eds. 1995. *Women Writing Culture*. Berkeley: University of California Press.

Benedict, Ruth. 1942 *Race and Racism*. London: Routledge and Kegan Paul.

Benjamin, Walter. 1969. *Illuminations*. New York: Schocken.

Benyshek, Daniel C. 2005. Type 2 Diabetes and Fetal Origins: The Promise of Prevention Programs Focusing on Prenatal Health in High Prevalence Native American Communities. *Human Organization* 64 (2):192–200.

Beurton, Peter J., Raphael Falk, and Hans-Jörg Rheinberger. 2000. *The Concept of the Gene in Development and Evolution: Historical and Epistemological Perspectives*. Cambridge: Cambridge University Press.

Black, S. A., K. S. Markides, and L. A. Ray. 2003. Depression Predicts Increased Incidence of Adverse Health Outcomes in Older Mexican Americans with Type 2 Diabetes. *Diabetes Care* 26 (10):2822–2828.

Blaffer Hrdy, Sara. 1986. Empathy, Polyandry, and the Myth of the Coy Female. In *Feminist Approaches to Science*, ed. Ruth Bleir. New York: Pergamon.

Bloor, David. 1999. "Anti-Latour." *Studies in History and Philosophy of Science* 30: 81–112.

Boas, Franz. 1940 [1888]. *Race, Language and Culture*. New York: Macmillan.
———. 1963 [1911]. *The Mind of Primitive Man*. New York: Free Reprint.
Bolnick, Deborah A. 2008. Individual Ancestry Inference and the Reification of Race as a Biological Phenomenon. In *Revisiting Race in a Genomic Age*, ed. Barbara A. Koenig, Sandra. S. Lee, and Sarah S. Richardson. New Brunswick, NJ: Rutgers University Press.
Bolnick, Deborah A., Duana Fullwiley, Troy Duster, et al. 2007. Genetics: The Science and Business of Genetic Ancestry Testing. *Science* 318 (5849):399.
Bonilla, Carolina, Lesley-Anne McDonald, Stacey Boxill, Tyisha William, et al. 2005. The 8818g Allele of the Agouti Signaling Protein (ASIP) Gene Is Ancestral and Is Associated with Darker Skin Color in African Americans. *Human Genetics* 116 (5):402–406.
Bourdieu, Pierre. 1977. *Outline of a Theory of Practice*. Translated by R. Nice. Cambridge: Cambridge University Press.
———. 1984. *Distinction*. Cambridge, MA: Harvard University Press.
Bourgois, Philippe, and Julie Bruneau. 2000. Needle Exchange, HIV Infection, and the Politics of Science: Confronting Canada's Cocaine Injection Epidemic with Participant Observation. *Medical Anthropology* 18 (4):325–350.
Bowker, Geoffrey, and Susan Leigh Star. 1999. *Sorting Things Out: Classifications and Its Consequences*. Cambridge, MA: MIT Press.
Braun, Lundy, Anne Fausto-Sterling, Duana Fullwiley, et al. 2007. Racial Categories in Medical Practice: How Useful Are They? *PLoS Medicine* 4 (9):e271.
Briggs, Laura. 2002. *Reproducing Empire: Race, Sex, Science, and U.S. Imperialism in Puerto Rico*. Berkeley: University of California Press.
Brues, Alice. 1993. The Objective View of Race. In *Race, Ethnicity, and Applied Bioanthropology*, ed. Claire C. Gordon. Arlington, VA: American Anthropological Association.
Burchell, G. (1993). "Liberal Government and Techniques of the Self." *Economy and Society* 22(3): 267–282.
Cain, Virginia, and Raynard Kington. 2003. Investigating the Role of Racial/Ethnic Bias in Health Outcomes (Editorial). *American Journal of Public Health* 93 (2):191–192.
Callon, Michel. 1986. Some Elements of a Sociology of Translation: Domestication of the Scallops and the Fishermen of St. Brieuc Bay. In *Power, Action, and Belief: A New Sociology of Knowledge?* ed. John Law. London: Routledge and Kegan Paul.
Callon, Michel, and Bruno Latour. 1981. Unscrewing the Big Leviathan: How Actors Macro-Structure Reality and How Sociologists Help Them to Do So. In *Advances in Social Theory and Methodology: Toward an Integration of Micro- and Macro-Sociologies*, ed. Karen Knorr-Cetina and Aaron V. Cicourel. London: Routledge and Kegan Paul.
Canguilhem, Georges. 1966 [1991]. *The Normal and the Pathological*. Translated by Carolyn Fawcett and Robert Cohen. New York: Zone.
Cartmill, Matt. 1998. The Status of the Race Concept in Physical Anthropology. *American Anthropologist* 100 (3):651–660.
Cavalli-Sforza, Luca, Paola Menozzi, and Alberto Piazza. 1994. *The History and Geography of Human Genes*. Princeton, NJ: Princeton University Press.

Centers for Disease Control and Prevention. 2000. Diabetes: A Serious Public Health Problem. Washington, DC: U.S. Department of Health and Human Services.

Chakraborty, R, and K. M. Weiss. 1988. Admixture as a Tool for Finding Linked Genes and Detecting That Difference from Allelic Association between Loci. *Proceedings of the National Academy of Sciences of the United States of America* 85 (23):9119.

Chaturvedi, N. 2001. Ethnicity as an Epidemiological Determinant—Crudely Racist or Crucially Important? *International Journal of Epidemiology* 30 (5):925–927.

Chaufan, Claudia. 2008. In Search of "Genetic Predispositions" to Common Diseases: Bang for Your Buck? Not Really. A Response to Robertson and Poulton, and Tuckson and Willard. *Social Science and Medicine* 67 (4):675–683.

Chavez, Leo R. 2001. *Covering Immigration: Popular Images and the Politics of the Nation.* Berkeley: University of California Press.

————. 2008. *The Latino Threat: Constructing Immigrants, Citizens, and the Nation.* Stanford, CA: Stanford University Press.

Checker, Melissa. 2005. *Polluted Promises: Environmental Racism and the Search for Justice in a Southern Town.* New York: New York University Press.

Cicourel, Aaron V. 1964. *Method and Measurement in Sociology.* New York Free Press.

Clarke, Adele, and Joan Fujimura 1992. What Tools? Which Jobs? Why Right? In *The Right Tools for the Job: At Work in Twentieth Century Life Sciences,* ed. Adele Clarke and Joan Fujimura. Princeton: Princeton University Press: 3–44.

Clifford, James. 1988. *The Predicament of Culture: Twentieth-Century Ethnography, Literature, and Art.* Cambridge, MA: Harvard University Press.

Cohen, Lawrence. 1999. Where It Hurts: Indian Material for an Ethics of Organ Transplantation. *Daedalus* 128 (4):135–164.

Cole, Luke W., and Sheila R. Foster. 2001. *From the Ground Up: Environmental Racism and the Rise of the Environmental Justice Movement, Critical America.* New York: New York University Press.

Cole, Simon 2007, "Is the 'Junk' DNA Designation Bunk?" *Northwestern University Law Review Colloquy* 102: 54–63.

————. 2001. *Suspect Identities.* Cambridge: Harvard University Press.

Collins, Francis S., Eric D. Green, Alan E. Guttmacher, et al. 2003. A Vision for the Future of Genomics Research. *Nature* 422 (6934):835–847.

Comaroff, John L., and Jean Comaroff. 2009. *Ethnicity, Inc.* Chicago: University of Chicago Press.

Condit, Celeste M. 2007. How Geneticists Can Help Reporters to Get Their Story Right. *Nature Reviews Genetics* 8 (10):815–820.

Cooper, Richard S., and Richard David. 1986. The Biological Concept of Race and Its Application to Public Health and Epidemiology. *Journal of Health Politics, Policy and Law* 11 (1):97–116.

Cooper, Richard S., Xuiqing Guo, Charles N. Rotimi, et al. 2000. Heritability of Angiotensin-Converting Enzyme and Angiotensinogen: A Comparison of U.S. Blacks and Nigerians. *Hypertension* 35 (5):1141–1147.

Corburn, Jason. 2005. *Street Science: Community Knowledge and Environmental Health Justice*. Cambridge, MA: MIT Press.

Cotera, Maria Eugenia. 2005. Jovita Gonzalez Mireles: A Sense of History. In *Latina Legacies: Identity, Biography, and Community*, ed. V. L. Ruiz and V. Sanchez Korrol. New York: Oxford University Press.

Cotera, Martha P. 1976. *Diosa Y Hembra: The History and Heritage of Chicanas in the U.S.* Austin, TX: Information Systems Development.

Cox, N. J., M. Frigge, and D. L. Nicolae, et al. 1999. Loci on Chromosomes 2 (Niddm1) and 15 Interact to Increase Susceptibility to Diabetes in Mexican Americans. *Nature Genetics* 21 (2):213–215.

De Genova, Nicholas. 1998. Race, Space, and the Re-Invention of Latin America in Mexican Chicago. *Latin American Perspectives* 25 (5):87–116.

———. 2005. *Working the Boundaries: Race, Space, and "Illegality" In Mexican Chicago*. Durham, NC: Duke University Press.

———. 2006. *Racial Transformations: Latinos and Asians Remaking the United States*. Durham, NC: Duke University Press.

De Genova, Nicholas, and Ana Y. Ramos-Zayas. 2003. *Latino Crossings: Mexicans, Puerto Ricans, and the Politics of Race and Citizenship*. New York: Routledge.

De León, Arnoldo. 1983. *They Called Them Greasers: Anglo Attitudes toward Mexicans in Texas 1821–1900*. Austin: University of Texas Press.

DeWitt, Thomas, and Samuel Scheiner, eds. 2004. *Phenotypic Plasticity: Functional and Conceptual Approaches*. Oxford: Oxford University Press.

DiGiacomo, S. M. 1999. Can There Be a "Cultural Epidemiology"? *Medical Anthropology Quarterly* 13 (4):436–457.

Dominguez, Virginia. 1986. *White by Definition: Social Classification in Creole Louisiana*. New Brunswick: Rutgers University Press.

Drysdale, Connie M., Dennis W. McGraw, Catharine B. Stack, et al. 2000. Complex Promoter and Coding Region ß2–Adrenergic Receptor Haplotypes Alter Receptor Expression and Predict in Vivo Responsiveness. Washington, DC: National Academy of Sciences.

DuBois, W. E. B. 1990 [1903]. *The Souls of Black Folk*. New York: Vintage/Library of America.

———, ed. 1906. *The Health and Physique of the Negro American*. A social study made under the direction of Atlanta University by the Eleventh Atlanta Conference. Atlanta University Publications, No. 11. Atlanta: Atlanta University Press.

Duggirala, R. et al. 1999. Linkage of Type 2 Diabetes Mellitus and of Age at Onset to a Genetic Location on Chromosome 10q in Mexican Americans. *American Journal of Human Genetics* 64 (4):1127–40.

Duggirala, R., J. Blangero, L. Almasy, et al. 2000. A Major Susceptibility Locus Influencing Plasma Triglyceride Concentrations Is Located on Chromosome 15q in Mexican Americans. *American Journal of Human Genetics* 66 (4): 1237–1345.

Durkheim, Emile, and Marcel Mauss. 1963 [1903]. *Primitive Classification*. Translated by Rodney Needham. Chicago: University of Chicago Press.

Duster, Troy. 1990. *Eugenics through the Backdoor*. New York: Routledge.

———. 2001a. The Chronicle Review. *Chronicle of Higher Education* 54 (11):B6.

———. 2001b. The Sociology of Science and the Revolution in Molecular Biology. In *Blackwell Companion to Sociology*. Oxford: Blackwell Publishers.

———. 2002. Sociological Stranger in the Land of the Human Genome Project. *Contexts* 1 (3):69–70.

Ehm, M. G., et al. 2000. Genomewide Search for Type 2 Diabetes Susceptiblity Genes in Four American Populations. *American Journal of Human Genetics* 66 (6):1871–1881.

Elbein, S. C., M. D. Hoffman, K. Teng, et al. 1999. A Genome-Wide Search for Type 2 Diabetes Susceptibility Genes in Utah Caucasians. *Diabetes* 48 (5):1175–1182.

Epstein, Steven. 2007. *Inclusion: The Politics of Difference in Medical Research*. Chicago: University of Chicago Press.

Escobar, Arturo. 1995. *Encountering Development: The Making and Unmaking of the Third World*. Princeton, NJ: Princeton University Press.

Evans, Patrick, Nitzan Mekel-Bobrov, J. Eric Vallender, et al. 2006. Evidence That the Adaptive Allele of the Brain Size Gene Microcephalin Introgressed into Homo Sapiens from an Archaic Homo Lineage. *Proceedings of the National Academy of Sciences* 103 (48):18178–18183.

Evans-Pritchard, E. E. 1940. *The Nuer*. Oxford: Clarendon.

Fabian, Johannes. 2001. *Anthropology with an Attitude: Critical Essays*. Stanford, CA: Stanford University Press.

Fairclough, Norman. 1995. *Critical Discourse Analysis: The Critical Study of Language*. London: Longman.

Farmer, Paul. 1992. *AIDS and Accusation: Haiti and the Geography of Blame*. Berkeley: University of California Press.

———. 1997. Social Scientists and the New Tuberculosis. *Social Science and Medicine* 44 (3):347–358.

———. 1999. *Infections and Inequalities: The Modern Plagues*. Berkeley: University of California Press.

———. 2005. *Pathologies of Power: Health, Human Rights, and the New War on the Poor. With a New Preface by the Author, California Series in Public Anthropology, 4*. Berkeley: University of California Press.

Fausto-Sterling, Anne. 1985. *Myths of Gender: Biological Theories about Women and Men*. New York: Basic Books.

———. 1989. Life in the Xy Corral. *Women's Studies International Forum* 12 (3):319–331.

———. 2008. The Bare Bones of Race. *Social Studies of Science* 38 (5):657–694.

Ferguson, James. 1994. *The Anti-Politics Machine:"Development," Depoliticization, and Bureaucratic Power in Lesotho*. Minneapolis: University of Minnesota Press.

Fisher, Jill A. 2009. *Medical Research for Hire: The Political Economy of Pharmaceutical Clinical Trials*. New Brunswick, NJ: Rutgers University Press.

Flores, William, and Rina Benmayor, eds. 1997. *Latino Cultural Citizenship: Claiming Identity, Space and Rights*. Boston: Beacon.

Flyvbjerg, Bent. 2001. *Making Social Science Matter: Why Social Inquiry Fails and How It Can Succeed Again.* Cambridge: Cambridge University Press.

Fortun, Kim. 2006. Cultural Critique in and of American Culture. *Cultural Anthropology* 21 (3):496–500.

Fortun, Mike. 2008. *Promising Genomics: Iceland and deCODE Genetics in a World of Speculation.* Berkeley: University of California Press.

Foucault, Michel. 1972. *The Archeology of Knowledge and the Discourse on Language.* Trans. A. M. Sheridan Smith. New York: Pantheon.

———. 1983. The Subject and Power. Afterword to *Michel Foucault: Beyond Structuralism and Hermeneutics*, ed. Hubert L. Dreyfus and Paul Rabinow.

———. 1991 [1978]. Governmentality. In *The Foucault Effect: Studies in Governmentality*, ed. Graham Burchell, Colin Gordon, and Peter Miller. Chicago: University of Chicago Press.

Francis, Darlene D., F. A. Champagne, D. Liu, et al. 2006. Maternal Care, Gene Expression, and the Development of Individual Differences in Stress Reactivity. *Annals of the New York Academy of Sciences* 896:66–84.

Francis, Darlene D., Josie Diorio, Paul M. Plotsky, et al. 2002. Environmental Enrichment Reverses the Effects of Maternal Separation on Stress Reactivity. *Journal of Neuroscience* 22 (18):7840–7843.

Francis, Darlene D., Kathleen Szegda, Gregory Campbell, et al. 2003. Epigenetic Sources of Behavioral Differences in Mice. *Nature Neuroscience* 6 (5):445–446.

Frankenberg, Ronald. 1993. Risk: Anthropological and Epidemiological Narratives of Prevention. In *Knowledge, Power, and Practice: The Anthropology of Medicine in Everyday Life*, ed. Shirley Lindenbaum and Margaret M. Lock. Berkeley: University of California Press.

Franklin, Sarah, and Margaret M. Lock, eds. 2003. *Remaking Life and Death: Toward an Anthropology of the Biosciences.* Santa Fe, NM: School of American Research Press.

Frayling, T. M., et al. 2000. No Evidence for Linkage at Candidate Type 2 Diabetes Susceptibility Loci on Chromosomes 12 and 20 in the United Kingdom Caucasians. *Journal of Endocrinological Metabolism* 85 (2):853–857.

Freire, Paulo. 1968. *Pedagogy of the Oppressed.* New York: Seabury.

———. 1970. Cultural Action and Conscientization. *Harvard Educational Review* 10:452–477.

Feudtner, Chris. 2003. *Bittersweet: Diabetes, Insulin, and the Transformation of Illness.* Durham, NC: University of North Carolina Press.

Fujimura, Joan H. 1987. Constructing Doable Problems in Cancer Research: Articulating Alignment. *Social Studies of Science* 17 (2):257–293.

———. 1996. *Crafting Science: A Sociohistory of the Quest for the Genetics of Cancer.* Cambridge, MA: Harvard University Press.

Fujimura, Joan H., Troy Duster, and Ramya Rajagopalan. 2008. Introduction: Race, Genetics, and Disease: Questions of Evidence, Matters of Consequence. *Social Studies of Science* 38 (5):643–656.

Fujimura, Joan H., and Michael Fortun. 1996. Constructing Knowledge across Social Worlds: The Case of DNA Sequence Databases in Molecular Biology. In *Naked Science: Anthropological Inquiry into Boundaries, Power, and Knowledge*, ed. L. Nader. New York: Routledge.

Fullwiley, Duana. 2007a. The Molecularization of Race: Institutionalizing Human Difference in Pharmacogenetics Practice. *Science as Culture* 16 (1): 1–30.

———. 2007b. Race and Genetics: Attempts to Define the Relationship. *BioSocieties* 2 (2):221–237.

———. 2008. The Biologistical Construction of Race: Admixture Technology and the New Genetic Medicine. *Social Studies of Science* 38 (5):695–735.

Garcia Canclini, Néstor. 1993. *Transforming Modernity: Popular Culture in Mexico*. Austin: University of Texas Press.

Gardner, L., M. Stern, et al. (1984). Prevalence of Diabetes in Mexican Americans. Relationship to Percent of Gene Pool Derived from Native American Sources. *Diabetes* 33(1): 86–92.

Garro, Linda. 1995. Individual or Societal Responsibility? Explanations of Diabetes in an Anishinaabe (Ojibway) Community. *Social Science and Medicine* 40 (1):37–46.

Ghosh, S., et al. 1998. A Large Sample of Finnish Diabetic Sib-Pairs Reveals No Evidence for a Non-Insulin-Dependent Diabetes Mellitus Susceptibility Locus at 2qter. *Journal of Clinical Investigation* 102 (4):704–709.

Gilroy, Paul. 1991. *"There Ain't No Black in the Union Jack": The Cultural Politics of Race and Nation*. Chicago: University of Chicago Press.

———. 1994. *The Black Atlantic*. Cambridge: Harvard University Press.

Ginsburg, Faye. 2006. Ethnography and American Studies. *Cultural Anthropology* 21 (3):487–495.

Glenn, David. 2006. Blood Feud: A Controversy over South American DNA Samples Held in North American Laboratories Ripples through Anthropology. *Chronicle of Higher Education* (http://chronicle.com/article/Blood-Feud/13242/, last accessed October 18, 2010).

Gluckman, P. D., M. A. Hanson, C. Cooper, et al. 2008. Effect of in Utero and Early-Life Conditions on Adult Health and Disease. *New England Journal of Medicine* 359 (1):61.

González Burchard, Esteban, Pedro C. Avila, Sylvette Nazario, et al. 2004. Lower Bronchodilator Responsiveness in Puerto Rican Than in Mexican Subjects with Asthma. *American Journal of Respiratory Critical Care Medicine* 169:386–392.

González Burchard, Esteban, Luisa N. Borrell, Shweta Choudhry, et al. 2005. Latino Populations: A Unique Opportunity for the Study of Race, Genetics, and Social Environment in Epidemiological Research. *American Journal of Public Health* 95:2161–2168.

González Burchard, Esteban, Elad Ziv, Natasha Cole, et al. 2003. The Importance of Race and Ethnic Background in Biomedical Research and Clinical Practice. *New England Journal of Medicine* 348 (12):1170–1175.

Goodman, Alan H. 1997. Bred in the Bone? *The Sciences* 37 (2):20–25.

————. 2001. Six Wrongs of Racial Science. In *Race in Twenty-First Century America*, ed. T. M. Curtis Stokes and Genice Rhodes-Reed. East Lansing: Michigan State University Press.

Goodman, Alan H., Deborah Heath, and Susan M. Lindee, eds. 2003. *Genetic Nature/Culture: Anthropology and Science beyond the Two-Culture Divide*. Berkeley: University of California Press.

Goodman, Alan H., and Thomas L. Leatherman. 1998. Traversing the Chasm between Biology and Culture. Introduction to *Building a New Biocultural Synthesis: Political-Economic Perspectives on Human Biology*, ed. Alan H. Goodman and Thomas L. Leatherman. Ann Arbor: University of Michigan Press.

————. 2005. Context and Complexity in Human Biological Research. In *Complexities: Beyond Nature and Nurture*, ed. Susan McKinnon and Sydel Silverman. Chicago: University of Chicago Press.

Gould, Stephen Jay. 1981. *The Mismeasure of Man*. New York: Norton.

————. 1993. American Polygeny and Craniometry before Darwin: Blacks and Indians as Separate, Inferior Species. In *The "Racial" Economy of Science: Toward a Democratic Future*, ed. Sandra Harding. Bloomington: Indiana University Press.

Grant, Struan F. A., Gudmar Thorleifsson, Inga Reynisdottir, et al. 2006. Variant of Transcription Factor 7-Like 2 (Tcf7l2) Gene Confers Risk of Type 2 Diabetes. *Nature Genetics* 38 (3):320–323.

Gravelle, Hugh. 1998. How Much of the Relation Between Population Mortality and Unequal Distribution of Income Is a Statistical Artefact? *British Medical Journal* 316 (7128):382–385.

Graves, Joseph L. 2001. *The Emperor's New Clothes: Biological Theories of Race at the Millennium*. New Brunswick, NJ: Rutgers University Press.

Gravlee, Clarence C. 2009. How Race Becomes Biology: Embodiment of Social Inequality. *American Journal of Physical Anthropology* 139 (1):47–57.

Greenhalgh, Susan. 2008. *Just One Child: Science and Policy in Deng's China*. Berkeley: University of California Press.

Gregory, Steven, and Roger Sanjek, eds. 1994. *Race*. New Brunswick, NJ: Rutgers University Press.

Griffiths, Anthony, Jeffrey Miller, David Suzuki, et al. 1993. *An Introduction to Genetic Analysis*. Fifth ed. New York: Freeman and Co.

Guerrero Mothelet, Veronica, and Stephan Herrera. 2005. Mexico Launches Bold Genome Project. *Nature Biotechnology* 23(9): 1030.

Guo, Guang, Michael Roettger, and Jean Shih. 2006. Contributions of the Dat1 and Drd2 Genes to Serious and Violent Delinquency among Adolescents and Young Adults. *Human Genetics* 121 (1):125–136.

Gupta, Akhil, and James Ferguson, eds. 1997. *Anthropological Locations: Boundaries and Grounds of a Field Science*. Berkeley: University of California Press.

Hacking, Ian. 1999. *The Social Construction of What?* Cambridge, MA: Harvard University Press.

Hahn, Beth A. 1995. Children's Health: Racial and Ethnic Differences in the Use of Prescription Medications. *Pediatrics* 95 (5):727–732.

Hahn, Robert A. 1992. The State of Federal Health Statistics on Racial and Ethnic Groups. *Journal of American Medical Association* 267:268–71.

———. 1995. Anthropology and Epidemiology: One Logic or Two? In *Sickness and Healing: An Anthropological Perspective*, ed. R. Hahn. New Haven, CT: Yale University Press.

Hahn, Robert A., Joseph Mulinare, and Steven M. Teutsch. 1992. Inconsistencies in Coding of Race and Ethnicity between Birth and Death in U.S. Infants: A New Look at Infant Mortality, 1983 through 1985. *Obstetrical and Gynecological Survey* 47 (7):486.

Hahn, Robert A., Scott F. Wetterhall, George A. Gay, Dorothy S. Harshbarger, Carol A. Burnett, Roy Gibson Parrish, and Richard J. Orend. 2002. The Recording of Demographic Information on Death Certificates: A National Survey of Funeral Directors. *Public Health Reports* 117(1):37–43.

Hale, Charles R. 2006. Activist Research v. Cultural Critique: Indigenous Land Rights and the Contradictions of Politically Engaged Anthropology. *Cultural Anthropology* 21 (1):96–120.

———. 2008. *Engaging Contradictions: Theory, Politics, and Methods of Activist Scholarship*. Berkeley: University of California Press.

Hales, C. Nicholas, and David J. P. Barker. 1992. Type 2 (Non-Insulin Dependent) Diabetes Mellitus: The Thrifty Phenotype Hypothesis. *Diabetologia* 35:595–601.

Hall, Stuart. 2002. Race, Articulation, and Societies Structured in Dominance. In *Race Critical Theory*, ed. Philomena Essed and David Theo Goldberg. Malden, MA: Blackwell Publishers.

Haney López, Ian F. 1996. *White by Law*. New York: New York University Press.

Hanis, C. L., et al. 1996. A Genome-Wide Search for Human Non-Insulin-Dependent (Type2) Diabetes Genes Reveals a Major Susceptibility Locus on Chromosome 2. *Nature Genetics* 13 (2):161–166.

Hanson, R. L., M. G. Ehm, D. J. Pettitt, et al. 1998. An Autosomal Genomic Scan for Loci Linked to Type II Diabetes Mellitus and Body-Mass Index in Pima Indians. *American Journal of Human Genetics* 63 (4):1130–1138.

Haraway, Donna. 1988. Situated Knowledges: The Science Question in Feminism as a Site of Discourse on the Privilege of Partial Perspective. *Feminist Studies* 14 (3):575–599.

———. 1989. *Primate Visions: Gender, Race, and Nature in the World of Modern Science*. London: Routledge.

———. 1991. *Simians, Cyborgs, and Women: The Reinvention of Nature*. New York: Routledge.

———. 1997. *Modest_Witness@Second_Millenium.Femaleman(C)_Meets_Oncomouse(Tm): Feminism and Technoscience*. New York: Routledge.

———. 2003. For the Love of a Good Dog. In *Genetic Nature/Culture: Anthropology and Science beyond the Two-Culture Divide*, ed. Alan H. Goodman, Deborah Heath and Susan M. Lindee. Berkeley: University of California Press.

Harding, Sandra. 1986. *The Science Question in Feminism*. Ithaca, NY: Cornell University Press.

———, ed. 1993. *The "Racial" Economy of Science: Toward a Democratic Future*. Bloomington: Indiana University Press.

Harrell, Jules, Sadiki Hall, and James Taliaferro. 2003. Physiological Responses to Racism and Discrimination: An Assessment of Evidence. *American Journal of Public Health* 93 (2):243–248.

Harrison, Faye V. 1995. The Persistent Power of "Race" in the Cultural and Political Economy of Racism. *Annual Review of Anthropology* 24:477–474.

Harvey, David. 1990. *The Condition of Postmodernity: An Enquiry into the Origins of Cultural Change*. Cambridge: Blackwell.

Hayden, Cori. 2003. *When Nature Goes Public: The Making and Unmaking of Bioprospecting in Mexico*. Princeton, NJ: Princeton University Press.

———. 2007. Taking as Giving: Bioscience, Exchange, and the Politics of Benefit-Sharing. *Social Studies of Science* 37 (5):729–758.

Health and Human Services. 2001. Report on the Diabetes Prevention Trial Issued August 7, 2001.

Heath, Deborah. 1998. Bodies, Antibodies and Modest Interventions. In *Cyborgs and Citadels: Anthropological Interventions in Emerging Sciences and Technologies*, ed. Gary. L. Downey and Joe. Dumit, 67–82. Santa Fe, NM: School of American Studies Press.

Heath, Deborah, Erin Koch, Barbara Ley, and Michael Montoya. 1999. Nodes and Queries: Linking Locations in Networked Fields on Inquiry. *American Behavioral Scientist* 43 (3):450–463.

Heath, Deborah, Rayna Rapp, and Karen Sue Taussig. 2004. Genetic Citizenship. In *A Companion to the Anthropology of Politics*, ed. David Nugent and Joan Vincent. London: Blackwell.

Hegele, R. A., B. Zinman, A. J. Hanley, et al. 2003. Genes, Environment, and Oji-Cree Type 2 Diabetes. *Clinical Biochemistry* 36 (3):163–170.

Helmreich, Stefan. 2003. Torquing Things Out: Race and Classification in Geoffrey C. Bowker and Susan Leigh Star's Sorting Things Out: Classification and Its Consequences. *Science, Technology, and Human Values* 28 (3):435–440.

———. 2008. Species of Biocapital. *Science as Culture* 17 (4):463–478.

Hill, Jane. 1993. Hasta La Vista Baby: Anglo Spanish in the American Southwest. *Critique of Anthropology* 13 (2):145–176.

Hinkes, Madeline. 1993. Realities of Racial Determination in a Forensic Setting. In *Race, Ethnicity, and Applied Bioanthropology*, ed. Claire C. Gordon. Arlington, VA: American Anthropological Association.

Hogle, L. 1995. Standardization across Non-Standard Domains: The Case of Organ Procurement. *Science, Technology, and Human Values* 20 (4):482–501.

———. 1999. *Recovering the Nation's Body: Cultural Memory, Medicine, and the Politics of Redemption*. New Brunswick, NJ: Rutgers University Press.

Hood, L., J. R. Heath, M. E. Phelps, et al. 2004. Systems Biology and New Technologies Enable Predictive and Preventative Medicine. *Science Signaling* 306 (5696):640.

Horikawa, Y., N. Oda, N. J. Cox, et al. 2000. Genetic Variation in the Gene Encoding Calpain-10 Is Associated with Type 2 Diabetes Mellitus. *Nature Genetics* 26 (2):163–175.

Horsman, Reginald. 1998. Anglo-Saxons and Mexicans. In *The Latino Condition*, ed. Richard Delgado and Jean Stefancic. New York: New York University Press.

Hostetler, John, and Gertrude Enders Huntington 1967. *The Hutterites in North America.* New York: Holt, Rinehart and Winston.

Hubbard, Ruth. 1990. Genes as Causes. In *The Politics of Women's Biology.* New Brunswick, NJ: Rutgers University Press.

Hubbard, Ruth, and Elijah Wald. 1993. *Exploding the Gene Myth: How Genetic Information Is Produced and Manipulated by Scientists, Physicians, Employers, Insurance Companies, Educators, and Law Enforcers.* Boston: Beacon.

Hunt, Linda M., Miguel A. Valenzuela, and Jacqueline A. Pugh. 1998. Porque Me Tocó a Mi? Mexican American Diabetes Patients' Causal Stories and Their Relationship to Treatment Behaviors. *Social Science and Medicine* 46 (8):959–969.

Ignatiev, Noel. 1995. *How the Irish Became White.* New York: Routledge.

Imperatore, G., W. C. Knowler, R. G. Nelson, and R. L. Hanson. 2001. Genetics of Diabetic Nephropathy in the Pima Indians. *Current Diabetes Report* 1 (3): 275–281.

Inhorn, Marcia C. 1995. Medical Anthropology and Epidemiology: Divergences or Convergences? *Social Science and Medicine* 40 (3):285–290.

Inhorn, Marcia C., and K. Lisa Whittle. 2001. Feminism Meets the "New" Epidemiologies: Toward an Appraisal of Antifeminist Biases in Epidemiological Research on Women's Health. *Social Science and Medicine* 53 (5):553–567.

Institute of Medicine. 2003. *Unequal Treatment: Confronting Racial and Ethnic Disparities in Health Care,* ed. Brian D. Smedley, Adrienne Y. Stith and Alan R. Nelson. Washington, D.C: National Academy Press.

Jackson, Fatima L. C. 2004. Human Genetic Variation and Health: New Assessment Approaches Based on Ethnogenetic Layering. *British Medical Bulletin* 69 (1):215–235.

Jacobson, Matthew F. 1998. *Whiteness of a Different Color: European Immigrants and the Alchemy of Race.* Cambridge, MA: Harvard University Press.

Jasanoff, Sheila, ed. 2004. *States of Knowledge: The Co-Production of Science and Social Order.* London: Routledge.

Jasanoff, Sheila, and Brian Wynne. 1998. Science and Decisionmaking. *Human Choice and Climate Change* 1:1–87.

Jezewski, M., and J. Poss. 2002. Mexican Americans' Explanatory Model of Type 2 Diabetes. *Western Journal Nursing Research* 24 (8):840–858.

Johannsen, Robert. 1985. *To the Halls of the Montezumas: The Mexican War in the American Imagination.* New York: Oxford University Press.

Jones, James 1981 *Bad Blood.* New York: Free Press.

Jordinova, Ludmilla. 1989. *Sexual Visions: Images of Gender in Science and Medicine Between the Eighteenth and Twentieth Centuries.* Madison: University of Wisconsin Press.

Kahn, Jonathan. 2003. Getting the Numbers Right. *Perspectives in Biology and Medicine* 46 (4):473–483.

———. 2004. How a Drug Becomes "Ethnic": Law, Commerce, and the Production of Racial Categories in Medicine. *Yale Journal of Health Policy, Law, and Ethics* 4:1–46.

———. 2005. From Disparity to Difference: How Race-Specific Medicines May Undermine Policies to Address Inequalities in Health Care. *Southern California Interdisciplinary Law Journal* 15:105.

———. 2006. Harmonizing Race: Competing Regulatory Paradigms of Racial Categorization in International Drug Development. *Santa Clara Journal of International Law* 5:34–56.

Kaufman, Jay S., and Richard S. Cooper. 2001. Commentary: Considerations for Use of Racial/Ethnic Classification in Etiologic Research. *American Journal of Epidemiology* 154 (4):291–298.

Kaufman, Jay S., Richard S. Cooper, and Daniel L. McGee. 1997. Socioeconomic Status and Health in Blacks and Whites: The Problem of Residual Confounding and the Resiliency of Race. *Epidemiology* 8 (6):621–628.

Keane, Webb. 2003. Self-Interpretation, Agency, and the Objects of Anthropology: Reflections on a Genealogy. *Comparative Studies in Society and History* 45 (2):222–248.

Keller, Evelyn Fox. 2000. *The Century of the Gene.* Cambridge, MA: Harvard University Press.

Kennedy, Kenneth. 1995. But Professor, Why Teach Race Identification If Races Don't Exist? *Journal of Forensic Sciences* 40 (5):797–800.

Kitano, Hiroaki. 2002. Systems Biology: A Brief Overview. *Science* 295 (5560):1662–1664.

Kittles, Rick A., and Kenneth M. Weiss. 2003. Race, Ancestry, and Genes: Implications for Defining Disease Risk. *Annual Review of Genomics and Human Genetics* 4 (1):33–67.

Kleinman, Arthur. 1988. *The Illness Narratives: Suffering, Healing, and the Human Condition.* New York: Basic Books.

Knoppers, Bartha Maria. 1999. Status, Sale, and Patenting of Human Genetic Material: An International Survey. *Nature Genetics* 22 (May):23–26.

Knorr-Cetina, Karin. 1999. *Epistemic Cultures: How the Sciences Make Knowledge.* Cambridge, MA: Harvard University Press.

Kong, Auge, and Nancy Cox. 1997. Allele-Sharing Models: Lod Scores and Accurate Linkage Tests. *American Journal of Human Genetics* 61:1179–1188.

Kopytoff, Igor. 1986. The Cultural Biography of Things: Commodification as Process. In *The Social Life of Things: Commodities in Cultural Perspective*, ed. A. Appadurai. New York: Cambridge University Press.

Kraut, Alan. 1994. *Silent Travelers: Germs, Genes, and the "Immigrant Menace."* Baltimore: Johns Hopkins University Press.

Kress, G. 1988. *Linguistic Processes in Sociocultural Practice.* Oxford: Oxford University Press.

Krieger, Nancy. 1999. Embodying Inequality: A Review of Concepts, Measures, and Methods for Studying Health Consequences of Discrimination. *International Journal of Health Services* 29 (2):295–352.

———. 2003. Does Racism Harm Health? Did Child Abuse Exist before 1962? On Explicit Questions, Critical Science, and Current Controversies: An Ecosocial Perspective. *American Journal of Public Health* 93 (2):194–199.

———. 2005. Embodiment: A Conceptual Glossary for Epidemiology. *Journal of Epidemiology and Community Health* 59:350–355.

Krieger, Nancy, and Elizabeth Fee. 1994a. Man Made Medicine and Women's Health: The Biopolitics of Sex/Gender and Race Ethnicity. *International Journal of Health Service* 24:265–283.

———. 1994b. Social Class: The Missing Link in U.S. Health Data. *International Journal of Health Services: Planning, Administration, Evaluation* 24 (1):25.

Kuzawa, Christopher W. 2007. Developmental Origins of Life History: Growth, Productivity, and Reproduction. *American Journal of Human Biology* 19 (5):654–661.

LaDuke, Winona. 2005. *Recovering the Sacred: The Power of Naming and Claiming*. Cambridge, MA: South End Press.

Landecker, Hannah 1999. Between Beneficence and Chattel: The Human Biological in Law and Science. *Science in Context* 12:203–225.

———. 2000. Immortality, in Vitro: A History of the Hela Cell Line. In *Biotechnology and Culture: Bodies, Anxieties, Ethics*, ed. Paul Brodwin. Bloomington: Indiana University Press.

Langford, Jean. 2002. *Fluent Bodies: Ayurvedic Remedies for Postcolonial Imbalance*. Durham, NC: Duke University Press.

Latour, Bruno. 1987. *Science in Action: How to Follow Scientists and Engineers through Society*. Cambridge, MA: Harvard University Press.

———. 1988. *The Pasteurization of France*. Trans. Alan Sheridan. Cambridge, MA: Harvard University Press.

Latour, Bruno, and S. Woolgar. 1986. *Laboratory Life: The Social Construction of Scientific Facts*. Beverly Hills, CA: Sage.

Lee, Sandra Soo-Jin, Joanna Mountain, and Barbara Koenig. 2001. The Meanings of "Race" in the New Genomics: Implications for Health Disparities Research. *Yale Journal of Health Policy, Law, and Ethics* 1 (1):33–75.

Leon, David A. 2004. Biological Theories, Evidence, and Epidemiology. *International Journal of Epidemiology* 33 (6):1167–1171.

Lewontin, Richard C. 1972. The Apportionment of Human Diversity. *Evolutionary Biology* 6:381–398.

———. 1991. *Biology as Ideology: The Doctrine of DNA*. New York: Harper Collins.

———. 2000. *The Triple Helix: Gene, Organism, and Environment*. Cambridge, MA: Harvard University Press.

Lewontin, Richard C., Steven Rose, and Leon J. Kamin. 1984. *Not in Our Genes: Biology, Ideology, and Human Nature*. New York: Pantheon.

Leys Stepan, Nancy. 1991. *"The Hour of Eugenics": Race, Gender, and Nation in Latin America*. Ithaca, NY: Cornell University Press.

Limón, José. 1994. *Dancing with the Devil: Society and Cultural Poetics in Mexican American South Texas*. Madison: University of Wisconsin Press.

Lindenbaum, Shirley. 2001. Kuru, Prions, and Human Affairs. *Annual Review of Anthropology* 30:363–385.

Lippman, Abby. 1993. Prenatal Genetic Testing and Geneticization: Mother Matters for All. *Fetal Diagnosis and Therapy* 8:175–178.

Lock, Margaret M. 1993. Cultivating the Body: Anthropology and Epistemologies of Bodily Practice and Knowledge. *Annual Review of Anthropology* 22:133–155.

———. 2001. The Alienation of Body Tissue and the Biopolitics of Immortalized Cell Lines. *Body & Society* 7(2–3): 63.

———. 2005. Eclipse of the Gene and the Return of Divination 1. *Current Anthropology* 46:47–70.

Lock, Margaret M., and Judith Farquhar. 2007. *Beyond the Body Proper: Reading the Anthropology of Material Life, Body, Commodity, Text*. Durham, NC: Duke University Press.

Lupton, Deborah. 1999. *Risk*. London: Routledge.

Macpherson, Crawford B. 1962. *The Political Philosophy of Possessive Individualism. Hobbes to Locke*. Oxford: Clarendon.

Marcus, George. 1988. The Constructive Uses of Deconstruction in the Ethnographic Study of Notable American Families. *Anthropological Quarterly* 61: 3–16.

Marcus, George, and Michael M. J. Fischer. 1986. *Anthropology as Cultural Critique*. Chicago: University of Chicago Press.

Maril, Robert Lee. 1989. *The Poorest of Americans: The Mexican Americans of the Lower Rio Grande Valley of Texas*. Notre Dame, IN: University of Notre Dame Press.

Marks, Jonathan. 1995. *Human Biodiversity: Genes, Race, and History*. New Brunswick, NJ: Transaction.

———. 1996a. The Legacy of Serological Studies in American Physical Anthropology. *History and Philosophy of Life Sciences* 18:345–362.

———. 1996b. Science and Race. *American Behavioral Scientist* 40 (2):123–133.

———. 1998. Replaying the Race Card. *Anthropology Newsletter* 39 (5).

Marmot, Michael. 2005. Social Determinants of Health Inequalities. *Lancet* 365 (9464):1099–1104.

Martin, Emily. 1987. *The Woman in the Body*. Boston: Beacon.

———. 1992. The Egg and the Sperm: How Science Has Constructed a Romance Based on Stereotypical Male-Female Roles. *Signs* 16 (3):485–501.

———. 1994. *Flexible Bodies: The Role of Immunity in American Culture from the Days of Polio to the Age of AIDS*. Boston: Beacon.

Martin, John, et al. 2000. Nutritional Origins of Insulin Resistance: A Rat Model for Diabetes-Prone Human Populations. *Journal of Nutrition* 130:741–744.

Marx, Karl. 1976. *Capital*. Vol. 1. Trans. Ben Fowkes. New York: Vintage Books.

Maty, Siobhan C., Susan A Everson-Rose, Mary N. Haan, et al. 2005. Education, Income, Occupation, and the 34-Year Incidence (1965–99) of Type 2 Diabetes in the Alameda County Study. *International Journal of Epidemiology* 34 (6):1274–1281.

Maty, Siobhan C., John W. Lynch, Trivellore E. Raghunathan, et al. 2008. Childhood Socioeconomic Position, Gender, Adult Body Mass Index, and Incidence of Type 2 Diabetes Mellitus over 34 Years in the Alameda County Study. *American Journal of Public Health* 98 (8):1486–1494.

Maty, Siobhan C., John W. Lynch, J. L. Balfour, et al. 2002. Interaction between Childhood Socioeconomic Position, Adult Body Mass Index, and 34-Year Incidence of Type 2 Diabetes Mellitus. *Annals of Epidemiology* 12 (7):501.

Maugh II, Thomas. 2000. Mutated Gene Tied to Diabetes in Some Groups. *Los Angeles Times*, September 27:1.

Maurer, Bill. 2005. *Mutual Life, Limited: Islamic Banking, Alternative Currencies, Lateral Reason*. Princeton, NJ: Princeton University Press.

Mauss, Marcel. 1990. *The Gift: The Form and Reason for Exchange in Archaic Societies*. Trans. W. D. Halls. London: Routledge.

McAfee, Kathleen. 2003. Neoliberalism on the Molecular Scale: Economic and Genetic Reductionism in Biotechnology Battles. *Geoforum* 34 (2):203–219.

McDermott, Robyn. 1998. Ethics, Epidemiology, and the Thrifty Gene: Biological Determinism as a Health Hazard. *Social Science and Medicine* 47 (9):1189–1195.

McHughen, Stephanie A., Paul Rodriguez, Jeffrey A. Kleim, et al. 2010. BDNF Val66met Polymorphism Influences Motor System Function in the Human Brain. *Cerebral Cortex* 20(5) 1254–1262.

Menchaca, Martha. 1993. Chicano Indianism: A Historical Account of Racial Repression in the United States. *American Ethnologist* 20 (3):583–603.

Mi, Jie, et al. 2000. Effects of Infant Birthweight and Maternal Body Mass Index in Pregnancy on Components of the Insulin Resistance Syndrome in China. *Annals of Internal Medicine* 132 (4):253–260.

Micklos, David, and Greg Freyer. 1990. *DNA Science: A First Course in Recombinant DNA Technology*. Burlington, NC: Cold Springs Harbor Laboratory Press and Caroline Biological Supply Company.

Miles, Robert, and Malcolm Brown. 2003. *Racism*. London: Routledge.

Minkler, Meredith, and Nina Wallerstein. 2003. *Community Based Participatory Research for Health*. San Francisco, CA: Jossey-Bass.

Mintz, Sidney. 1985. *Sweetness and Power*. New York: Penguin.

Mitchell, B. D., S. A. Cole, W. C. Hsueh, et al. 2000. Linkage of Serum Insulin Concentrations to Chromosome 3p in Mexican Americans. *Diabetes* 49 (3):513–516.

Mitchell, B. D., S. Williams-Blangero, R. Chakraborty, et al. 1993. Comparison of Three Methods for Assessing Amerindian Admixture in Mexican Americans. *Ethnicity and Disease* 3 (1):22–31.

Mol, Annemarie. 2002. *The Body Multiple: Ontology in Medical Practice*. Durham, NC: Duke University Press.

Molina, Natalia. 2003. Illustrating Cultural Authority: Medicalized Representations of Mexican Communities in Early-Twentieth-Century Los Angeles. *Aztlan* 28 (1):129–143.

———. 2006. Medicalizing the Mexican: Immigration, Race, and Disability in the Early-Twentieth-Century United States. *Radical History Review* 94:22–37.

Molnar, Stephen. 1998. *Human Variation: Races, Types, and Ethnic Groups*. Upper Saddle River, NJ: Prentice Hall.

Montagu, Ashley. 1997 [1942]. *Man's Most Dangerous Myth: The Fallacy of Race*. Walnut Creek, CA: AltaMira Press.

Montejano, David. 1997 [1987]. *Anglos and Mexicans in the Making of Texas, 1936–1986*. Austin: University of Texas Press.

Montoya, Michael J. 2007. Bioethnic Conscription: Genes, Race, and Mexicana/o Ethnicity in Diabetes Research. *Cultural Anthropology* 22 (1):94–128.

Montoya, Michael J., and Benjamin Howard. 2008. Dangerous Implications of Racial Genetics Research. *American Journal of Obstetrics and Gynecology* 198 (4):483.

Montoya, Michael J., and Erin Kent. 2010. Correspondence Re: Racial Disparities in Cancer Survival among Randomized Clinical Trials of the Southwest Oncology Group. *Journal of the National Cancer Institute* 102 (4):277–278.

———. forthcoming. Dialogical Action: From Community Based to Community Driven Action Research. *Qualitative Health Research*.

Moore, Donald S., Jake Kosek, and Anand Pandian, eds. 2003. *Race, Nature, and the Politics of Difference*. Durham, NC: Duke University Press.

Morgan, Lynn M. 2001. Community Participation in Health: Perpetual Allure, Persistent Challenge. *Health Policy and Planning* 16 (3):221–230.

Nader, Laura. 1972. Up the Anthropologist: Perspectives from Studying Up. In *Reinventing Anthropology*, ed. Dell Hymes. New York: Random House.

———, ed. 1996. *Naked Science: Anthropological Inquiry into Boundaries, Power, and Knowledge*. New York: Routledge.

National Institute of Diabetes and Digestive and Kidney Disease, NIDDK. 2006. *Diabetes Dictionary*. National Institutes of Health. Available at http://diabetes.niddk.nih.gov/dm/pubs/dictionary/index.htm.

Nature, Genetics. 2000. Census, Race and Science. *Nature Genetics Editorial* 24 (2):97–98.

Navarro, Vicente. 2004. The Politics of Health Inequalities Research in the United States. *International Journal of Health Services* 34 (1):87–99.

Nazroo, James. 2003. The Structuring of Ethnic Inequalities in Health: Economic Position, Racial Discrimination, and Racism. *American Journal of Public Health* 93 (2):277–284.

Neel, James V. 1962. Diabetes Mellitus: A "Thrifty" Genotype Rendered Detrimental by Progress? *American Journal of Human Genetics* 14:353–362.

———. 1976. Diabetes Mellitus—A Geneticist's Nightmare. In *The Genetics of Diabetes Mellitus*, ed. W. Creutzfeldt, J. Kobberling, and J. V. Neel. New York: Springer-Verlag.

———. 1982. The Thrifty Gene Revisited. In *The Genetics of Diabetes Mellitus*, ed. J. Kobberling and R. Tattersall. New York: Academic Press.

———. 1999. The "Thrifty Genotype" in 1998. *Nutrition Reviews* 57 (5):S2–S9.

Nelson, Alondra. 2008. Bio Science: Genetic Genealogy Testing and the Pursuit of African Ancestry. *Social Studies of Science* 38:759–783.

Nestle, Marion. 2002. *Food Politics: How the Food Industry Influences Nutrition and Health*. Berkeley: University of California Press.

Oakes, Michel J., and Peter H. Rossi. 2003. The Measurement of SES in Health Research: Current Practice and Steps toward a New Approach. *Social Science and Medicine* 56 (4):769–784.

Omi, Michael, and Howard Winant. 1994. *Racial Formation in the United States: From the 1960s to the 1980s*. New York: Routledge and Kegan Paul.

———. 1996. The Racialization of a Debate: The Charreada as Tradition or Torture. *American Anthropologist* 98 (3):505.

Ong, Aihwa. 1992. Limits to Cultural Accumulation: Chinese Capitalists on the American Pacific Rim. *Annals of the New York Academy of Sciences* 645: 125–143.

Ong, Aihwa, and Stephen J. Collier, eds. 2005. *Global Assemblages: Technology, Politics, and Ethics as Anthropological Problems*. Malden, MA: Blackwell Publishing.

Osborne, Newton, and Marvin Feit. 1992. Commentary: The Use of Race in Medical Research. *JAMA* January 8(267) 2:275–279.

Palsson, Gisli. 2007. *Anthropology and the New Genetics*. Cambridge: Cambridge University Press.

Paradies, Yin C., Michael J. Montoya, and Stephanie M. Fullerton. 2007. Racialized Genetics and the Study of Complex Diseases. *Perspectives in Biology and Medicine* 50 (2):203–227.

Parry, Bronwyn. 2004. *Trading the Genome: Investigating the Commodification of Bio-Information*. New York: Columbia University Press.

Payne, Perry W., Jr., Charmaine Royal, and Sharon L. R. Kardia. 2007. Genetic and Social Environment Interactions and Their Impact on Health Policy. *Journal of the American Academy of Orthopaedic Surgeons* 15 (suppl. 1):S95.

Pellow, David N., and Robert J. Brulle, eds. 2005. *Power, Justice, and the Environment: A Critical Appraisal of the Environmental Justice Movement*. Cambridge, MA: MIT Press.

Perkins, Jimmy L., Antonio N. Zavaleta, Gia Mudd, et al. 2001. The Lower Rio Grande Valley Community Health Assessment. Houston: University of Texas Health Science Center.

Permutt, M. A. 2001. A Genome Wide Scan for Type 2 Diabetes Susceptibility Loci in a Genetically Isolated Population. *Diabetes* 50 (3):681–685.

Pettit, D. J., R. Nelson, M. Saad, et al. 1993. Diabetes and Obesity in the Offspring of Pima Indian Women with Diabetes during Pregnancy. *Diabetes Care* 16:310–314.

Phelan, Jo C., Bruce G. Link, Ana Diez-Roux, et al. 2004. "Fundamental Causes" of Social Inequalities in Mortality: A Test of the Theory. *Journal of Health and Social Behavior* 45 (3):265–285.

Pierce, I. 1996. Traditional Epidemiology, Modern Epidemiology, and Public Health. *American Journal of Public Health* 86:678–683.

Pollan, Michael. 2006. *The Omnivore's Dilemma: A Natural History of Four Meals*. New York: Penguin.

Pritchard, J. K., M. Stephens, and P. Donnelly. 2000. Inference of Population Structure Using Multilocus Genotype Data. *Genetics* 155 (2):945.

Rabinow, Paul. 1992. Artificiality and Enlightenment. In *Incorporations*, ed. Jonathan Crary and Sanford Kwinter. New York: Urzone.

———. 1996a. *Essays on the Anthopology of Reason*. Princeton, NJ: Princeton University Press.

———. 1996b. *Making PCR: The Story of Biotechnology*. Chicago: University of Chicago Press.

———. 1999. *French DNA: Trouble in Purgatory*. Chicago: University of Chicago Press.

————. 2005. Amidst Anthropology's Problems. In *Global Assemblages: Technology, Politics, and Ethics and Anthropological Problems*, ed. Aihwa Ong and Stephen J. Collier. Malden, MA: Blackwell.

Rabinow, Paul, and Talia Dan-Cohen. 2005. *A Machine to Make a Future: Biotech Chronicles*. Princeton, NJ: Princeton University Press.

Raphael, Dennis 2006. Social Determinants of Health: Present Status, Unanswered Questions, and Future Directions. *International Journal of Health Services* 36 (4):651–677.

Rapp, Rayna. 1995. Accounting for Amniocentesis. In *Knowledge, Power, and Practice: The Anthroplogy of Medicine in Everyday Life*, ed. Shirley Lindenbaum and Margaret Lock. Berkeley: University of California Press.

————. 1999. *Testing Women, Testing the Fetus: The Social Impact of Amniocentesis in America*. New York: Routledge.

Rapp, Rayna, Deborah Heath, and Karen Sue Taussig. 2001. Genealogical Dis-Ease: Where Hereditary Abnormality, Biomedical Explanation, and Family Responsibility Meet. In *Relative Matters: New Directions in the Study of Kinship*, ed. Sarah Franklin and Susan MacKinnon. Durham, NC: Duke University Press.

Rasmussen, Kathleen M. 2001. The "Fetal Origins" Hypothesis: Challenges and Opportunities for Maternal and Child Nutrition. *Annual Review of Nutrition* 21 (1):73–95.

Reardon, Jenny. 2001. The Human Genome Diversity Project: A Case Study in Coproduction. *Social Studies of Science* 31 (3):357–388.

————. 2005. *Race to the Finish: Identity and Governance in an Age of Genomics*. Princeton, NJ: Princeton University Press.

Reverby, Susan. 2009. *Examining Tuskegee: The Infamous Syphilis Study and Its Legacy*. Chapel Hill, NC: University of North Carolina Press

Rheinberger, Hans-Jörg. 1994. *Modes of Reasoning in Genetic Engineering and Molecular Biology*. Salzburg, Austria: Institute for Genetics and General Biology, University of Salzburg.

————. 2000. Gene Concepts: Fragments from the Perspective of Molecular Biology. In *The Concept of the Gene in Development and Evolution*, ed. Peter Beurton, Raphael Falk, and Hans-Jörg Rheinberger. Cambridge: Cambridge University Press.

Rhine, Stanley. 1990. Non-Metric Skull Racing. In *Skeleton Attribtion of Race: Methods for Forensic Anthropology. Anthropological Papers No. 4.* ed. G. W. Gill and S. Rhine. Albuquerque, NM: Maxwell Museum of Anthropology.

Riles, Annelise. 2006. Anthropology, Human Rights, and Legal Knowledge: Culture in the Iron Cage. *American Anthropologist* 108 (1):52–65.

Risch, Neil, Esteban González Burchard, Elad Ziv, and Hua Tang. 2002. Categorization of Humans in Biomedical Research: Genes, Race and Disease. *Genome Biology* 3 (7):1–12.

Rock, Melanie. 2003. Sweet Blood and Social Suffering: Rethinking Cause-Effect Relationships in Diabetes, Distress, and Duress. *Medical Anthropology* 22 (2):131–174.

Roediger, David R. 1991. *The Wages of Whiteness: Race and the Making of the American Working Class*. New York: Verso.

Romero, Mary. 1997. *Challenging Fronteras: Structuring Latina and Latino Lives in the U.S.: An Anthology of Readings*. New York: Routledge.

Rosaldo, Michelle Z. 1974. Woman, Culture, and Society: A Theoretical Overview. In *Woman, Culture, and Society*, ed. Michelle Z. Rosaldo and Louise Lamphere. Stanford, CA: Stanford University Press.

Rosaldo, Renato. 1997. Cultural Citizenship, Inequality, and Multiculturalism. In *Latino Cultural Citizenship: Identity, Space, and Rights*, ed. William Flores and Rina Benmayor. Boston: Beacon.

Rose, Nikolas, and Carlos Novas. 2005. Biological Citizenship. In *Global Assemblages: Technology, Politics, and Ethics as Anthropological Problems*, ed. Aihwa Ong and Stephen J. Collier. Malden, MA: Blackwell.

Rosenberg, N. A., J. K. Pritchard, J. L. Weber, H. M. Cann, K. K. Kidd, L. A. Zhivotovsky, and M. W. Feldman. 2002. Genetic Structure of Human Populations. *Science* 298 (5602):2381.

Rosmond, Roland. 2005. Role of Stress in the Pathogenesis of the Metabolic Syndrome. *Psychoneruroendocrinology* 30 (1):1–10.

Ruiz, Vicki L. 1998. *From out of the Shadows: Mexican Women in Twentieth-Century America*. New York: Oxford University Press.

Ruiz, Vicki L., and Virginia Sanchez Korrol, eds. 2005. *Latina Legacies: Identity, Biography, and Community*. New York: Oxford University Press.

Rylko-Bauer, Barbara, Merrill Singer, and John Van Willigen. 2006. Reclaiming Applied Anthropology: Its Past, Present, and Future. *American Anthropologist* 108 (1):178–190.

Sacks, Karen. 1994. How Did Jews Become White Folks. In *Race*, ed. Steven Gregory and Roger Sanjek. New Brunswick, NJ: Rutgers University Press.

Sanford, Victoria, and Asale Angel-Ajani. 2006. *Engaged Observer: Anthropology, Advocacy, and Activism*. New Brunswick, NJ: Rutgers University Press.

Sankar, Pamela. 2006. Hasty Generalisation and Exaggerated Certainties: Reporting Genetic Findings in Health Disparities Research. *New Genetics and Society* 25 (3):249–264.

Sauer, Norman. 1992. Forensic Anthropology and the Concept of Race: If Races Don't Exist, Why Are Forensic Anthropologists So Good at Identifying Them? *Social Science and Medicine* 34 (2):107–111.

Sauer, Uwe, Matthias Heinemann, and Nicola Zamboni. 2007. Getting Closer to the Whole Picture. *Science (Washington)* 316 (5824):550–551.

Scheper-Hughes, Nancy, and Margaret Lock. 1987. The Mindful Body: Prolegomenon to Future Work in Medical Anthropology. *Medical Anthropology Quarterly* 1 (1):6–41.

Schiebinger, Londa L. 1993. *Nature's Body: Gender in the Making of Modern Science*. Boston: Beacon.

Schlosser, Eric. 2001. *Fast Food Nation: The Dark Side of the All-American Meal*. New York: Houghton Mifflin Harcourt.

Schneider, Anne, and Helen Ingram. 1993. Social Construction of Target Populations: Implications for Politics and Policy. *American Political Science Review*:334–347.

Schoenberg, Nancy E., Elaine M. Drew, Eleanor Palo Stoller, et al. 2005. Situating Stress: Lessons from Lay Discourses on Diabetes. *Medical Anthropology Quarterly* 19 (2):171–193.

Schulman, Kevin A., et al. 1999. The Effect of Race and Sex on Physicians' Recommendations for Cardiac Catheterization. *New England Journal of Medicine* 340 (8):618–626.

Schulz, Amy J., Shannon Zenk, Angela Odoms-Young, et al. 2005. Healthy Eating and Exercising to Reduce Diabetes: Exploring the Potential of Social Determinants of Health Frameworks within the Context of Community-Based Participatory Diabetes Prevention. *American Journal of Public Health* 95 (4):645–651.

Schwartz, Robert, S. 2001. Racial Profiling in Medical Research. *New England Journal of Medicine* 344 (18):1392–1393.

Seguin, Beatrice, Billie Jo-Hardy, Peter A. Singer, and Abdallah S. Daar. 2008. Genomics, Public Health and Developing Countries: The Case of the Mexican National Institute of Genomic Medicine (INMEGEN). *Nature Reviews.* October Supplement: S5-S9.

Serre, David, and Svante Pääbo. 2004. Evidence for Gradients of Human Genetic Diversity Within and Among Continents. *Genome Research* 14 (9):1679.

Serres, Michel. 1980. *Le Passage Du Nord-Ouest.* Paris: Editions de Minuit.

———. 1994. *Atlas.* Paris: Julliard.

Sharp, Leslie. 2001. Commodified Kin: Death, Mourning, and Competing Claims on the Bodies of Organ Donors in the United States. *American Anthropologist* 103 (1):112–133.

Shoelson, Steven E., Jongsoon Lee, and Allison B. Goldfine. 2006. Inflammation and Insulin Resistance. *Journal of Clinical Investigation* 116 (7):1793–1801.

Shriver, Mark D., Michael W. Smith, Li Jin, et al. 1997. Ethnic-Affiliation Estimation by Use of Population-Specific DNA Markers. *American Journal of Human Genetics* 60 (4):957–964.

Simmons, Kimberly E. 2008. Navigating the Racial Terrain: Blackness and Mixedness in the United States and the Dominican Republic. *Transforming Anthropology* 16 (2):95–111.

Singer, Merrill. 2005. New Drugs on the Street: An Introduction. *Journal of Ethnicity in Substance Abuse* 4 (2):1.

———. 2006. What Is the "Drug User Community"? Implications for Public Health. *Human Organization* 65 (1):72–80.

Smay, Diana, and George Armelagos. 2000. Galileo Wept: A Critical Assessment of the Use of Race in Forensic Anthropology. *Transforming Anthropology* 9 (2):19–29.

Smith-Morris, Carolyn. 2004. Reducing Diabetes in Indian Country: Lessons from the Three Domains Influencing Pima Diabetes. *Human Organization* 63 (1):34–46.

Spero, David. 2006. *Diabetes: Sugar-Coated Crisis: Who Gets It, Who Profits and How to Stop It.* Gabriola Island: New Society Publishers.

Star, Susan L., and James R. Griesemer. 1989. Institutional Ecology, "Translations," and Boundary Objects: Amateurs and Professionals in Berkeley's

Museum of Vertebrate Zoology, 1907–1939. *Social Studies of Science* 19 (3):387–420.

Stern, Alexandra M. 1999. Buildings, Boundaries, and Blood: Medicalization and Nation-Building on the U.S.-Mexico Border, 1910–1930. *Hispanic American Historical Review* 79 (1):41–81.

Stern, Michael P. 1999. Genetic and Environmental Influences on Type 2 Diabetes Mellitus in Mexican Americans. *Nutrition Reviews* 57 (5):S66–S70.

Stern, Michael P., R. Duggirala, B. D. Mitchell, et al. 1996. Evidence for Linkage of Regions on Chromosomes 6 and 11 to Plasma Glucose Concentrations in Mexican Americans. *Genome Research* 6 (8):724–734.

Stocking, George W., Jr. 1968. On the Limits of "Presentism" and "Historicism" in the Historiography of the Behavioral Sciences. In *Race, Culture, and Evolution: Essays in the History of Anthropology*. ed. George W. Stocking. New York: Free Press.

Strathern, Marilyn 1991. *Partial Connections*. Savage, MD: Rowman and Littlefield.

———. 1996. Potential Property: Intellectual Rights and Property in Persons. *Social Anthropology* 41:17–32.

Subramanian, G., Adams, Mark D., Venter, J. Craig, and Broder, Samuel. 2001. Implications of the Human Genome for Understanding Human Biology and Medicine. *JAMA* 286:2296–2307.

Sunder Rajan, Kaushik. 2003. Genomic Capital: Public Cultures and Market Logics of Corporate Biotechnology. *Science as Culture* 12 (1):87–121.

———. 2006. *Biocapital: The Constitution of Postgenomic Life*. Durham, NC: Duke University Press.

Swarup, Vikas. 2005. *Q and A (Slumdog Millionaire)*. New York: Scribner.

Tallbear, Kimberly. 2007. Narratives of Race and Indigeneity in the Genographic Project. *Journal of Law, Medicine, and Ethics* 35 (3):412–424.

———. 2008. Native-American-DNA.Com: In Search of Native American Race and Tribe. In *Revisiting Race in a Genomic Age*, ed. Barbara A. Koenig, Sandra S. Lee, and Sarah S. Richardson. New Brunswick, NJ: Rutgers University Press.

Tang, Hua, et al. 2005. Genetic Structure, Self-Identified Race/Ethnicity, and Confounding in Case-Control Association Studies. *American Journal of Human Genetics* 76, 268–275.

Tang, Hua, Eric Jorgenson, Maya Gadde, et al. 2006. Racial Admixture and Its Impact on BMI and Blood Pressure in African and Mexican Americans. *American Journal of Human Genetics* 119 (6):624–633.

Tapper, Melbourne. 1995. Interrogating Bodies: Medico-Racial Knowledge, Politics, and the Study of a Disease. *Comparative Studies in Society and History* 37 (1):76–93.

———. 1999. *In the Blood: Sickle Cell Anemia and the Politics of Race*. Philadelphia: University of Pennsylvania Press.

Taussig, Karen Sue. 2009. *Ordinary Genomes*. Durham, NC: Duke University Press.

Taussig, Karen Sue, Rayna Rapp, and Deborah Heath. 2003. Flexible Eugenics: Technologies of the Self in the Age of Genetics. In *Genetic Nature/Culture:*

Anthropology and Science beyond the Two-Culture Divide, ed. Alan H. Goodman, Deborah Heath, and Susan M. Lindee. Berkeley: University of California Press.

Taussig, Michael. 1992. *The Nervous System*. New York: Routledge.

Taylor, Janelle S. 2003. Confronting "Culture" in Medicine's "Culture of No Culture." *Academic Medicine* 78 (6):555–559.

Templeton, Alan R. 1998. Human Races: A Genetic and Evolutionary Perspective. *American Anthropologist* 1001 (2):632–650.

———. 2003. Human Races in the Context of Recent Human Evolution. In *Genetic Nature/Culture: Anthropology and Science beyond the Two-Culture Divide*, ed. Alan H. Goodman, Deborah Heath, and Susan M. Lindee. Berkeley: University of California Press.

Tesh, Sylvia N. 2001. *Uncertain Hazards: Environmental Activists and Scientific Proof*. Ithaca, NY: Cornell University Press.

Thacker, Eugene. 2004. *Biomedia*. Vol. 11, *Electronic Mediations*. Minneapolis: University of Minnesota Press.

Tierney, Patrick. 2000. *Darkness in El Dorado*. New York: Norton.

Traweek, Sharon. 1988. *Beamtimes and Lifetimes: The World of High Energy Physicists*. Cambridge: Harvard University Press

Trostle, James A. 2005. *Epidemiology and Culture*. Cambridge, UK: Cambridge University Press.

Trostle, James, and Johannes Sommerfeld. 1996. Medical Anthropology and Epidemiology. *Annual Review of Anthropology* 25:253–74.

Truett, Samuel, and Elliott Young. 2004. *Continental Crossroads: Remapping U.S.-Mexico Borderlands History*. Durham, NC: Duke University Press.

Tutton, Richard. 2007. Constructing Participation in Genetic Databases. *Science, Technology & Human Values* 32(2): 172–195.

Van Ryn, Michelle, and Steven S. Fu. 2003. Paved with Good Intentions: Do Public Health and Human Service Providers Contribute to Racial/Ethnic Disparities in Health? *American Journal of Public Health* 93 (2):248–255.

Vargas, Deborah R. 2007. Brown Country: Johnny Rodriguez. *Aztlán: A Journal of Chicano Studies* 32 (1):219–228.

Vélez-Ibáñez, Carlos G. 1996. *Border Visions: Mexican Cultures of the Southwest United States*. Tucson: University of Arizona Press.

Visweswaran, Kamala. 1998. Race and the Culture of Anthropology. *American Anthropologist* 100 (1):70–83.

Wagner, Roy. 2001. *An Anthropology of the Subject: Holographic Worldview in New Guinea and Its Meaning and Significance for the World of Anthropology*. Berkeley: University of California Press.

Wailoo, Keith. 2003. *Inventing the Heterozygote: Molecular Biology, Racial Identity, and the Narratives of Sickle Cell Disease, Tay-Sachs, and Cystic Fibrosis*. In *Race, Nature, and the Politics of Difference*, ed. Donald S. Moore, Jake Kosek and Anand Pandian. Durham, NC: Duke University Press.

Wallace, Douglas C. 2005. A Mitochondrial Paradigm of Metabolic and Degenerative Diseases, Aging, and Cancer: A Dawn for Evolutionary Medicine. *Annual Review of Genetics* 39:359–407.

Weber, Karl. 2009. *Food, Inc: How Industrial Food Is Making Us Sicker, Fatter, and Poorer—and What You Can Do About It*. New York: Public Affairs.

Weber, Max. 2002. *The Protestant Ethic and the" Spirit" of Capitalism and Other Writings*. New York: Penguin.

Weiss, Kenneth M., and Joseph D. Terwilliger. 2000. How Many Diseases Does It Take to Map a Gene with SNPs? *Nature Genetics* 26 (2):151–157.

Weiss, Kenneth M., Robert F. Ferrell and Craig Hanis 1984. A New World Syndrome of Metabolic Diseases with a Genetic and Evolutionary Basis. *Yearbook of Physical Anthropology* 27: 153–178.

Whitmarsh, Ian. 2008. *Biomedical Ambiguity: Race, Asthma, and the Contested Meaning of Genetic Research in the Caribbean*. Ithaca, NY: Cornell University Press.

WHO, Commission on Social Determinants of Health. 2008. *Closing the Gap in a Generation: Health Equity through Action on the Social Determinants of Health. Final Report*. Geneva, Switzerland: World Health Organization, Commission on Social Determinants of Health.

Wiegman, Robyn. 2000. Feminism's Apocalyptic Futures. *New Literary History* 31 (4):805–825.

Wilkinson, R. G. 1992. Social Class Differences in Infant Mortality. *British Medical Journal* 305:1227–1228.

Williams, Brackette. 1995. Classification Systems Revisited: Kinship, Caste, Race, and Nationality as the Flow of Blood and the Spread of Rights. In *Naturalizing Power: Essays in Feminist Cultural Analysis*, ed. Sylvia Yanagisako and Carol Delaney. New York: Routledge.

Williams, David R., and Chiquita Collins. 1995. U.S. Socioeconomic and Racial Differences in Health: Patterns and Explanations. *Annual Review of Sociology* 21 (1):349–386.

Williams, David R., Harold W. Neighbors, and James S. Jackson. 2003. Racial/Ethnic Discrimination and Health: Findings from Community Studies. *American Journal of Public Health* 93 (2):200–208.

Willis, Paul. 1977. *Learning to Labor: How Working Class Kids Get Working Class Jobs*. New York: Columbia University Press.

Wilson, William J. 1980. *The Declining Significance of Race*. Chicago: Chicago University Press.

Yanagisako, Sylvia. 2002. *Producing Culture and Capital: Family Firms in Italy*. Princeton: Princeton University Press.

Yanagisako, Sylvia, and Carol Delaney. 1995. *Naturalizing Power: Essays in Feminist Cultural Analysis*. New York: Routledge.

Zavella, Patricia. 1991. Reflections on Diversity among Chicanas. *Frontiers: A Journal of Women Studies*:73–85.

Zimmet, Paul. 1997. The Challenge of Diabetes: Diagnosis, Classification, "Coca-Colonization," and the Diabetes Epidemic. In *The Medical Challenge*, ed. Ernst Fischer and Gerald Möller. Munich: Piper Verlag.

Zuberi, Tukufu. 2001. *Thicker Than Blood: How Racial Statistics Lie*. Minneapolis: University of Minnesota Press.

Index

Italicized *f* or *t* next to page numbers indicate figures or tables, respectively.

semiotic processes, and genetics of
chronic, 65. *See also specific diseases*
DNA (deoxyribonucleic acid), 195, 206n21
DNA donors/samples: biogenetics and, 176;
circulation of, 36, 142–43; commodification of Mexicanas/os bodies and,
144–47, 149–52, 155, 156, 216n38;
coproduction between field office data
collection and, 78, 137; ethics and,
147–50, 155–56, 188; ethnic homogeneity and, 92–93; ethnic purity and, 97,
109; exchanges/value of and, 147–50,
149–50, 155–56, 188; farmworkers in
California and, 140–41; gene/s and,
77–78; genetic epidemiology and, 11;
hierarchies and, 99–100; life history
of, 145–47, 149, 156; marketing and,
144–45, 149–50, 151–52, 155, 216n38;
racialized property and, 144–45, 154;
racialized property/ and, 144–45, 154;
risk of illness and, 102–4; social
relations and, 37–38, 76, 83–84,
154–55, 158; sociohistorical context
and, 105–7, 109; U.S.-Mexico border
diabetes research and, 13, 70, 71f,
72, 78
DNA labels, xiv, xix, xx, 6, 62, 146,
151–52, 161. *See also* DNA donors/
samples
dominance/subordination. *See* Anglo-
Mexican relations; biopolitics/
governmentality
Durkheim, Émile, 182
Duster, Troy: on ethics, 15; on inequalities,
23, 34–35, 110, 177; on race/ethnicity
relations, 58, 219n42; on scientific claim/
medical problem circular reasoning, 53,
59–60, 62–64, 187, 207n49; on
SNPs-based research, 58, 66

ELSI (ethical, legal, and social implications)
working group, 15–16
embryology, 29, 204n100
environment: genes/environments
comparisons, 4, 158, 159–61, 217n7;
health and, 77, 159; racial classifications/
labels and, 22, 175; risk of diabetes and,
3, 22, 33, 35, 44, 132, 158; social
determinants and, 34, 160–61; thrifty
genotype hypothesis and, 48, 160. *See
also* diet hypothesis
epidemiology of race, 89, 158, 159–61,
217n7. *See also* genetic epidemiology;
social epidemiology analysis

epistemic approach, xvi–xvii, 28, 33, 102,
195, 204n116
epistemological critique, 89, 181, 195
Epstein, Steven, 85–86
equitable exchanges, 141, 144–45, 155. *See
also* inequalities
Escobar, Arturo, 99
essentialism, 90, 94, 108, 195
ethics: DNA donors/samples and, 147–50,
155–56, 188; ELSI working group
and, 15–16; exchanges/value of
DNA donors/samples and, 147–50,
155–56, 188; knowledge production
and, 22
ethnic homogeneity: about and, 92, 94,
96–97, 110–11; admixture estimates
and, 62, 93–96, 98, 104, 169; Asians
and, 62; bioethnic conscription and,
162–63, 178; DNA donors/samples
and, 92–93; Europeans and, 93; gene/s
and, 92; individual as representative
of group and, 92; Mexicanas/os and,
5, 57, 91–94, 97, 99, 104, 159,
183; nature/culture and, 98, 104;
population-based research and, 211n4;
racial discourse and, 57; racism and,
96; SNPs and, 92–93; sociohistorical
context and, 95–96; threat narratives
and, 92. *See also* ethnic purity;
individual
ethnicity, 7, 13, 14, 43, 195. *See also* race/
ethnicity
ethnic purity: about, 37, 91–92, 96–97,
110–11; admixture estimates and,
91–92, 111, 211n10; Anglo-Mexican
relations and, 99–100; articulation work
and, 102–3; bioethnic conscription and,
107–8; biological/social binaries and,
97–99, 102, 212n37; bipolitics/
governmentality and, 100–101, 106,
110, 111, 212n58; diet hypothesis and,
97–98; DNA donors/samples and, 97,
109; interpellation/hailing and, 99,
107; Mexicanas/os and, 5, 91–94, 97,
99, 159, 183; risk of illness for
biosocial groups and, 100–105; social
classification/hierarchies and, 97, 98–99;
sociohistorical context and, 36, 104–10,
111; threat narratives and, 37, 103–4,
106, 108, 212n58. *See also* ethnic
homogeneity; individual
ethnographies, 74, 126–29, 128, 144–45,
214n21, 214n24, 215n11. *See also*
anthropology

ontology *(continued)*
182; difference and, 30, 32, 204n113;
ethnorace and, 102; participation
ideology/humanist subjectification and,
100; of race and genes, 17; risk of
diabetes and, 101; totiontology, 32, 197;
transnational protogenetic subjects and,
104. *See also* biological/social binaries;
material and semiotic processes; nature/
culture
Other, the, xix, 21f, 88, 108
out-of-Africa replacement hypothesis, 54,
206n31

Palsson, Gisli, 3, 204n16
Paradies, Yin C., 160
partiality, xviii, 32, 112, 138, 213n2
participation ideology/humanist subjectification, 37, 81–87, 96–100, 104, 107–8
patent, for polygene, 152, 155, 216n39
PCOS (polycystic ovarian syndrome),
41–42
pharmaceutical industries: ADA and,
152–54, 169–73, *171f*; Amaryl ad
campaign and, 158, 169–74, *171f*, 175,
187; collaborations and, 152; diabetes
defined, 4; financial/social interests and,
146–47, 209n14; polygene patent and,
152, 216n39; race/ethnicity and,
169–70, 175; race/ethnicity in drug
marketing campaigns and, 36–37, 157,
158–59, 169–74, 218n37, 219n42,
219n44, 219n46
phenotype: about, 197; collaborative data
creation and, 133; genetic epidemiology
and, 124–26; genetics and, 44–45;
health/disease gene research and, 130;
polygene and, 44; race/ethnicity and, 14,
53, 125
physiological conditions, xvii, 2, 17–18,
129–32, 186, 200n3, 215n53
political economy: of body/health, 22–25,
202n62; race/ethnicity and, 13; racism
and, 75; U.S.-Mexico border and, 24,
27, 74–76, 77, 87, 141, 184, 209n14
political values of inclusion, and recruitment, 79, 80, 82, 85–87, 106, 109
polycystic ovarian syndrome (PCOS), 41–42
polygene: about, 131, 197; causation/
susceptibility and, 44, 76–77, 92, 106,
117, 191; chromosomes and, 44, 163,
167; knowledge production and,
163–64; patent for, 152, 155, 216n39;
phenotype and, 44; U.S.-Mexico border

diabetes research and, 78, 106. *See also*
gene/s
population-based research: about, 19–20,
151–52, 157–58, 162; advantages, 20,
186; allelic variation and, 53, 93;
biogenetics and, 57, 110; ethnic homogeneity and, 211n4; geoterritorial/
geopolitical space and, 18–19, 20, 21f,
22; hybrid subjects and, 76, 96–97;
knowledge production and, 18–20, 21f,
22, 202n59; race or ethnicity and, 7,
56–58; scientific claim/medical problem
circular reasoning and, 184; taxonomies
and, xvi, xx, 163, 182; within-group
comparisons and, 18, 26
Pritchard, J. K., 207n49
public health: diabetes as problem and, 3–5,
159, 200n8, 200n10; environment and,
77, 159; ethnorace/ethnoracial and, 1;
inequalities and, 25, 202n62; knowledge
production and, 22–25; political
economy of body/health and, 22–25,
202n62. *See also* health/disease gene
research
Puerto Rican populations, 68, 95, 162,
218n19
purity. *See* ethnic purity

Rabinow, Paul, xvii, 6–7, 100–101, 110,
126–29, 174
race: AAA on, 19, 63; about, 35, 56–57, 67,
197; Amerindians' cultural distinctions
and, 68; anthropology, and debates over,
xviii; as biological taxonomic system,
14–16, 22–23, 31–32, 181; epidemiology of, 89, 158, 159–61, 217n7;
Europeans and, 54, *54f*; forensic
sciences and, 60–61; genetic diversity
and, 53–54, *54f*; genome/s and, 59, 152,
200n3, 200n16; knowledge production,
and theories about, 22–25; as lively
cultural form, 33, 204n117; nature and,
179–80; ontology and, 17; population-
based research, and ethnicity or, 7,
56–58; race-no-race debates, 14–18, 23,
25, 30, 43, 62–64, 66–67, 191; racial
discourse and, 43, 47, 56–57, 65–66,
205n9; as social construct, 7, 13–16, 29,
31–32, 43, 63; sociohistorical context
and, 33; as totiontology, 32. *See also*
ethnorace/ethnoracial
race/ethnicity: about, 39, 57, 200n2;
biogenetics and, 14, 100, 102, 180,
218n36; diabetes enterprise and, xiv,

TEXT
10/13 Sabon

DISPLAY
Sabon

COMPOSITOR
Westchester Book Group

INDEXER
J. Naomi Linzer Indexing Services

PRINTER AND BINDER
Maple-Vail Book Manufacturing Group